PRAISE FOR BUSTING BREAST CANCER: FIVE SIMPLE STEPS TO KEEP BREAST CANCER OUT OF YOUR BODY

"This bold, superbly researched book is a clarion call and prescription for all women who seek to PREVENT—rather than eventually treat—this devastating female Emperor of All Maladies."

—Joseph C. Maroon, MD, FACS
Clinical Professor, Heindl Scholar in Neuroscience, and Vice Chairman of the Department of Neurological Surgery at University of Pittsburgh School of Medicine; Author of Square One—The Secret to a Balanced Life

"Busting Breast Cancer helps draw attention to the growing number of women facing a breast cancer diagnosis not just once, but twice and beyond. Susan asks some tough questions and stimulates our curiosity to dig deeper for the answers, while offering tangible steps to change breast cancer outcomes. This is an excellent resource for patients and practitioners alike."

—Dr. Nasha Winters, ND, FABNO
Founder and CEO, drnasha.com; Co-Author of The Metabolic Approach to Cancer

"As a breast cancer survivor, I found Busting Breast Cancer to be an eye-opening read. How I wish I had access to this book 30 years ago; I feel certain I would have avoided a traumatic diagnosis and treatment regimen."

—Shannon Lea Pickering, MS
Health Restoration Advocate and Founder of Autoimmune Foodie in Austin, TX

"In Busting Breast Cancer, Susan Wadia-Ells outlines strategies for reducing risk and improving outcomes. I love how she includes the detailed research and science to back it all up!"

—Maria Emmerich
International Best-Selling Author of The 30-Day Ketogenic Cleanse and many other ketogenic cookbooks

"Susan Wadia-Ells' book has a trove of information on little-known ways to reduce the risk of breast cancer. The information is scientifically based, but not generally accepted by the medical establishment that makes income and profit from treating diseases, not preventing them."

—William B. Grant, PhD
Director, Sunlight, Nutrition, and Health Research Center

"Susan Wadia-Ells has put all her passion and energy into this book. Busting Breast Cancer empowers each reader with the information and knowledge needed to control one's own health and destiny. We must have more authors like Wadia-Ells, who are able to bridge the gap of information about the actual causes of cancer to the general public. Researchers and medical doctors are only a small part of the momentum needed to push this new knowledge beyond question!"

—George Yu, MD,
YuFoundation.org and Clinical Professor of Urologic and Pelvic Surgery, George Washington Medical Center, Washington, DC

"Susan should be congratulated for effectively breaking down the complexities of cancer physiological biochemistry for the general public. I highly recommend Busting Breast Cancer! It is entertaining, revealing and full of useful information."

—Dr. Michael J. Gonzalez
Professor, University of Puerto Rico Medical Sciences Campus, School of Public Health, Department of Human Development

"Eloquently written, must-read, eye-opener book for my patients, relatives and fellow doctors. As a former conventional clinical oncologist and now an integrative/Functional Medicine Clinical Oncologist, I was intrigued to look at her references...and really, my mind was blown away–so much excellent data!"

—Dr. Wafaa Abdel-Hadi, MD
Functional Medicine Clinical Oncologist and Founder, AWARE clinic, Giza, Egypt

"Kudos to Dr. Susan Wadia-Ells for holding a mirror to us in the medical profession who have not dared to debunk the establishment. She has succinctly dissected the shortcomings of the 'Standard of Care' in cancers, namely, surgery, chemotherapy and radiation."

—Dr. Janak Nathan, MD
Neurologist and Founder, Asian Institute of India (AIKD),
Mumbai, India

"Today we need to integrate ancient wisdoms (Get some sun!) with the work of contemporary scientists (Reduce those carbs!). Let Busting Breast Cancer be your starting guide to the new world of Integrative Healthcare, where you can act to control your destiny."

—Diane Weissman
Noakes Foundation Nutrition Coach, Fountain Hills, AZ

"Finally, someone has practical help for breast cancer. This is a must-read if you want to prevent this diagnosis. Your oncologists don't know this information. But, by reading this book, you can help them to help you! I encourage you to read Busting Breast Cancer now."

—Dr. David Minkoff, MD
Founder and Medical Director, LifeWorks Wellness, Clearwater, FL

"Busting Breast Cancer's five simple prevention steps can become a virtual lifeline for all women; but especially for those on the African continent who can't afford the expensive treatments."

—Rehmah Kasule:
Founder-CEDA International, Kampala Uganda; Harvard
University-Advanced Leadership Initiative Senior Fellow 2020

"I firmly believe that breast cancer IS preventable! Had I known this information years ago myself, I know I could have prevented my own diagnoses."

—Layce Murray, LMT
Cancer Support Coach, Board Certified Drugless Practitioner,
Certified Integrative Nutrition Coach, Boise, Idaho

"The breast cancer industry is controlled by big businesses who profit by your illness not by your health. It doesn't have to be this way. In fact, it shouldn't be this way. There are many nutritional and lifestyle interventions that have been scientifically proven to intercept and reverse a breast cancer diagnosis. Cancer is a metabolic disease, which means its progression or reversal is strongly influenced by lifestyle issues (food, stress, exercise, sleep, etc.). And who controls your lifestyle? You do. That means you are in charge of your healing. Not the drug companies. But you need a road map and someone to guide you. Busting Breast Cancer is your road map and Susan Wadia-Ells, PhD is your guide. Susan has written a masterpiece that is both easy to read and scientifically compelling. Her research references include such luminaries as Nobel Prize winners Dr. Otto Warburg and Dr. James Watson, and Dr. Thomas Seyfried, Biology Professor at Boston College and author of Cancer as a Metabolic Disease. If you have breast cancer or know someone who does, please learn the truth about the cause, management and prevention of breast cancer. Knowledge is empowering. Take back your power by reading this book—it could save your life or someone you love."

—Catharine Arnston
Founder, CEO and Chief Scientific Officer, ENERGYbits Inc.

"As a ten-year pancreatic cancer survivor who turned my illness over to my spiritual guide, I appear to have been intuitively guided to avoid biopsies, toxic chemicals, radiation and surgery. My doctor said the odds were half of one percent survival. I used a no-sugar organic diet and other detoxification practices. I started meditating and allowing the divine energy to heal me. This approach apparently helped rid my mind of its forever crucially high cortisol levels, enabling my entire body and mind to move toward my ongoing optimal health. Thank you, Susan, for writing this book for me and for so many other women who continue to question today's cancer authorities in order to truly nurture and effectively protect ourselves."

—Marleny Franco
author: Gardening the Organic Way

BUSTING BREAST CANCER

FIVE SIMPLE STEPS
TO KEEP BREAST CANCER
OUT OF YOUR BODY

SUSAN WADIA-ELLS, PhD

Foreword by Thomas N. Seyfried, PhD

Busting Breast Cancer: Five Simple Steps to Keep Breast Cancer Out of Your Body
Copyright © 2020, Susan Wadia-Ells

Important Warning and Disclaimer
The contents of this book are for informational purposes only and are not intended to diagnose, treat, cure, or prevent any condition or disease. You understand that this book is not intended as a substitute for consultation with a licensed practitioner. The author is not a medical professional. All the information contained in this book is based on the research or experience of others, along with some of the author's personal experience. This book is not intended to supplement nor replace the advice or guidance of a healthcare professional. The author specifically disclaims any liability, loss, or risk, personal or otherwise, that is incurred as a consequence, directly or indirectly, of the use and application of any of the contents of this book. The use of this book implies your acceptance of this disclaimer.

Published by Busting Breast Cancer©, Manchester by-the-Sea, MA
www.bustingbreastcancer.com

Editorial: Nancy Brandwein, Emilie Sandoz-Voyer and Judith Bloch (Girl Friday Productions); Albert M. Liberatore, Jr. (Edits Made Easy); Kate Victory Hannisian (Blue Pencil Consulting)

Interior, Cover Design and Graphics: Tessa Magnuson (Align Graphic Design, LLC)

ISBN 978-1-7345324-0-1 (paperback)
ISBN 978-1-7345324-1-8 (e-book)
LCCN 2020922057

First Edition

Printed in the United States of America

TO MY MANY TEACHERS:

Anne Janeway, Joan Loomis Hastings, Freda Gould Rebelsky, Linda B. Haltinner, Jeroo Eduljee, Jane L. Gardiner, Stephen LaPierre and Jo Sephus

TABLE OF CONTENTS

FIGURES & TABLES

ACRONYMS & ABBREVIATIONS

ACS	American Cancer Society
ACS	American College of Surgeons
AHA	American Heart Association
AMA	American Medical Association
ATP	Adenosine triphosphate
BC	Boston College
BCA	Breast Cancer Action
BCRP	Breast Cancer Research Program
BMI	body mass index
BPA	bisphenol A
BRCA1	BReast CAncer gene 1
BRCA2	BReast CAncer gene 2
BSE	breast self-exam
CAGR	compound annual growth rate
CARE	Women's Contraceptive and Reproductive Experience study
CBE	clinical breast exam
CCK	cholecystokinin
CDC	Centers for Disease Control
COC	combination oral contraceptives
CRADAs	Cooperative Research and Development Agreements
CRP	C-reactive protein
d3	vitamin D3
DCIS	ductal carcinoma in situ
DCIS411	DCIS blog
DGAs	Dietary Guidelines for Americans
DMPA	depot medroxyprogesterone acetate
DNA	deoxyribonucleic acid
dnMBC	de novo metastatic breast caner
DON	glutamine antagonist 6-diazo-5-oxo-L-norleucine
DRIs	Dietary Reference Intakes

DTC	direct-to-consumer (advertising)
GKI	glucose ketone index
GMO	genetically modified organism
HER2	human epidermal growth factor receptor 2
HHS	US Department of Health and Human Services
HRT	hormone replacement therapy
HR Positive	types of breast cancer cells that contain hormone receptors
HR Negative	types of breast cancer that do not contain hormone receptors
HPV	human papillomavirus
I-fluid	interstitial fluid
IMBA	Institute of Molecular Biotechnology (Vienna, Austria)
IUs	international units
IOM	Institute of Medicine (renamed National Academy of Medicine (NAM) in 2015)
IUDs	intrauterine devices
MBC	metastatic breast cancer
MBCN	Metastatic Breast Cancer Network
MPA	medroxyprogesterone acetate
MtNBC	metastatic triple-negative breast cancer
NAACCR	North American Association of Central Cancer Registries
NAM	National Academy of Medicine (known as Institute of Medicine IOM, until 2014)
NCDB	National Cancer Database (American College of Surgeons)
NCI	National Cancer Institute
Ng/ml	nanograms per milliliter
NHI	National Health Initiative
NIH	National Institutes of Health
NPR	National Public Radio
NSAIDs	nonsteroidal anti-inflammatory drugs
OCs	organochlorides
OCs	oral contraceptives
ODS	ozone depleting substances
OSAS	obstructive sleep apnea syndrome

P53	tumor suppressor gene
PCBs	polychlorinated biphenyls
PDR	Physicians' Desk Reference
PET	positron emission tomography
PMS	premenstrual syndrome
POPs	persistent organic pollutants
RADs	units of radiation
RANK/RANKL	Receptor activator of nuclear factor B; Not to be confused with RANKL, the osteoblast cell-surface receptor that binds to RANK.
rMBC	recurrent metastatic breast cancer
ROS	reactive oxygen species
SEER	Surveillance, Epidemiology, and End Results (SEER) Program (NCI)
SEER 9	SEER database that includes 9 cancer registries and about 9% of population
SEER 13	SEER database that includes 13 cancer registries
SOC	standard of care
SPF	sun protection factor
Stage 0	DCIS (ductal carcinoma in situ)
Stage I	early invasive breast cancer
Stage II	early invasive breast cancer
Stage III	early invasive breast cancer
Stage IV	metastatic breast cancer
SUNARC	Sunlight, Nutrition, and Health Research Center
SWC	Smart Women's Choice contraceptive cream
TNBC	triple-negative breast cancer
USDA	United States Department of Agriculture
USPSTF	US Preventive Services Task Force
UVA	Ultraviolet A Rays
UVB	Ultraviolet B Rays
UVM	University of Vermont
UT	University of Texas
VDR	vitamin D receptor

"Breast cancer and mastectomy are not unique experiences, but ones shared by thousands of American women. Each of these women has a particular voice to be raised in what must become a female outcry against all preventable cancers."

—Audre Lorde (1934–1992)
The Cancer Journals

FOREWORD

I am delighted to write the foreword to Dr. Susan Wadia-Ells' important book, *Busting Breast Cancer*. Cancer in general, and breast cancer specifically, is a devastating disease that continues to produce physical and emotional distress for those affected. Despite enormous resources directed to cancer treatment, the incidence of new cases and death rates continues to climb. A fundamental misunderstanding of cancer biology is responsible in large part for the failure to effectively manage this disease. Cancer is currently viewed as a type of genetic disease, causing uncontrolled growth of cells in various tissues. This view has led to radical approaches to cancer therapy, including surgical mutilation, damaging radiation, and poisonous chemicals. Some of the newer cancer immunotherapies, which are supposed to target gene-linked checkpoints, are inordinately expensive, marginally effective, and unacceptably toxic. It has been my view that no major advances in cancer management will be realized as long as cancer is viewed as a genetic disease.

Emerging evidence shows that cancer is primarily a *metabolic disease*. The large numbers of gene mutations found in cancer cells arise as secondary effects of destabilized cellular energy metabolism. Cancer is caused from damage to the mitochondria, a cytoplasmic organelle network responsible for maintaining energy homeostasis through cellular respiration. Damage to the mitochondria produces reactive oxygen species (ROS) that are carcinogenic and mutagenic. It is the ROS that produce the plethora of mutations seen in the various forms of the disease. Cancer is not many diseases but is a singular disease of disturbed energy metabolism. The view of cancer as a mitochondrial metabolic disease can now explain the *oncogenic paradox*, which has puzzled cancer researchers for decades. The oncogenic paradox addressed the difficulty in linking various cancer-provoking causes (for example, viruses, chemicals, radiation, rare inherited mutations, and age) to a common pathophysiological mechanism. This oncogenic puzzle was also highlighted in Dr. Siddhartha Mukherjee's book, *The Emperor of All Maladies: A Biography of Cancer*. It now appears that each of these different cancer-associated agents causes damage to the mitochondria and, therefore, the ability of the cell to obtain energy through respiration. Cancer arises only in those cells that can transition from respiration energy to fermentation energy. Fermentation is a primitive form of cellular energy production that existed on our planet before oxygen appeared in the atmosphere. Fermentation is, therefore, the signature defect seen in all cancer cells, and is often referred to as the Warburg Effect. It is now clear that cancer originates from damage to the mitochondria in the cytoplasm, rather than from damage to the genome in the nucleus. The genomic damage in tumor cells follows, rather than precedes, the disturbances in cellular respiration. A lay account of this information was also recently highlighted in Travis Christofferson's provocative book, *Tripping Over the Truth: How the Metabolic Theory of Cancer Is Overturning One of Medicine's Most Entrenched Paradigms.* New, nontoxic and cost-effective therapeutic strategies for cancer management and prevention become apparent once cancer becomes recognized as a mitochondrial metabolic disease.

Dr. Wadia-Ells addresses key issues related to the incidence, management, and prevention of breast cancer. I was surprised to learn from her research that current information on breast cancer incidence in the US is poorly understood and likely inaccurate. Why should women in the US be left in the dark regarding information that can impact their health? Hopefully, Dr. Wadia-Ells' exposure of the increasing breast cancer epidemic will lead to greater attention among government and private agencies that monitor this disease. All women should have unbiased information regarding the incidence of a disease that primarily affects them. Dr. Wadia-Ells also describes a number of simple steps that can help women prevent breast cancer. It is important to recognize that some of her recommendations (for example, tips to maintain the health and vitality of cellular mitochondria) are relevant not only to breast cancer, but to all types of cancer. Many of her recommendations are simple and practical and might not be known to most women. For example, systemic inflammation can contribute to the occurrence of cancer, and the procedures she mentions to reduce systemic inflammation will go far in reducing breast cancer, as well as other cancers. She also addresses the potential causes of triple-negative breast cancer and questions whether surgical amputation is really necessary to prevent gene-linked breast cancers. This information will be important for helping women make informed decisions regarding their health. I applaud Dr. Wadia-Ells in boldly tackling the underlying causes of the breast cancer epidemic and in providing practical solutions to reduce this epidemic. All women, and anyone interested in preventing cancer, will benefit from reading this book.

Thomas N. Seyfried, PhD

Professor of Biology, Boston College | Author, *Cancer as a Metabolic Disease: On the Origin, Management, and Prevention of Cancer*

INTRODUCTION
OUR UNNECESSARY BREAST CANCER EPIDEMIC

This is a book about women taking charge of our own health. It's also a book that finally offers women a recipe for effective breast cancer prevention. So, this is a book you should read.

In 2012, the *metabolic approach* to cancer was first brought to light through the publication of Dr. Thomas N. Seyfried's landmark work, *Cancer as a Metabolic Disease: On the Origin, Management and Prevention of Cancer*. Until this time, neither biologists nor doctors had ever been given a complete scientific understanding of why one woman develops breast cancer while another woman never does. Previously, oncologists and breast surgeons could do little more than smile weakly and tell a woman, "Maybe it was just your turn," or "I guess you were just the unlucky one."

And there wasn't much that women themselves could do. They could run for the cause or wear pink headscarves over their bald heads and try to put on a brave smile. It was sad, but true. Oncologists and breast surgeons had no biologically based answers for our most burning questions:

"Why me?"

"How did I develop breast cancer?"

"How can I get rid of it—and prevent it from coming back again?"

Today, we finally understand. And it's the kind of understanding that makes everything look different than it did before—like discovering that the earth isn't flat, after all! Today, we take it for granted that the earth is round; and one day, we'll take for granted these newfound insights into how cancer works. But for now, it's all still new.

What's new? Biologists have finally put together all the pieces of this cancer puzzle. We're finally able to trace the logical, straightforward, biological path a healthy breast cell takes as it moves forward...or backwards. Thanks to these biologists, people like you and me can actually understand how and why a normal, healthy cell is able to turn itself into that first destructive cancer cell.

In his groundbreaking 2012 textbook, Dr. Seyfried lays out this revolutionary approach to cancer. Drawing on dozens of published, peer-reviewed laboratory and clinical studies spanning the past century, Dr. Seyfried finally makes sense out of the development of that first cancer cell. Armed with this information, individual cancer patients, medical schools, healthcare practitioners, and both government and private organizations can now work together to stop today's worldwide cancer epidemic from continuing at its terrifying pace. Published by the leading medical and scientific publishing house John Wiley & Sons, Dr. Seyfried's book has now put mainstream cancer centers on notice. It's time to change the way they do business.

Today, in the US alone, there is no longer a need for 1,600 people to die each day from cancer. Today, in the US alone, there is no longer a need for untold thousands more individuals to die each day from heart attacks, blood diseases, lung infections, liver failure, and suicides—too often the tragic side effects of today's toxic, mutilating, and misinformed cancer treatments. One of our many imperfect sources of national breast cancer statistics tells us that an estimated 276,480 new invasive breast tumors will be diagnosed in an unknown number of women in 2020; while another 48,550 women will be told, based on their mammogram report, that they have atypical cells in one or more ducts of their breast tissue, called *stage 0 breast cancer*, and urged to begin invasive breast cancer treatment.[1] Another national database puts the total number of women diagnosed in 2017 with invasive breast cancer cases at 350,000, with stage 0 or *in situ* cases at 84,367.[2] All of these women are then encouraged to begin toxic treatments for invasive breast cancer.

Clinicians treating metastatic breast cancer patients in the US sometimes share another national statistic that is not yet well publicized: the estimated number of women each year who are treated for an early-stage invasive breast cancer diagnosis (stages I, II, and III) who suffer a recurrence of their original diagnosis. One statistic from this recurrence group that stands out, above all, is the number of women treated who go on to develop metastatic breast cancer within months, years or decades.

As numerous clinical studies tell us, "Despite advances in the treatment of breast cancer, approximately 20–40% of women initially diagnosed with earlier stages of breast cancer eventually develop recurrent advanced or metastatic disease."[3] Metastatic or stage IV breast cancer is the terminal stage of this disease. This means that 3 women in every 10 who are treated in the US today for an early-stage invasive breast cancer will receive an early death sentence. These are horrific odds.

In 2019, an estimated 41,760 women in the US died from this stage 4 disease.[4] Estimates for earlier years, and for 2020, all show similar reported breast cancer mortality figures.[5] Today's "slash, burn and poison"[6] approach to breast cancer treatment (as breast cancer surgeon Dr. Susan Love has long described it) is not doing a very good job of protecting many breast cancer patients' long-term optimal health. Today's mainstream toxic treatments must be seen for what they are: *outdated, simply not good enough*. Yes, it is certainly best to find ways to stop breast cancer before it can develop in your body.

Busting Breast Cancer, the book you are holding, is a book for every woman. That's because *Busting Breast Cancer* describes the groundbreaking metabolic approach to cancer in easy-to-understand terms. The five simple lifestyle changes, based on this modern-day approach to understanding cancer and described in the pages ahead, are simple daily habits that can keep our metabolism, our bodies' operating systems, moving forward in such a way as to effectively keep breast cancer from beginning to develop in our bodies. Who knew?

Many of the studies you'll read about in this book make it clear how, once a sufficient number of women in the US are following these five prevention steps, the incidence of breast cancer in our country can decrease by anywhere from 50 to 80 percent. Take a moment to take that in: It's possible for individual women to reduce the incidence of breast cancer in the United States by 50 to 80 percent! That's astounding. Sadly, however, there is a major obstacle: a woman's internal resistance to change. It's that resistance that will make some of you read about these prevention steps, slam the book shut, and walk away.

Are you someone who doesn't like to rock the boat? Are you someone who becomes really uncomfortable when asked to question authority? Is change difficult for you? Are you someone who's afraid to take action or to speak up? If so, *Busting Breast Cancer* may be a real challenge.

I mention this fact because *Busting Breast Cancer* calls into question some of what you've believed in, up to this point. This book will show the outdated, incorrect, even damaging information that's coming out of such trusted institutions as the American Cancer Society, Susan G. Komen for the Cure, Planned Parenthood, the National Cancer Institute, the National Academy of Medicine and even the US Department of Agriculture's "food pyramid." That's going to be hard to digest.

In her best-selling book, *Women, Food and God*, Geneen Roth writes about "The Voice." If you're like most women, then you know "The Voice" only too well. It's that internal critic that never seems very far away. It always comes alive when it's time to try something new; something daring, something exhilarating, something possibly even lifesaving—like the lifestyle changes you'll read about in this book.

So, you've been warned: as you learn new things in the pages ahead, "The Voice" is going to tell you to put the book down and stick with what's familiar. I hope you won't do that. Because what's familiar isn't working—far too many women are developing and dying every day from a disease they don't have to have. I hope you'll tell "The Voice" to be quiet and let you read on, discovering the basics of this new metabolic, transparent and *lifestyle-based* understanding of cancer.

Once you've read through Chapter 1, it might become much easier to make your own decisions about how best to protect yourself from developing that first breast cancer cell. By the time you finish reading this book, I hope you'll also understand why every woman must stop being passive when it comes to the possibility of developing breast cancer. I hope you'll come to see why each of us can—and *must*—take control of our own health. And that means changing many of our daily habits. In their place, you'll learn to substitute new habits that will keep your breast cells' power batteries, known as *mitochondria*, healthy and cancer free throughout the course of your life.

Today, US women of all ages face the highest breast cancer rates the world has ever known. And sadly, those statistics are getting worse, not better. This is because our mainstream breast cancer industry does not yet understand what this book will teach you: why one woman develops breast cancer and another woman does not. So, they go on telling us to let mammography machines smash our breasts and shoot radiation into our soft tissue in search of a tumor or irregular cells. They call this barbaric practice "breast cancer screening" and "breast cancer prevention." You may be shocked to discover (in Chapter 5) that it is neither of these things.

Fortunately, this book on the new metabolic understanding of cancer clearly answers that one critical question: Why does one woman develop breast cancer while another woman never does? This new approach to cancer can also guide each of us as we take the nourishing, inexpensive, and incredibly effective prevention steps described in the chapters ahead. But watch out! There will be pushback from every voice of authority out there! This is because as these prevention steps begin to reduce the incidence of breast cancer, women's success will damage the breast cancer industry's booming financial projections.

By 2027, reports tells us, the worldwide breast cancer treatment market is expected to reach $22.4–38.4 billion. This means that industry leaders and investors in pharmaceutical, radiology, and cancer centers are counting on record-breaking breast cancer drug sales, combined with other record-breaking cancer treatment income, to create an 8.3–10.7% percent compound annual growth rate (CAGR) over this forecast period.[7] Over one-third of these dollars is expected to be generated by the US market. Of course, this term "US market" refers to you, me, and every other woman alive today in the United States. Yes, this industry is *counting* on you and me, and more than a quarter-million other American women, to develop more and more breast cancer each and every coming year.[8] One particular market research firm's press release from 2018 says it frighteningly well: "Breast Cancer Market: Elegant Growth at a CAGR of 9.2%." The article goes on to say, "As no absolute treatment is available, there is a scope for developing the market across the world."[9]

Yes, today's breast cancer industry represents a true conflict of interests—especially for women who own pharmaceutical and radiology stocks. The very industry women rely on to prevent and cure breast cancer makes its ever-expanding profits from *not* preventing and *not* curing breast cancer! Let that sink in.

Figure I.1: Global Breast Cancer Drugs Market Share, 2017(%)

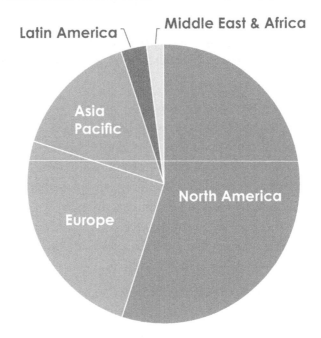

US women pay out over 50% of all revenues received by the worldwide breast cancer industry.

Grand View Research "Breast Cancer Drugs Market Size, Share & Trends Analysis Report by Type (Hormonal Receptors, Mitotic Inhibitors, HER2 Inhibitors), By Region, And Segment Forecasts, 2019-2025" press release February 2019.

Remember, American women represent only 4.3 percent of the world's female population.[10] But, according to at least one market research report, we continue to contribute more than 50 percent of all income generated worldwide by the breast cancer treatment industry.[11] American women need this breast cancer epidemic to end! This can only happen as individual women decide to make a few significant lifestyle changes. Without taking the steps described in this book, too many women will not be able to keep breast cancer out of their bodies. It will only be when enough individual women ignore current-day authorities and instead, embrace these new habits. This is the only way that individual women will be able to shrink today's expanding breast cancer industry within the next five to ten years and beyond.

Here is a quote from another world market report; this one predicts even greater worldwide breast cancer income growth if women refuse to change many of their current lifestyle habits. "The breast cancer therapeutics market is set to exceed USD 28 billion by 2024...rising shift(s) towards adoption of western lifestyles...rising prevalence of obesity in women after menopause will drive the industry size...rising use of hormone replacement therapy (HRT) and oral birth control pills ...will boost the business size over the forecast period. Growing exposure to certain carcinogens and endocrine disrupters, for example in the workplace, working night shifts (also) results in increased risks (that) are surging up the global market...US market accounted for the highest regional share in 2018."[12]

Our Subservient Federal Cancer Agencies

It's easy to understand why private interests tend to engage only in research aimed at developing expensive drugs and other treatments, since those are far more profitable than most lifestyle-based prevention methods. But our national cancer agencies are taxpayer-funded organizations. These agencies, established to protect all citizens' health, should not be helping develop expensive cancer treatment drugs that pharmaceutical companies can eventually sell at inflated prices, reaping billions for a select few.[13] Yet, for decades, most taxpayer dollars earmarked for breast cancer research have been spent on encouraging more women to have more mammograms, and on developing newer, more expensive and usually more profitable drugs and radiation procedures to treat this disease; never on helping women actually prevent breast cancer in the first place.[14] But why?

Our federal cancer agencies continue to be led by individuals, appointed by both Democratic and Republican administrations. These individuals remain connected—attached for life—to today's highly profitable cancer treatment industry. These policymakers often move back and forth between corporate and government decision-making positions, using public funds to expand the mainstream industry; often favoring the development of new drugs and diagnostic practices, even, we are told, if such drugs and tests are not always innovative or needed, but will be profitable. Much of the time these government agencies, controlled or influenced by corporate lobbying groups, misinform the public, ignore, or even ban inexpensive and available prevention options (many of which you'll find discussed in the chapters ahead).[15]

We Must Each Take Charge

This is a very personal book. I didn't decide to spend the past dozen years of my life studying and writing about breast cancer prevention because of some isolated intellectual curiosity. Nor did I receive a massive research grant out of the blue. I am not a scientist, by any stretch of the imagination—my first and last biology course was during sophomore year of high school, and I quickly vowed never to touch another dead frog again! But once this merciless disease killed my friend Jerilyn in 2007, when she was only 57 years old, I became determined to find out where all of this breast cancer came from in the first place. I didn't want to end up like my good friend and too many others: sick, unable to work, bankrupt, and then dead from this dread disease. The greatly loved director of a small, private East Coast school for children with learning differences, Jerilyn spent well over $75,000 out of pocket—and her insurance company spent well over $300,000—before her death. Totally trusting today's mainstream cancer industry, Jerilyn died less than five years after her first diagnosis, despite the over quarter-million dollars spent trying to manage her cancer.

Call it ignorance, innocence, insanity, or pure arrogance on my part, but for some reason Jerilyn's death stirred up my investigative journalism juices, and with the ongoing support of hundreds of concerned individuals and a few small foundations over these past years, I became determined to see if I could uncover published, but ignored, peer-reviewed, evidence-based research that could answer my three burning questions: Why do some women develop breast cancer? How exactly does this disease develop? And what can I do to prevent breast cancer from starting up in my own body?

Yes, American women are clearly under an unnecessary siege, as pharmaceutical and radiology companies continue to assure their investors that breast cancer is not going away anytime soon—at least not in the United States, where they triumphantly project those 7 to 10 percent compound annual growth rates, called CAGRs,[16] in breast cancer treatment income for the coming decade. As if such estimates are not bad enough, some of these numbers appear to be partially based on the 2015 calculations of a leading statistician at the National Cancer Institute, predicting that American women will experience a huge surge—a *50 percent* increase—in breast cancer diagnoses in the coming decade. What is the major cause of this projected storm of new breast cancer cases? It's the baby boomers, we're told. Women born between 1946 and 1964 will have all reached retirement age during that time period.[17]

Yes, both institutional and individual pharmaceutical drug investors may be smacking their lips as they anticipate increasing breast cancer treatment profits, at more and more women's expense. But American women no longer need to stand by and silently suffer under this onslaught. Remember, breast cancer treatment centers and drug companies need more and more clients (think: women) to satisfy their investors' financial goals. Stopping breast cancer before it starts is just not the cancer industry's job, and it's never going to be their priority. This means individual women, each taking the five effective prevention steps described in this book, will create the only group in the United States that can slow down and eventually end this unnecessary epidemic. Remember, individual women comprise the only group in the US today that has the self-interest to stop most breast cancer before it starts. And thanks to the information you'll find in the pages of this book, we now have the knowledge, too. We'll do it ourselves—one woman at a time.

Welcome to our very personal revolution.

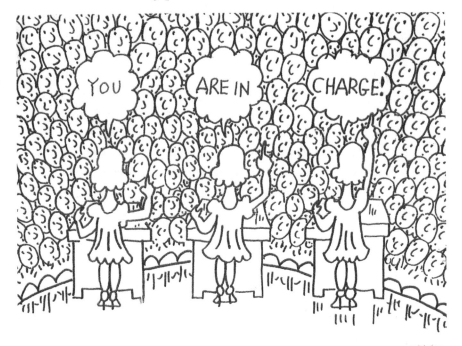

Phyllis Yampolsky ©2014

INTRODUCTION ENDNOTES

1   R.L. Siegal, K.D. Miller and A. Jemal, "Cancer Statistics, 2020," *CA: A Cancer Journal for Clinicians* 70, no.1 (January/February 2020): 7-30, https://doi.org/10.3322/caac.21590; The American College of Surgeons' National Cancer Database calculates much higher rates of breast cancer than the above 2017 state-based cancer registry data and NCI SEER 2016 sources. See Chapter 5 and Chapter 9.

2   Figure based on the 70% figure recorded by the American College of Surgeons, "National Database: 2017."

3   Joyce O'Shaughnessy, "Extending Survival with Chemotherapy in Metastatic Breast Cancer," (October 2005) https://doi.org/10.1634/theoncologist.10-90003-20. also see: Takeshita et al.,"Late Recurrence of Breast Cancer Is Associated with Pro-cancerous Immune Microenvironment in the Primary Tumor," *Scientific Reports* 9, no.16942 (2019), https://doi.org/10.1038/s41598-019-53482-x.

4   American Cancer Society, Breast Cancer Facts and Figures, 2019–2020, https://www.cancer.org/content/dam/cancer-org/research/cancer-facts-and-statistics/breast-cancer-facts-and-figures/breast-cancer-facts-and-figures-2019-2020.pdf.

5   Siegal, Miller and Jamal, "Cancer Statistics, 2020," *CA: A Cancer Journal for Clinicians* 70, no.1 (January/February 2020); American Cancer Society, "Breast Cancer Facts and Figures, 2019–2020, https://www.cancer.org/content/dam/cancer-org/research/cancer-facts-and-statistics/breast-cancer-facts-and-figures/breast-cancer-facts-and-figures-2019-2020.pdf.

6   Susan Bolotin, "Slash, Burn and Poison," Books, *The New York Times on the Web*, April 13, 1997.

7   iHealthcareAnalyst, Inc., "Global Breast Cancer Therapeutics Market $22.4 Billion by 2027," April 21, 2020, https://www.ihealthcareanalyst.com/higher-incidence-rising-prevalence-drive-breast-cancer-therapeutics-market/. Grand View Research, "Breast Cancer Drug Market Worth $38.4 Billion By 2025 | CAGR: 10.7%," Feb 2019, https://www.grandviewresearch.com/press-release/global-breast-cancer-drugs-market.

8   Research and Markets, "Global Breast Cancer Treatment Market 2017–2025," Research and Markets.com, https://www.businesswire.com/news/home/20170928005543/en/Global-Breast-Cancer-Treatment-Market-2017-2025—.

9   Market Research Futures, "Breast Cancer Market Elegant Growth at a CAGR of 9.2% by Types & Treatment—Asserts MRFR," June 26, 2018, https://www.abnewswire.com/pressreleases/breast-cancer-market-2018-share-elegant-growth-at-a-cagr-of-92-by-treatment-chemotherapy-surgery-radiation-therapy-etc-avail-at-marketreseacrhfuturecom_233852.html.

10 Amanda K. Baumle editor, *Demography In Transition: Emerging Trends in Population Studies*, Cambridge Scholars Publishing; Unabridged edition (October 1, 2006).

11 Grand View Research, "Breast Cancer Drugs Market Size, Share & Trends Analysis Report by Type (Hormonal Receptors, Mitotic Inhibitors, HER2 Inhibitors), By Region, And Segment Forecasts, 2019-2025," press release, February 2019, https://www.grandviewresearch.com/industry-analysis/breast-cancer-drugs-market.

12 Market Watch, "Breast Cancer Therapeutics Market Set for Rapid Growth and Trend by 2027," April 28, 2020, https://www.marketwatch.com/press-release/breast-cancer-therapy-market-2020-2027-top-manufacturers-competitive-landscape-growth-rate-2020-08-17?tesla=y.

13 Matt Richtel and Andrew Pollack, "Harnessing the US Taxpayer to Fight Cancer & Make Profits," December 19, 2016, *The New York Times*, https://www.nytimes.com/2016/12/19/health/harnessing-the-us-taxpayer-to-fight-cancer-and-make-profits.html.

14   See: Marcia Angell, *The Truth About the Drug Companies: How They Deceive Us and What to Do About It* (New York: Random House, 2004); Samuel A. Epstein, *National Cancer Institute and American Cancer Society: Criminal Indifference to Cancer Prevention and Conflicts of Interest* (Bloomington, IN: Xlibris, 2011).

15   See Carl Elliott, *White Coats, Black Hats: Adventures on the Dark Side of Medicine* (Boston: Beacon, 2010); Devra Davis, *The Secret History of the War on Cancer* (New York: Basic Books, 2007); Samuel A. Epstein, *National Cancer Institute and Criminal Indifference*, 2011.

16   Investopedia defines compound annual growth rate (CAGR) as the rate of return that would be required for an investment to grow from its beginning balance to its ending balance, assuming the profits were reinvested at the end of each year of the investment's lifespan. https://www.investopedia.com/investing/compound-annual-growth-rate-what-you-should-know/.

17   Philip Rosenberg, National Cancer Institute, "U.S. Breast Cancer Cases Expected to Increase by as Much as 50 Percent by 2030," presentation to the annual meeting of the American Association for Cancer Research, Philadelphia, PA, April 18, 2015 (unpublished). Press release: https://mb.cision.com/Public/3069/9755232/81b414b4ec298479.pdf.

PART I.
THEORY

THE METABOLIC APPROACH TO CANCER:
Finally Understanding the Earth is Round

"In principle, there are few chronic diseases more easily preventable than cancer...the origin of carcinogenesis resides with the mitochondria in the cytoplasm, not with the genome in the nucleus."

—Thomas N. Seyfried,
Cancer as a Metabolic Disease

My friend Marissa was 61 years old in August 2013 when she was diagnosed with invasive breast cancer. A mammogram detected a pea-size 1.3 cm (1/2-inch) mass in her left breast, and a fine needle aspiration determined the tumor contained triple-negative cancer cells. Marissa refused further diagnostic tests. She also declined surgery, radiation, and drugs. Like more and more cancer patients today, Marissa was determined to avoid the industry's highly imperfect—and highly toxic—treatments. She wanted to find nourishing ways to begin healing her own body.

A month later, Marissa's research led us both to attend the first national Cure to Cancer Summit. This free, ten-day, online audio event included interviews with thirty international health practitioners, cancer researchers, and cancer patients who all had personal experience with various nontoxic, noninvasive cancer treatments. These innovative treatments included the use of hyperbaric oxygen, heat therapies, and dietary therapies. One naturopathic doctor insisted that today's mainstream invasive treatments are barking up the wrong tree; she said that instead of trying to destroy each and every duplicating cancer cell with a variety of harsh frontal attacks, it's more important to cut off the fuels that feed the cancer cells.

During these hopeful Cure to Cancer Summit sessions, Marissa and I heard other speakers also describe cancer as a *metabolic* disease. We learned that a healthy cell becomes a cancer cell once its mitochondria—think of them as the cell's power batteries—are severely damaged. When that happens, those cells are no longer able to process oxygen to make energy. "Cancer," that same holistic physician said, "does not begin when one of your genes spontaneously mutates, for some unknown or assumed reason, into a nasty cancer cell. These genetic mutations are always a second, third, or fourth step in the life of a cancer cell—not that key first step."

As Marissa and I continued to listen each day to the online cancer summit's speakers, we heard things that fundamentally changed the way we understood cancer. The naturopathic doctor told us about a Boston College biologist, Dr. Thomas Seyfried, who had recently published a book laying out a metabolic approach to cancer. According to this new approach, all types of cancer have the same biological beginning. The disease of cancer happens when our body's operating system (its metabolism) malfunctions. Dr. Seyfried's book describes how that first breast cancer cell is born when the mitochondria (or power batteries) within a breast duct or milk lobe cell suffocate. And the process is the same for liver cells, lung cells, brain cells, blood cells—it turns out that different types of cancer aren't so different, after all! If Dr. Seyfried was right, then that would mean that breast cancer (indeed, *all* cancer) might actually be *preventable*! It would mean that women don't have to be sitting ducks, waiting passively for the dreaded diagnosis—that women could *do* something, could take charge of their own health. By caring for the precious mitochondria in their breast cells, women have the power to actually keep breast cancer out of their bodies!

As I complete this manuscript in the spring of 2020, it's been more than six years since my friend Marissa bucked the mainstream cancer authorities and decided to use only noninvasive, nontoxic, metabolic therapies to treat her cancer. And she continues winning the battle against that 2013 cancer diagnosis—in fact, Marissa's tumor can no longer even be detected on her biannual ultrasound tests! She also continues to enjoy better health than when she was first diagnosed. Having maintained her hundred-pound weight loss since that initial diagnosis, Marissa has also continued to keep her vitamin D3 blood level around 100 nanograms per milliliter (ng/ml); that's a far cry from her low D3 blood level of 9 ng/ml at the time she was diagnosed. Today, Marisa no longer uses her favorite placenta-based skin cream,[1] and she continues to say "No!" to her life-long love, sugar. She also remains faithful to new daily habits that have proven helpful in battling her recurrent bouts of immobilizing stress. Clearly, Marissa made the right choice when she opted for a metabolic approach to her cancer.

A Solution to the Oncogenic Paradox: How Cancer Really Works

Before we turn our attention to the concrete steps you can take to prevent a breast cancer diagnosis, it is important to know about the dozens of small organelles within each of our breast cells, called mitochondria. It is also important to understand each tiny mitochondrion's relationship to breast cancer; actually, to all cancers.

The central insight of the metabolic approach to cancer has to do with what happens when a cell's mitochondria begin to suffocate. It turns out that suffocating mitochondria don't always self-destruct and die. Instead, these clever "power batteries" within our cells are sometimes able to switch their oxygen-based generating systems back to their original, prehistoric fermenting (glucose-powered) energy systems.

The insight that our mitochondria evolved from prehistoric, fermenting, single-cell bacteria was first described in the late 1960s by Dr. Lynn Margulis, a biologist at Boston University. Challenging the view of the top biology scholars of her day, Dr. Margulis stuck by her unique theory of mitochondrial evolution—all while having to endure her peers' ridicule for decades. Today, she is lauded as the scientist who firmly established the now-accepted *endosymbiotic theory of eukaryotic cell development.*[2] In fact, a decade before her death in 2011, she was awarded the National Medal of Science for this discovery.[3] In non-science speak, her theory explains how the power batteries (mitochondria) in mammals and the power batteries (chloroplasts) in plants were both created when two different types of bacteria joined together.

Revolutionary as this theory (and the metabolic approach to cancer that develops from it) may be, it's important to acknowledge right at the outset that there is at least one area of agreement among virtually everyone who studies or treats cancer. On the one side, we have mainstream medical schools, most cancer centers and most cancer researchers who continue to adhere to the genetic theory of cancer. On the other side, we have biologists and a growing number of clinicians who now understand that cancer is a metabolic disease.[4] But on both sides of the issue, virtually all agree on this: There are at least seven different ways in which our lifestyles, life choices, and life events are directly connected to the development of cancer. Mainstream oncologists call this the oncogenic *paradox*.[5] Dr. Seyfried often begins his talks about the metabolic approach to cancer with this question: *How is it possible that so many different phenomena cause the same disease?* Today, biologists, beginning with Professor Seyfried, who first pieced together the complete metabolic approach to cancer, and others say that it's not a paradox at all. Given the metabolic understanding of how cancer begins, there are any number of lifestyles, life choices, life events, and even a few inherited mutated tumor suppressor genes[6] that have one thing in common: they all can help cause the mitochondria in cells to suffocate, initiating the development of that first cancer cell.

What follows in much of this book is a look at various ways each of us can protect our mitochondria—especially the mitochondria in our breast cells—so that they won't become damaged by, and suffocate from, any or many of these seven causes. Taking steps to protect these all-important power batteries in our breast cells so that they can process lots of oxygen each day, ultimately means taking steps to keep breast cancer out of our bodies forever.

The Seven Causes of Cancer

Since it's a point on which virtually everyone agrees, let's take a look at these seven lifestyles, life choices and life events that can contribute to the development of cancer.

Cause #1: Chronic, whole-body inflammation

This type of inflammation may originate from a wide range of substances or conditions.[7] The list includes some prescription drugs, autoimmune conditions, obesity, chronically high levels of toxic (free or unbalanced) estrogen, excessive alcohol consumption, smoking, lack of exercise, allergies, asthma, poor oral health, and high cortisol levels that stem from unrelenting stress.[8] Chronically experiencing *unbalanced* levels of a sex hormone, such as having more estrogen than progesterone in your body, is a major factor in many women's breast cancer diagnoses. This is because excess levels of animal and chemical estrogens and chemical progestins are toxic to a woman's breast cells; damaging the mitochondria and accelerating the duplication of existing cancer cells in the breast. In Chapter 2 we'll discuss how natural estrogen from a woman's fat cells (or adipose tissue) can raise her breast cancer risk. In Chapter 4 we'll discuss the breast cancer risk posed by a chemical called progestin, used in birth control drugs and some hormone replacement drugs. In Chapter 6 we'll discuss how to prevent the accumulation of unbalanced/excess estrogens, including estrogen-like chemicals called *xenoestrogens*.

Cause #2: Radiation (ionizing or ultraviolet)

Ironically, much of the radiation women encounter comes from the mainstream cancer industry's efforts to diagnose and treat breast cancer! Mammography and other types of medical diagnostic tests, along with certain cancer treatments, used in cancer clinics today, bombard breast cells with the radiation that can, itself, be a major culprit in suffocating our mitochondria and causing cancer.[9]

Cause #3: Specific viral infections

HIV-AIDS,[10] hepatitis C,[11] HPV,[12] and some types of herpes[13] are known to damage cells' mitochondria and contribute to cancer development.

Cause #4: Intermittent hypoxia (sleep apnea)

Several studies now find that obstructive sleep apnea syndrome (OSAS) causes oxidative stress and systemic whole-body inflammation.[14] Such inflammation, as we have already described, is a contributor to the development of cancer.

Cause #5: Chemical carcinogens

Harmful chemicals include glyphosate (in such products as Roundup) and atrazine, found in GMO foods and some public water supplies in the US and West Africa. These will be discussed in more detail in Chapters 6 and 7.[15]

Figure 1.1: The Oncogenic Paradox: Seven Causes of Cancer

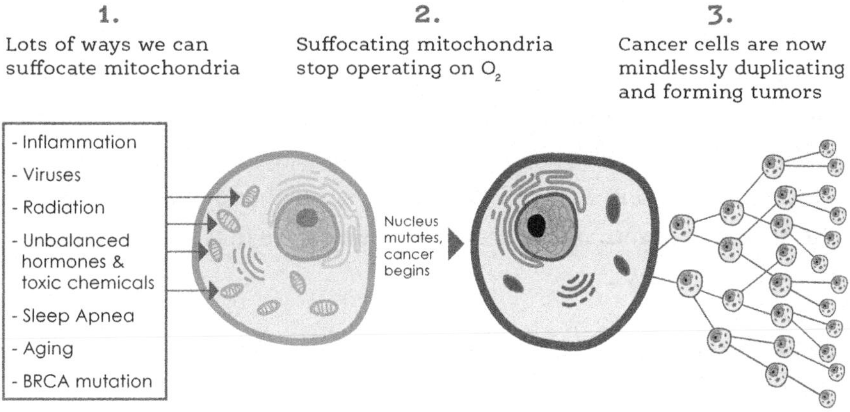

1.	**2.**	**3.**
Lots of ways we can suffocate mitochondria	Suffocating mitochondria stop operating on O_2	Cancer cells are now mindlessly duplicating and forming tumors

- Inflammation
- Viruses
- Radiation
- Unbalanced hormones & toxic chemicals
- Sleep Apnea
- Aging
- BRCA mutation

Nucleus mutates, cancer begins

The oncogenic paradox asks, "how can there be at least seven ways to create the same disease called 'cancer'?"

Adapted from Thomas N. Seyfried, Cancer as a Metabolic Disease: On the Origin, Management, and Prevention of Cancer, p. 254.

Cause #6: Inherited gene mutations

Women born with a damaged or mutated BRCA1 or BRCA2 gene have inherited one or more unique breast cancer risk factors within each damaged gene. It's important to remember, though, that a damaged or mutated BRCA1 or BRCA2 gene *does not directly cause breast cancer* all by itself. Instead, such a gene can sometimes damage, instead of protect breast cells' mitochondria, giving that woman an extra risk factor or two for developing breast cancer.[16] This is why only 40 percent of women worldwide who are born with a mutated BRCA1 or BRCA2 gene, eventually go on to develop breast cancer. Meanwhile, the remaining 60 percent of women born with a mutation in either of these two genes are somehow able to protect their breast cells' mitochondria. Therefore, they never develop the disease.[17] Chapter 8 describes some ways a damaged or mutated BRCA gene can increase a woman's vulnerability to the development of breast cancer. This same chapter also describes how women can actively help mitigate some of these vulnerabilities or risk factors, using specific lifestyle practices.

Cause #7: Aging

Statistics tell us that the risk of developing breast cancer increases with a woman's age. But why? We know that the cartilage in our knees and hip joints can wear out with age, especially if we've experienced an injury or failed to give our bodies adequate nutrition over the years to create new cartilage. In similar fashion, if we neglect the nutritional needs of our mitochondria, and if we rarely detoxify the mitochondria in our breast cells, they will eventually suffocate. And that's the first step in the cancer-creation process.[18]

How Some Boston College Mice Made World History

In his 2014 book, science writer Travis Christofferson chronicles Dr. Seyfried's amazing adventure as the biology professor uncovered, and then pieced together, all the steps that create that first cancer cell. According to Christofferson's stunning narrative, Seyfried's unbelievable journey began when the professor had a chance encounter with some mice that were given a drug that made them lose their appetite. The mice simply stopped eating. Lo and behold, their cancerous tumors quickly shrank! After trying out a few more reduced-calorie experiments on a bunch of other cancerous mice, Dr. Seyfried realized that if you stopped feeding mice much of anything, similar to putting a human on a water-only fast, these rodents' cancerous tumors would shrink...and shrink quickly![19]

In the course of conducting research, teaching and mentoring both undergrads and graduate students at Yale and Boston College since the 1970s, Dr. Seyfried and his lab members had published research on any number of genetic diseases. For a long time, Seyfried's labs had focused on unraveling the complexities behind rare genetic-based diseases, such as Tay-Sachs and Sandhoff;[20] on using the ketogenic diet to manage childhood epilepsy; and on developing laboratory models of metastatic cancer cells. No wonder those fasting mice and their shrinking tumors were such a startling phenomenon. The shrinking tumors in those underfed mice raised lots of questions for this genetics-trained biologist. Did Dr. Seyfried's discovery mean that a cancer cell's growth was not initiated by a mutating gene in a cell's nucleus, but instead had something to do with diet, with a mouse's or a person's metabolism? Did it mean that cancer is somehow or actually a rather straightforward and understandable disease? Might it be possible for people to learn how to prevent and manage a cancer diagnosis with some combination of metabolic adjustments focused on food or nourishment, cellular cleansing, and immune-strengthening lifestyles?

If so, then the mainstream cancer treatment industry has been barking up the wrong tree—with tragic results. Every day 1,600 or more people die from cancer in the United States alone.[21] And possibly three times that number die from heart attacks, strokes, liver failure, and suicides that stem from today's highly imperfect, highly toxic, and often mutilating cancer treatments.[22] It seems pretty clear that the genetic approach to cancer isn't working very well.

Dr. Seyfried's mice made him consider that, perhaps, cancer might *not* be the complex, genetics-based, uncontrollable and complex horror show that everyone seemed to presume it is. He began to wonder whether other scientists had ever documented anything like those fasting mice and their rapidly shrinking tumors. Was there published research, hidden away in scientific journals? Had important studies been ignored, left unfunded, or brushed off as simplistic, irrelevant, or even ridiculous? Was there documented knowledge out there that supported a biologically-grounded metabolic origin of that first cancer cell? Seyfried put on his well-worn Sherlock Holmes cap and decided to find out.

By 2000, Dr. Seyfried and his laboratory team had come across Nobel Prize-winning biologist Otto Warburg's finding that all cancer cells have something fascinating in common: cancer cells no longer respire or process oxygen to create their cell's energy; instead, all cancer cells ferment. In other words, all cancer cells use glucose, not oxygen, to create the energy to keep their fermenting cells duplicating. This discovery, showing how cancer cells each break down or ferment glucose as a major source of energy, is known today as the Warburg effect."[23]

Encouraged by these findings, Professor Seyfried and his team continued their research. They found a collection of papers published by Dr. Peter L. Pedersen, a determined researcher at Johns Hopkins Medical

School. Since the 1970s, Professor Pederson has been studying and describing "in elegant detail" how cancerous mitochondria operate.[24] This, in turn, led Dr. Seyfried to uncover published papers documenting two incredibly basic, yet stunning, lab experiments, both conducted in the mid-1990s by graduate students at the University of Vermont (UVM) and at the University of Texas (UT).[25] As Christofferson tells the story, each of these student lab teams, unaware of the other's research, created reconstituted cells—what biology students call *recons*.[26] In this case they transplanted the cancerous nucleus from a cancerous mouse cell into the healthy cytoplasm (the rest of the cell, located outside the nucleus) of a healthy mouse cell.[27] Presto! When the students injected this cancerous nucleus into their healthy cell that included healthy mitochondria, their new recon (laboratory-constructed cell) did not become cancerous! That cancerous nucleus was not able to control the operation of its new, healthy cellular home. Those students had found something startling. When it comes to the origin of cancer, those cellular power batteries, our cells' mitochondria (located outside a cell's nucleus), control their cell's nucleus.

The Warburg Effect

"Cancer, above all other diseases, has countless secondary causes. But, even for cancer, there is only one prime cause. Summarized in a few words, the prime cause of cancer is the replacement of the respiration of oxygen in normal body cells by a fermentation of sugar.

Just as there are many remote causes of plague: heat, insects, rats, but only one common cause, the plague bacillus, there are a great many remote causes of cancer: tar, rays, arsenic, pressure, urethane—but there is only one common cause into which all other causes of cancer merge, the irreversible injuring of respiration."

Otto Warburg, The Prime Cause and Prevention of Cancer, Lecture, delivered to Nobel Laureates, Lindau, Lake Constance, Germany, June 30, 1966.

The UVM students kept going, this time doing their recon experiment in reverse: They added a healthy nucleus from a mouse cell into the cytoplasm of a cell filled with cancerous mitochondria. Presto, that cancerous cell remained cancerous. Yes, that healthy nucleus was clearly impotent; it could not redirect those cancerous mitochondria. These students' experiments showed that when it comes to causing and controlling cancer, our mitochondria are in charge.

Summarizing these experiments, and adding his own surprise discovery involving the fasting lab mice, Dr. Seyfried told Christofferson in 2013, "The beauty of it is that none of these people were doing these experiments specifically to test the (Warburg) hypothesis. It was tested unknowingly by the person doing the experiments, so you couldn't ask for anything less biased."[28]

Figure 1.2: Role of the nucleus and mitochondria in the origin of tumors

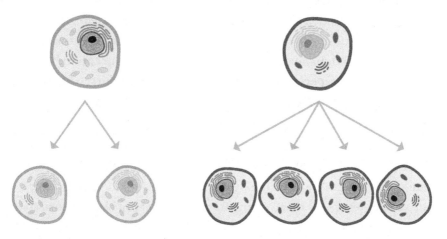

Experiment #1	Experiement #2
Healthy mitochondria + cancerous nucleus = healthy cells	Cancerous mitochondria + healthy nucleus = cancerous cells

The mitochondria run the show.

Adapted from T.N. Seyfried, Cancer as a Metabolic Disease: On the Origin, Management and Prevention of Cancer, 2012, 203 (Figure 11.3).

UVM professor William Schaeffer and UT professor Jerry Shay each published their graduate students' startling recon experiments. But both papers were completely ignored.[29] It appears that not one person at the National Institutes of Health (which includes the National Cancer

Institute) was willing to fund any follow-up studies. "Rather than shaking the foundation of cancer biology, the claim was ignored—even worse than being argued against," Christofferson concludes in his book.[30]

Linda Nebeling: A Nutritionist Questions Authority

Next in his journey of discovery, Dr. Seyfried uncovered the PhD dissertation of Dr. Linda Nebeling. Back in 1995, Linda Nebeling was an open-minded PhD candidate in nutrition at Case Western Reserve in Cleveland. Nebeling was interested in exploring nutritional therapies for treating cancer. This was also the same time when a new type of cancer diagnostic test, nicknamed the PET scan, began to be used.

PET is an acronym for positron emission tomography.[31] As many cancer patients know all too well, a PET scan enables radiologists to identify, locate, and measure tumors throughout a person's body. Patients are asked to fast for at least twelve hours prior to their scan. This is because oncologists actually do realize that all cancer cells consume tons more glucose (sugar) than healthy cells do. So, when any cancer patient does not eat any food (specifically, no glucose) for twelve hours, whatever cancer cells are growing within their bodies become very hungry.

When a PET scan is conducted, the fasting patient is first injected with radioactive glucose. Then, using a full-body scanner, technicians can track the radioactive glucose as it flows through the patient's body. As hungry cancer cells move quickly to gobble up the radioactive sugar, the scan notes where these eating frenzies are taking place. These spots help identify the existence, the location, and the size of any tumors. As Christofferson describes the creation of the PET scan as it evolved during the late 1970s and early 1980s, "The process of a PET scan was a dramatic visualization of cancer's grotesquely voracious appetite for glucose. The scan was evidence of cancer's perverted metabolism... Oncologists all over the globe read millions of PET scans, staring at the quality that Warburg and Pedersen had claimed defined cancer... ...staring at it every day.[32]

Linda Nebeling's dissertation goal was straightforward. According to her interviews with Christofferson in 2013, could she affect the growth of a person's cancer cells by changing the food they ate? Specifically, if patients ate a no-glucose/high-fat diet for a period of time, would the growth of their tumors be affected? This was an unheard-of idea for oncologists.

In order to carry out this experiment, Nebeling would have to find one or more patients who had been sent home to die—patients who had gone through all the treatments that cancer centers had to offer, but to no avail.

Nebeling eventually began working with two very young girls, both facing near-term death from advancing brain tumors. Each girl had been diagnosed with a different type of tumor, and each had been unsuccessfully treated with surgery, radiation, and/or chemotherapy. Both had been left neurologically damaged before being sent home to die. Trying Linda Nebeling's low-glucose/high-fat ketogenic diet was their families' last hope.

Within a week of beginning the rigorous diet, PET scans showed that tumor growth had slowed in both girls. This slower level of growth continued throughout the research study's 8-week duration. Both families also found each child to have an improved quality of life once they began the low-glucose diet therapy.[33]

Nebeling published her dissertation findings in 1992.[34] A few years later, she published an article describing her work in the *Journal of the Academy of Nutrition and Dietetics*.[35] However, just like the UVM and UT students before her, Nebeling, also, was not able to find any funding for follow-up research. She was therefore unable to continue her promising work with the girls—or with any other cancer patients.

Years later, Dr. Nebeling called her research breakthrough "a blending of nutrition with pediatric oncology with PET scanning." And she described her work with the girls as "a perfect collision of theory and technology."[36]

In my personal correspondence with Dr. Nebeling in early 2019, the nutritionist wrote, "One subject in the ketogenic diet study was lost to follow-up within a year from the completion of the study, the second subject remained a patient at the oncology clinic up to five years post study before lost to follow-up. One subject did live significantly longer than was originally expected."[37]

Miriam Kalamian: The Mother Who Could

Miriam Kalamian first discovered the concept that a ketogenic diet could starve cancer cells in 2005, after stumbling upon one of Dr. Seyfried's early published papers online. Kalamian's four-year-old son Raffi was facing an uphill battle with an extremely aggressive brain tumor. Suddenly, the desperate mother had found a ray of hope. Reading Dr. Seyfried's work, which included a description of Dr. Nebeling's earlier success in slowing the growth of the two girls' brain tumors, Kalamian contacted Dr. Seyfried. Courageously questioning cancer authorities who could only offer her son more neurologically destructive therapies, Kalamian instead began using this very-high-fat/very-low-glucose diet to help slow the growth of, or hopefully even shrink, the tumor in her son's brain. Her courage in questioning authority and opting for a metabolic treatment enabled her child to enter his teens, while also enjoying a fairly high quality of life for much of that time.[38]

Soon after beginning this nutritional treatment with her son, Kalamian began formal nutrition training, with the pioneering goal of helping her son and other cancer patients use dietary therapies for managing and healing their cancerous tumors. Today, Kalamian's work directly contributes to Dr. Seyfried's research, as she is now a part of his international team of laboratory researchers, clinicians, and others who continue to develop and immediately use metabolic protocols for all types of cancer diagnoses. Kalamian's 2017 book, *Keto for Cancer*, has become the bible for health practitioners and individual patients using the low-glucose ketogenic diet as a targeted dietary therapy,[39] as a medicine to extend their patients' or their own lives.

Our All-Important Mitochondria

Why or how, exactly, do low-glucose (also called low-carbohydrate) diets help slow or stop the growth of cancerous tumors? It all begins, with our breast cells' tiny mitochondria.

Each of our breast duct cells and breast lobe cells apparently contains over 100 mitochondria. For most women, breast cancer develops in either a breast duct or lobe. In contrast, each brain cell and each liver cell contains thousands of these tiny power batteries.[40] This is because our brain and our liver require much more energy to function on our behalf—much more energy than it takes for a dormant, or even a lactating, breast duct or lobe to function.

Here is another important biological fact. Dr. Lynn Margulis, the Boston University biologist credited with first understanding the prehistoric origin of our mitochondria, realized that each of these mitochondria, these little princesses, had been self-supporting, glucose-loving, single cell bacteria back in prehistoric time. This is illustrated by the fact that, even today, each tiny mitochondrion comes equipped with its own operating DNA, containing its own unique set of 37 genes. But why do I call our mitochondria *little princesses*?

Figure 1.3: In prehistoric times, the mitochondrion was a single cell bacterium

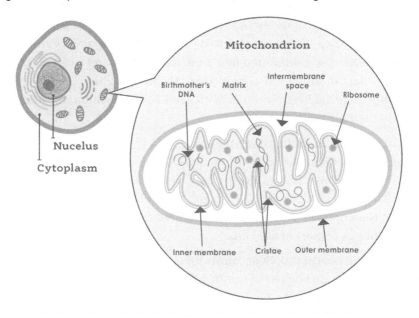

Each of the 100+ mitochondria in each of our breast duct cells and breast lobe cells contains its own unique set of genes. In prehistoric times the mitochondria were fueled by glucose because there wasn't enough oxygen in the atmosphere. When our mitochondria become damaged and can no longer process oxygen, they die or begin to process glucose instead, which is a hallmark of every cancer cell.

It turns out that each of us inherits all of our unique mitochondrial DNA from our birth mothers![41] This means the millions or trillions of mitochondrial genes within the mitochondria of our cells today are identical to those of our birth mothers'![42] As an aside, our birth mothers' DNA within our mitochondrial-based genes affects a variety of our body's functions. These include regulating how much cholesterol our body produces[43] and how efficiently our body can naturally kill off any cancer cells that decide to form.[44] Who knew?[45]

Our Birth Mothers Live Within Our Mitochondria!

"It's well known that the transfer of mitochondrial DNA from mother to offspring, often called maternal inheritance, occurs in humans and most multicellular organisms. Maternal inheritance is what allows genetic testing services like 23andMe to trace our maternal ancestries. You inherited your mitochondrial DNA from your mother, who inherited hers from her mother, and so forth. Maternal inheritance also gave rise to the idea that there exists a 'Mitochondrial Eve,' a woman from whom all living humans inherited their mitochondrial DNA.[45]

For a long time, biologists thought our DNA resided only in the control center of our cells, the nucleus. Then, in 1963, a couple at Stockholm University discovered DNA outside the nucleus. Looking through an electron microscope, Margit Nass-Edelson and Sylvan Nass noticed DNA fibers in structures called mitochondria, the energy centers of our cells.[46]

Our mitochondrial DNA accounts for a small portion of our total DNA. It contains just 37 of the 20,000 to 25,000 protein-coding genes in our body. But it is notably distinct from DNA in the nucleus. Unlike nuclear DNA, which comes from both parents, mitochondrial DNA comes only from the mother."

Steph Yin, "Why Do We Inherit Mitochondrial DNA Only from Our Mothers?" The New York Times, June 23, 2016, https://www.nytimes.com/2016/06/24/science/mitochondrial-dna-mothers.html

Preventing Recurrent Metastatic Breast Cancer: Understanding the Inherent Danger in Each Breast Biopsy

Breast cancer cells that have evolved into their most dreaded form, *metastatic cells*, are able to travel into vital organs and into the bones of a woman's body[47] This is called stage IV or metastatic breast cancer. This is a terminal stage, the cause of virtually all deaths from the uncontrolled growth of breast cancer cells.[48]

It is highly unusual for an early-stage (stages I, II or III) breast tumor to kill you. The breast is not a vital organ in the body. Current-day breast surgeons often amputate a woman's entire breast (called a "mastectomy") as a preferred form of both prevention and treatment. But for too many breast cancer patients, this radical treatment option, this mutilating surgery, does not make the cancer disappear. In fact, oncologists report that 20–40 percent of all women treated for an early-stage invasive breast tumor in the US go on to develop metastatic breast cancer. Oncologists call this recurrent or second breast cancer diagnosis *recurrent metastatic breast cancer or rMBC*.[49] Each such rMBC diagnosis means that the mainstream cancer industry's protocols, used to treat the woman's early-stage breast tumor, months, years or decades earlier, were not effective. A diagnosis of rMBC is a terminal diagnosis, resulting in an early death sentence.

Less than five percent of women initially diagnosed with breast cancer each year are immediately diagnosed with stage IV or metastatic breast cancer.[50] This diagnosis is called *de novo metastatic breast cancer or dnMBC*. This means the vast majority of metastatic breast cancer patients diagnosed each year are those who have experienced failed treatment protocols for their stage I, II or III earlier breast cancer diagnoses.[51] Although neither the government, nor the cancer industry releases any statistics on the number of women in the US who develop rMBC each year, researchers and clinicians, nevertheless, consider the 20–40 percent figure as accepted clinical knowledge.[52] The National Cancer Institute currently allocates hundreds of millions each year for metastatic breast cancer drug research, while the industry's largest drug companies and numerous startups are funding hundreds of millions more dollars in potential drugs and immunotherapies for metastatic breast cancer therapies. "North America accounts for the largest revenue followed by Europe, due to increased diagnosis of disease and enhanced healthcare infrastructure," is how one breast cancer market analyst describes the growing financial boom around the metastatic breast cancer situation in the US today.[53]

For now, however, the important questions are: How or why is recurrent metastatic breast cancer happening in the first place? How can we prevent it?

Tumor Biopsies and the "Seed and Soil" Theory of Metastatic Breast Cancer

Did you know that many clinicians, biologists and epidemiologist now believe that today's high rate of recurrent metastatic breast cancer is being caused by the frequent practice of breast tumor biopsies?[54] What is a tumor biopsy? Why is it done?

Once a tumor is found and suspected to be cancerous, surgeons begin their treatment plan by first diagnosing what kinds of cells comprise the tumor, using a biopsy procedure. They may puncture this teeming mass of loosely connected cancerous cells with a needle (called a *fine needle aspiration*). If they want more definitive information about the tumor's cells, they take a chunk out of the tumor (called a *core biopsy*). Both of these practices create a wound, increasing existing inflammation around the tumor or the clump of atypical breast cells as immune cells arrive to try and heal the tissue damage from the biopsy.[55] Dr. Seyfried describes another concern. "Needle biopsies increase tumor cells' access to glucose and glutamine, the main drivers of cancer."[56] Biopsies also carry the risk of dislodging a single cell or two from the tumor.[57] One meta study of tumor biopsies (a type of study where researchers compile findings from a number of individual studies on the same subject) estimates that breast biopsies carry the highest risk of all types of tumor biopsies, when it comes to the possibility of surgeons "seeding" a cell from the breast tumor, outside of the patient's breast. This meta study calculated this risk to be 94 percent.[58]

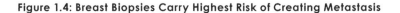

Figure 1.4: Breast Biopsies Carry Highest Risk of Creating Metastasis

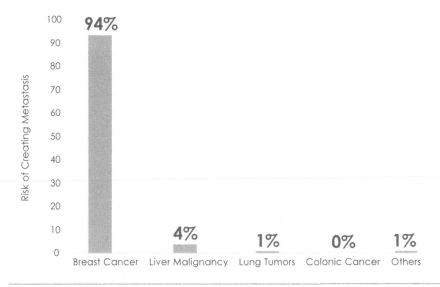

Statistical studies continue to show that biopsies of the breast carry the highest risk of allowing an early stage cancer cell to escape and transform into a metastatic cancer cell.

K. Shyamala, H.C. Girish, and S. Murgod, "Risk of Tumor Cell Seeding Through Biopsy and Aspiration Cytology," *Journal of the International Society of Preventative and Community Dentistry 4, no. 1 (January 2014), p. 11.*

Once dislodged, the renegade tumor cell can catch a free ride throughout a woman's body by fusing to a macrophage. Our macrophages are the most powerful cells in our body's immune system. Macrophages are the first to arrive on the scene once a biopsy takes place. Their job is to help heal the patient's newly created biopsied breast wound. But it is also possible for the macrophage to fuse with a renegade cancer cell, now freed from the tumor. The newly fused tumor cell and macrophage move around the body as a single cell, able to now lodge in the "soil" (the bone, the brain, the lungs and/or the liver). This hybrid cell can now begin to duplicate in its new location, creating those deadly metastatic tumors.[59]

Virtually all women who agree to be treated for a suspected breast tumor or with atypical cells that can only be discovered by a regular screening mammogram are first given biopsies. Is this why clinicians tell us that twenty to forty percent of all women "successfully treated" for an early-stage tumor in the US today go on to develop recurrent metastatic breast cancer?

Two Descriptions: How A Breast Biopsy Is Able to Cause Metastatic Cancer

1. "Metastasis involves the spread of cancer cells from the primary tumor to surrounding tissues and to distant organs and is the primary cause of cancer morbidity and mortality. In order to complete the metastatic cascade, cancer cells must detach from the primary tumor, intravasate into the circulatory and lymphatic systems, evade immune attack, extravasate at distant capillary beds, and invade and proliferate in distant organs. Currently, several hypotheses have been advanced to explain the origin of cancer metastasis. Many of the properties of metastatic cancer cells are also seen in normal macrophages. A macrophage origin of metastasis can also explain the long-standing "seed and soil" hypothesis and the absence of metastasis in plant cancers. The view of metastasis as a macrophage metabolic disease can provide novel insight for therapeutic management."

T.N. Seyfried and L.C. Huysentruyt, "On the Origin of Cancer Metastasis," Critical Views in Oncogenesis, vol. 18, no.1, 2013

2. "Cancer cells, besides reproducing uncontrollably, lose the cohesiveness and orderliness of normal tissue, invade and get detached from the primary tumor to travel and set up colonies elsewhere. Dislodging neoplastically altered cells from a tumor during biopsy or surgical intervention or during simple procedures like needle aspiration is a possibility because they lack cohesiveness, and they attain the capacity to migrate and colonize. Considering the fact that every tumor cell is bathed in interstitial fluid, which drains into the lymphatic system and has an individualized arterial blood supply and venous drainage like any other normal cell in our body, inserting a needle or a knife into a tumor creates the danger of dislodging a loose tumor cell into either the circulation or into the tissue fluid. Tumor cells are easier to dislodge due to lower cell-to-cell adhesion. This theory about the possibility of seeding of tumor cells is supported by several case studies that have shown that

after diagnostic biopsy of a tumor, many patients developed
cancer at multiple sites and showed the presence of circulating
cancer cells in the bloodstream on examination."

K. Shymala, H.C. Girish and Sanjay Murgod, "Risk of Tumor Cell Seeding Through Biopsy and Aspiration Cytology," Journal of International Society of Preventive and Community Dentistry, 4, no. 1, 2014.

Why Biopsies Are No Longer Needed

As earlier described, laboratory or pre-clinical research now affirms
the evolutionary biology behind the recently completed understanding that cancer is a singular disease; a metabolic disease that begins in
the mitochondria of our cells. While Dr. Warburg proved that all cancer cells require glucose to survive and thrive, Dr. Seyfried's more recent
work describes something Dr. Warburg missed. Dr. Seyfried discovered
that cancerous mitochondria also need to process the amino acid glutamine in order to survive and thrive.[60] Some metastatic tumors and triple-negative breast cells, we are now learning, process more glutamine
than glucose.[61]

This metabolic understanding of cancer means there is no need to biopsy
a tumor to figure out what kinds of mutations are present on a patient's
cancer cells, before beginning treatment. This is because such genetic
information is actually irrelevant to successfully stop the growth of the
cancer. On the other hand, mainstream oncologists continue to believe
that the genetic makeup of a cancer cell is incredibly important in understanding how to destroy that cell. They feel compelled to gather all of the
possible genetic information that a biopsy can provide.

In contrast, as you will see from a case study of recurrent triple-negative
MBC, included in Chapter 7, oncologists designed the patient's cocktail
of nontoxic therapies based on the unique metabolism of the patient, not
on the kinds of chaotic mutations within her metastatic tumors. A
recent study describes how such metabolic therapies can be used as
an alternative or complementary approach for managing all stages of
breast cancer.[62]

Why is the US public not told how many women are developing rMBC each year? If 20–40% of all women treated each year for stages I, II or III breast cancer is truly the number of women who now go on to develop rMBC, this means, for example, that an estimated 97,000 women in the US in 2017 who were treated for early stage breast cancer will go on to develop rMBC at some later point in their lives.[63] Would ending the practice of breast biopsies diminish or curtail today's hush-hush epidemic of recurrent metastatic breast cancer?[64]

The Metabolic Approach to Cancer: A Summary

Before moving on, a quick review will help to ensure that we've grasped the most important points within the metabolic approach to cancer. Simply put, Dr. Seyfried found that a cancer cell is actually a sugar-loving zombie cell that should have died, but instead now moves forward on its own, mindlessly replicating itself like crazy, thus creating and growing cancerous tumors that are each made up of a mass of sugar-guzzling, glutamine-loving, ever-mutating cancer cells.[65] This is why metabolic cancer clinics in Turkey, Egypt, and Hungary, and those springing up elsewhere in the world, are now able to help patients effectively manage metastatic triple-negative breast tumors, glioblastomas, renal and other types of stage IV tumors, all by using similar cocktails of nontoxic metabolic therapies tailored to each person's unique metabolism.[66] Pre-clinical research now finds that combining ongoing metabolic therapies, including strict personalized therapeutic ketogenic diets, hyperbaric oxygen treatments, glutamine inhibitor drugs such as DON (Diazo-5-oxo-L-nor-leucine) and other nontoxic protocols that continue to strengthen healthy cells and decrease or eliminate the glucose and the glutamine that fuel cancer cells, can be effective in managing metastatic cancer cases, including late-stage experimental (laboratory-created) glioblastoma.[67]

The Cancer Industry Still Believes the Earth is Flat

Mainstream breast cancer treatment procedures, tests, and drugs continue to fuel a thriving and expanding industry in the US and worldwide. The global metastatic cancer treatment market was calculated to have a value of $54.11 billion in 2017. Estimates indicate this market will almost double, as it grows to $98.24 billion by 2025.[68] As a recent market research report tells us, "The global metastatic cancer treatment market, segmented based on therapeutic application, was dominated by breast cancer."[69] Meanwhile, as mentioned, the entire global breast cancer drug market is expected to be worth $30.4 billion by 2025, with US women contributing over half of this revenue.

At this same time, some leaders within today's traditional or mainstream cancer industry may quietly be beginning to acknowledge that cancer might somehow, in some ways, be a logical metabolic disease, not the complex genetic mystery occupying cancer centers today. Dr. Craig Thompson is CEO of the largest and oldest cancer hospital in the United States, the Memorial Sloan Kettering Cancer Center in New York City. He is also a cancer researcher and the controversial founder of Agios, a cancer drug development company in Cambridge, Massachusetts, that specializes in immunotherapies that can fight against specific gene mutations in cancer cells.[70]

In 2010, Dr. Thompson gave a talk to high school students titled "How Do People Get Cancer?" In a YouTube video of this presentation, you can watch as Dr. Thompson proudly says, "This is the first time you are going to hear this when it comes to cancer: It matters where your calories come from. If you overfeed somebody with fat, you don't increase their cancer risk at all. If you overfeed somebody with carbs, you dramatically increase their cancer risk."[71]

Six years later, Bret Stetka, a reporter for National Public Radio (NPR), interviewed Dr. Seyfried and a different Dr. Thompson—Dr. E. Aubrey Thompson, a renowned cancer researcher at the Mayo Clinic.[72] When the NPR journalist asked why Mayo and other cancer centers were not yet using this very-low-carb/high-fat ketogenic therapy to treat their cancer patients, Dr. E. Aubrey Thompson's response was jaw-dropping: "The drug companies aren't going to fund these types of trials. They can't make money marketing a diet."[73]

When the same journalist asked Dr. Seyfried his opinion on the treatments now being used by mainstream cancer centers, he quietly responded, "Why spend all this money going after all these different [genetic] pathways involved in cancer, when you can simply go after the key fuels?"[74]

Think of it this way: Everybody used to believe the cultural and religious dogma that insisted "the world is flat." Then somebody did some calculations, and later people actually sailed around the world, and the dogma changed. Suddenly, the world was round. But, unless you had believed the original Greek astronomers' observations back in the sixth century BC, or you believed Magellan's and Christopher Columbus's later travel stories, you probably kept operating as if the earth were flat. How long will it be before enough cancer patients, our medical schools, and subsequently oncologists in our cancer centers, understand that the earth is actually round? How long, I wonder, will it be before the metabolic approach to cancer takes hold?

Even Dr. James Watson now believes that cancer is actually a metabolic (i.e., energy-based) disease. He no longer adheres to the still-mysterious genetic theory of cancer that drives today's mainstream worldwide cancer industry. This is the gene theory that says somehow that first cancer cell begins when a gene in the nucleus of a breast duct cell, a colon cell or a lung cell decides to mutate, creating crazed nonstop duplicating cells that form lethal tumors.

Who's Dr Watson? He is a 1963 Nobel Prize winner for his co-discovery of the double helix shape of DNA, and he's the founding director of the groundbreaking 1990 human genome project. Watson is clearly one of the most important biologists of the twentieth century. When asked, in 2013, why our federal cancer agencies continue to ignore even the possibility that cancer is actually a logical or biologically straightforward metabolic disease and not a genetically-based disease, Dr. Watson responded, "the inherently conservative nature of the cancer research establishment [is] the biggest obstacle today to moving forward towards a true war against cancer...[because they are] still too closely wedded to moving forward with cocktails of drugs targeted against the growth-promoting molecules."[75]

Reinforcing this same belief, a few years later, Watson told The *New York Times*, "Locating the genes that cause cancer has been remarkably unhelpful. The belief that sequencing your DNA is going to extend your life, a cruel illusion." He then added, "If I were going into cancer research today, I would study biochemistry rather than molecular biology."[76]

Molecular Biology and Biochemistry: How Are They Different?

Molecular biology deals with the structure and function of our four macromolecules (i.e., proteins, carbohydrates, lipids [fat] and nucleic acids) mainly found in each cell's nucleus.

Biochemistry looks at the big-picture chemical processes within and relating to living organisms. Biochemical processes give rise to the complexity of life.

Today Dr. Seyfried, focused on the biochemistry of cancer, is certainly not alone in working to uncover ways to better help cancer patients manage their disease using nontoxic metabolic therapies. In this effort, he's joined by a group of highly energized, very smart, and open-minded people. They are pharmacologists, biochemists, biologists, oncologists, functional medicine practitioners, nutritionists, veterinarians, science writers and individual cancer patients around the globe. They are in Egypt, Hungary and Turkey; throughout the US, from Tampa to Rapid City and El Segundo (home of the Keto Pet Sanctuary), in San Juan, and in Newton Highlands and Chestnut Hill, Massachusetts.[77] This ever-expanding group of researchers, clinicians, and cancer patients is focused on enabling people to successfully heal from their cancer diagnoses. Instead of undertaking expensive, irrelevant and time-consuming steps of running single-protocol clinical studies, pre-clinical metabolic researchers are able to quickly move their new laboratory findings into oncology clinics, immediately offering metabolic oncologists new cocktails of nontoxic therapies in order to treat metastatic cancer cases.

These biologists, clinicians, and a growing number of self-directed cancer patients are literally working together, sometimes on a daily basis, in order to help extend individual lives, both human and canine, today and tomorrow. These health practitioners, researchers and patients are also publishing their joint findings on open-source online platforms and creating YouTube videos, so that other pioneering and courageous health practitioners and patients can easily and immediately access and utilize this new, ongoing, inexpensive and lifesaving knowledge.[78]

Today, many early-stage and metastatic cancer patients are experiencing the longevity and optimal health that often accompanies a metabolic understanding and treatment of their cancer diagnoses.[79] No wonder Dr. Seyfried continues to say, during any number of interviews with journalists and health practitioners alike, "It is just a matter of time until enough cancer patients refuse current-day toxic treatments and request metabolic therapies instead."[80]

Adding a new chapter to the #MeToo movement, more women concerned about today's breast cancer epidemic can now embrace this documented understanding of the biology behind each initial and recurrent breast cancer diagnosis. More women can finally begin to question today's mainstream cancer industry and its expanding worldwide markets. More women can also begin to question the industry's current refusal to treat women non-toxically, and the US government's practice of not publicly sharing our state-based recurrent metastatic cancer data.[81] Women can also ask why today's cancer industry is able to only treat two thirds of early-stage breast cancer patients successfully, allowing the other estimated 97,000 early-stage US breast cancer patients each year to go on to suffer an early death sentence once they develop rMBC in the coming months, years or decades.[82] Yes, women can and must speak all of our known and emerging truths to power.[83] More and more of our lives are at stake if we don't.

With the new metabolic approach to cancer now front and center in our minds, it's time to look at *Busting Breast Cancer's* five prevention steps. These are each biologically based, inexpensive, and nourishing lifestyles or daily habits that can help keep our mitochondria and our immune systems as strong as possible. Yes, it is time to finally follow famed breast cancer surgeon Dr. Susan Love's advice, given almost thirty years ago: "It certainly would be better to truly prevent breast cancer with lifestyle changes, than to try and turn it around at a later stage with drugs."[84]

The next chapter describes Prevention Step 1, the importance of eating lots of natural fats and very few starches or sugars (including very little fruit!). Moving yourself slowly into this high-fat/low-starch and low-sugar lifestyle is actually much easier than you might think. And if you happen to be obese, or even more than ten pounds overweight; especially if you are over 50 years old, pay close attention! You'll find that taking *Busting Breast Cancer's* first prevention step can immediately reduce your breast cancer risk by at least 30 percent. Who knew?

CHAPTER ENDNOTES

1   See Chapter 6.

2   Michael W. Gray, "Lynn Margulis and the Endosymbiont Hypothesis: 50 Years Later," *Molecular Biology of the Cell* 28, no. 10 (2017): 1285–87. https://www.molbiolcell.org/doi/10.1091/mbc.e16-07-0509.

3   National Science & Technology Medals Foundation, "President Clinton Awards Nation's Highest Honor for Science and Technology," March 6, 2000, https://www.eurekalert.org/pub_releases/2000-03/NSTM-PCan-0603100.php.

4   Michael J. Gonzalez and Jorge Duconge, "A Metabolic Explanation of Cancer: The Bio-Energetic Theory of Carcinogenesis, *Townsend Letter* (August/September 2018, https://www.townsendletter.com/AugSept2018/AugSept2018.html.

5   Thomas N. Seyfried, "Cancer as a Mitochondrial Metabolic Disease," *Frontiers in Cell and Developmental Biology* 3, no. 43 (July 7, 2015): https://doi.org/10.3389/fcell.2015.00043; G.P. Szigeti, O. Szasz, and G. Hegyi, "Connections Between Warburg's and Szent-Gyorgyi's Approach About Causes of Cancer," *Journal of Neoplasm* 1, no. 2 (2017); also see Siddhartha Mukherjee, *The Emperor of All Maladies* (New York: Scribner, 2010).

6   Travis Christofferson, "Angelina Jolie's Mastectomy: How Genes Relate to the Metabolic Origin of Cancer," May 17, 2013, Single Cause Single Cure (blog). (Now renamed Foundation for Metabolic Cancer Therapies, https://foundationformetaboliccancertherapies.com/.)

7   A. Guo et al., "C-Reactive Protein and Risk of Breast Cancer, *Scientific Reports* 5, no.10508, https://doi.org/10.1038/srep10508.

8   Martin Picard and Bruce S. McEwen, "Psychological Stress and Mitochondria: A Systematic Review," *Psychosomatic Medicine* 80, no. 2 (2018): 141-53. https://doi.org/10.1097/PSY.0000000000000545.

9   Marianne C. Aznar et al., "Exposure of the Lungs in Breast Cancer Radiotherapy: A Systematic Review of Lung Doses Published 2010-2015," *Radiotherapy and Oncology: Journal of the European Society for Therapeutic Radiology and Oncology* 126, no.1 (2018): 148-54, https://doi.org/10.1016/j.radonc.2017.11.022; Zarko Barjaktarovic et al., "Radiation-Induced Signaling Results in Mitochondrial Impairment in Mouse Heart at 4 Weeks After Exposure to C-Rays," *Public Library of Science One* 6, no.12 (December 2011), https://doi.org/10.1371/journal.pone.0027811.

10 M. Casula et al., "Infection with HIV-1 Induces a Decrease in mtDNA," *Journal of Infectious Diseases* 191 (2005):1468–71, https://doi.org/10.1016/j.radonc.2017.11.022.

11 Charlène Brault, Pierre L. Levy, and Birke Bartosch, "Hepatitis C Virus-Induced Mitochondrial Dysfunctions," *Viruses* 5 (2013): 954–80, https://doi.org/10.3390/v5030954.

12 Deborah Lai et al., "Localization of HPV-18 E2 at Mitochondrial Membranes Induces ROS Release and Modulates Host Cell Metabolism," *Public Library of Science One* 8, no. 9 (Sept 24, 2013), https://journals.plos.org/plosone/article?id=10.1371/journal.pone.0075625.

13 Mohsin Khan et al., "Mitochondrial Dynamics and Viral Infections: A Close Nexus," *Biochimia et Biophysica Acta* 1853 (2015): 2822–33, https://doi.org/10.1016/j.bbamcr.2014.12.040.

14 J. Cao et al, "Obstructive Sleep Apnea Promotes Cancer Development and Progression: A Concise Review," *Sleep Breath* 19, no. 2 (2015): 453–57, https://doi.org/10.1007/s11325-015-1126-x; Donato Lacedonia et al., "Mitochondrial DNA Alteration in Obstructive Sleep Apnea," *Respiratory Research* 16, no. 1 (April 2015): 47, https://doi.org/10.1186/s12931-015-0205-7.

15 John Peterson Myers et al., "Concerns over Use of Glyphosate-based Herbicides and Risk Associated with Exposures: A Consensus Statement," *Environmental Health* 15, no. 19 (2016),

https://doi.org/10.1186/s12940-016-0117-0. Also see the work of Breast Cancer Prevention Partners (formerly Breast Cancer Fund), www.bcpp.org.

16 Thomas N. Seyfried, "Cancer as a Mitochondrial Metabolic Disease," Frontiers in Cell and Developmental Biology 3, no. 43 (January 2010), https://doi.org/10.1186/1743-7075-7-7; Also see Chapter 9.

17 D. Torres et al, "Prevalence and Penetrance of BRCA1 and BRCA2 Germline Mutations in Colombian Breast Cancer Patients," Scientific Reports 7, no. 4713 (2017), https://doi.org/10.1038/s41598-017-05056-y; Sining Chen and Giovanni Parmigiani, "Meta-analysis of BRCA1 and BRCA2 Penetrance," Journal of Clinical Oncology 25, no.11 (2007): 1329–33, https://doi.org/10.1200/JCO.2006.09.1066; also see Chapter 8.

18 Ana Bratic and Nils-Göran Larsson, "The Role of Mitochondria in Aging," Journal of Clinical Investigation 123, no.3 (March 2013), https://doi.org/10.1172/JCI64125; Claudio Franceschi and Judith Campisi, "Chronic Inflammation (Inflammaging) and its Potential Contribution to Age-associated Diseases," Journals of Gerontology: Biological Sciences 69, no. S1 (June, 2014):54–59, https://doi.org/10.1093/gerona/glu057; Also see Chapter 6.

19 Travis Christofferson, Tripping Over the Truth: The Metabolic Theory of Cancer, p. 170-171.

20 Hannah E. Rockwell et al., "AAV-mediated Gene Delivery in a Feline Model of Sandhoff Disease Corrects Lysosomal Storage in the Central Nervous System," ASN Neuro 13, no.2 (April 2015), https://doi.org/10.1177/1759091415569908; Joy Resmovits, "Tay-Sachs Research Receives Unprecedented NIH Grant," The Forward: News That Matters to American Jews, (August 26, 2009), https://forward.com/news/112913/tay-sachs-research-receives-unprecedented-nih-gran/.

21 Doru Paul and Lisa Fayed, "Basic Cancer Survival Statistics, December 1, 2019, verywellhealth.com, https://www.verywellhealth.com/how-many-people-die-of-cancer-each-day-513641.

22 Daniel de Araujo Buttros et al., "High Risk for Cardiovascular Disease in Postmenopausal Breast Cancer Survivors," Menopause 26, no.9 (September 2019):1024–30, https://doi.org/10.1097/GME.0000000000001348; Radiation Therapy News, "Researcher Investigates Eliminating Radiation for HER2-Positive Breast Cancer," July 2001, https://www.itnonline.com/content/researcher-investigates-eliminating-radiation-her2-positive-breast-cancer; A. Saad et al., "Suicidal Death Within a Year of a Cancer Diagnosis: A Population-based Study," Cancer 125, no.6 (January 7, 2019): 972-79,https://acsjournals.onlinelibrary.wiley.com/doi/epdf/10.1002/cncr.31876; Marianne C. Aznar et al., "Exposure of the Lungs in Breast Cancer Radiotherapy: A Systematic Review of Lung Doses Published 2010-2015," Radiotherapy and Oncology: Journal of the European Society for Therapeutic Radiology and Oncology 126, no.1 (2018):148-54, https://doi.org/10.1016/j.radonc.2017.11.022.

23 Matthew G. Vander Heiden et al., "Understanding the Warburg Effect: The Metabolic Requirements of Cell Proliferation," Science 324, no. 5930 (2009):1029-33, https://doi.org/10.1126/science.1160809.

24 P.L. Pedersen, "Tumor Mitochondria and the Bioenergetics of Cancer Cells," Progress in Experimental Tumor Research 22, (1978):190-274, https://doi.org/10.1159/000401202; Peter L. Pedersen, Ko H. Young, and S. Mathupala, "The Pivotal Roles of Mitochondria in Cancer: Warburg and Beyond and Encouraging Prospects for Effective Therapies," Biochimica et Biophysica Acta 1797, nos. 6-7 (June-July 2010):1225-30, https://doi.org/10.1016/j.bbabio.2010.03.025. Also see Travis Christofferson, Tripping Over the Truth, 69-79.

25 B.A. Israel and W.I. Schaeffer, "Cytoplasmic Suppression of Malignancy," In Vitro Cellular and Developmental Biology 23, no. 9 (September 23, 1987): 627-32, https://doi.org/10.1007/BF0262107; J.W. Shay and H. Werbin, "Cytoplasmic Suppression of Tumorigenicity in Reconstructed Mouse Cells," Cancer Research 48, no. 4 (February 15, 1988): 48830-33, PMID: 3123054.

26 Travis Christofferson, *Tripping Over the Truth: The Metabolic Theory of Cancer*, 175-180.

27 Cytoplasm is a thick solution that fills each cell and is enclosed by the cell membrane. All of the organelles in eukaryotic cells (such as the nucleus, endoplasmic reticulum, and mitochondria) are located in the cytoplasm. The cytoplasm of a cell is the material or protoplasm within that living cell, excluding the cell's nucleus.

28 Christofferson, *Tripping Over the Truth*, 179–80.

29 Israel and Schaeffer, "Cytoplasmic Suppression of Malignancy," and Shay and Werbin, "Cytoplasmic Suppression."

30 Christofferson, *Tripping Over the Truth*, 178.

31 A. Zhu, D. Lee, and H. Shim, "Metabolic Positron Emission Tomography Imaging in Cancer Detection and Therapy Response," *Seminars in Oncology* 38, no.1 (2011): 55–69, https://pubmed. ncbi.nlm.nih.gov/21362516/.

32 Christofferson, *Tripping Over the Truth*, 81.

33 Christofferson, *Tripping Over the Truth*, 196-200.

34 Linda Nebeling, "Effects of Dietary Induced Ketosis on Tumor Metabolism, Nutritional Status and Quality of Life in Pediatric Oncology Patients," (PhD dissertation, Case Western Reserve University, 1992), http://rave.ohiolink.edu/etdc/view?acc_num=case1056547926.

35 L.C. Nebeling and E. Lerner, "Implementing A Ketogenic Diet Based on Medium-chain Triglyceride Oil in Pediatric Patients with Cancer," *Journal of the Academy of Nutrition and Dietetics* 95, no. 6 (June 1995): 693–97, https://doi.org/10.1016/S0002-8223(95)00189-1.

36 Christofferson, *Tripping Over the Truth*, 197.

37 L.C. Nebeling, correspondence with author, April 11, 2019.

38 Miriam Kalamian, "Advocating for a Therapeutic Ketogenic Diet," February 28, 2018, TEDx Talk, Sedona, AZ, https://www.youtube.com/watch?reload=9&v=zYcjnGi5cOs.

39 Miriam Kalamian, *Keto for Cancer: Ketogenic Metabolic Therapy as a Targeted Nutritional Strategy* (White River Junction, VT: Chelsea Green, 2017); Also see: dietarytherapies.com.

40 National Institutes of Health, "Mitochondrial DNA: Your Guide to Understanding Genetic Conditions," https://ghr.nlm.nih.gov/mitochondrial-dna.

41 R.E. Giles et al. "Maternal Inheritance of Human Mitochondrial DNA," *Proceedings of the National Academy of Sciences of the United States of America* 77, no.11 (1980): 6715-9, https://doi. org/10.1073/pnas.77.11.6715.

42 DNA holds all of the information that is contained within all of our cells. Most of this DNA information sits in the nucleus of each cell. A very small, but significant amount of DNA, however, sits within each tiny mitochondrion.

43 Antonia Flaquer et al., "Mitochondrial GWA Analysis of Lipid Profile Identifies Genetic Variants to Be Associated with HDL Cholesterol and Triglyceride Levels," *Public Library of Science One* 10, no. 5 (May 2015), https://doi.org/10.1371/journal.pone.0126294; Also see: Chapter 2.

44 Chunxin Wang and Richard J. Youle, "The Role of Mitochondria in Apoptosis," *Annual Review of Genetics* 43 (2009): 95-118, https://doi.org/10.1146/annurev-genet-102108-134850.

45 "Mitochondrial Eve: Mother of All Humans Lived 200,000 Years Ago," *Science Daily*, August 17, 2010, https://www.sciencedaily.com/releases/2010/08/100817122405.htm.

46 H. Manev, S. Dzitoyeva, & H. Chen, "Mitochondrial DNA: A Blind Spot in Neuroepigenetics," *Biomolecular Concepts* 3, no.2 (2012): 107-15, https://doi.org/10.1515/bmc-2011-0058.

47 Mohammed Akhtar et al., "Paget's 'Seed and Soil' Theory of Cancer Metastasis: An Idea Whose Time has Come," *Advances in Anatomy and Pathology* 26, no. 1 (2019): 69-74, https://doi.org/10.1097/PAP.0000000000000219; T.N. Seyfried and L.C. Huysentruyt, "On the Origin of Cancer Metastasis," *Critical Reviews in Oncogenesis* 18, no. 1-2 (2013): 43-73, https://doi.org/10.1615/critrevoncog.v18.i1-2.40.

48 Angela B. Mariotto et al., "Estimation of the Number of Women Living with Metastatic Breast Cancer in the United States," *Cancer Epidemiology, Biomarkers & Prevention* 26, no.6, (2017): 809-15, https://doi.org/10.1158/1055-9965.EPI-16-0889.

49 Takeshita et al.,"Late Recurrence of Breast Cancer Is Associated with Pro-cancerous Immune Microenvironment in the Primary Tumor," *Scientific Reports* 9, no.16942 (2019), https://doi.org/10.1038/s41598-019-53482-x. Marc Hurlbert, "Where Is the Data? The Epidemiology of Metastatic Breast Cancer," October 5, 2016, *Huffington Post*, https://www.huffpost.com/entry/where-is-the-data-the-epi_b_12311030; Nick Mulcahy, "The Mystery of a Common Breast Cancer Statistic," Medscape, August 18, 2020, https://www.medscape.com/viewarticle/849644.

50 American College of Surgeons, National Cancer Database, "NCDB Public Hospital Comparison Benchmark Reports, Cases Diagnosed," http://oliver.facs.org/BMPub/index.cfm. This estimate was developed using the American College of Surgeons' reported stage I, II and III breast cancer diagnoses during 2017 as its basis. The surgeons' reported numbers represent 70 percent of all reported breast cancer cases.

51 Amye J Tevaarwerk et al., "Survival in Patients with Metastatic Recurrent Breast Cancer After Adjuvant Chemotherapy: Little Evidence of Improvement Over the Past 30 Years," *Cancer* 119, no. 6 (2013):1140-8, https://doi.org/10.1002/cncr.27819.

52 T. Takeshita et al., "Late Recurrence of Breast Cancer Is Associated with Pro-cancerous Immune Microenvironment in the Primary Tumor," *Scientific Reports* 9, no.16942 (2019), https://doi.org/10.1038/s41598-019-53482-x. Metastatic Breast Cancer Network, "Statistics for Metastatic Breast Cancer," http://mbcn.org/statistics-for-metastatic-breast-cancer/; Joyce O'Shaughnessy, "Extending Survival with Chemotherapy in Metastatic Breast Cancer," *The Oncologist* 10, no. suppl. 3 (2005):20-9, https://doi.org/:10.1634/theoncologist.10-90003-20.

53 Infinium Global Research, "Metastatic Breast Cancer Treatment Market (Treatment Type-Chemotherapy, Radiation Therapy, Biologic Targeted Therapy, Breast Surgery, and Hormone Therapy; End user- Hospitals, Clinics, and Other Users): Global Industry Analysis, Trends, Size Share and Forecasts to 2025," May 2019, https://www.infiniumglobalresearch.com/healthcare-medical-devices/global-metastatic-breast-cancer-treatment-market; Also see: Chapter 9.

54 Mohammed Akhtar et al., "Paget's 'Seed and Soil Theory' of Cancer Metastasis: Jan 2019.; I.J.Fidler, "The Pathogenesis of Cancer Metastasis: The 'Seed and Soil' Hypothesis Revisited," *Nature Reviews Cancer* 3,(2003): 453–58, doi:10.1038/nrc1098.; TN Seyfried and LC Huysentruyt, "On the Origin of Cancer Metastasis," *Critical Reviews in Oncogenesis* 18, no. 1-2 (2013): 43–73, https://doi.org/10.1615/critrevoncog.v18.i1-2.40.

55 Gabriela Szalayova et al., "Human Breast Cancer Biopsies Induce Eosinophil Recruitment and Enhance Adjacent Cancer Cell Proliferation," *Breast Cancer Research and Treatment* 157, no. 3 (2016): 461-74, https://doi.org/10.1007/s10549-016-3839-3.

56 Dr Thomas N. Seyfried, personal email to the author, February 14, 2019.

57 C.F. Loughran, "Seeding of Tumour Cells Following Breast Biopsy: A Literature Review," *The British Journal of Radiology* 84 (2011):869-874, https://doi.org/10.1259/bjr/77245199; 1993, https://doi.org/10.1002/jso.2930530313; Mora M. Hansen et al., "Manipulation of the Primary Breast Tumor and the Incidence of Sentinel Node Metastases From Invasive Breast Cancer," *Archives of Surgery* 139 (June 2004) https://doi.org/10.1001/archsurg.139.6.634; JG Fortner, "Inadvertent Spread of Cancer at Surgery," *Journal of Surgical Oncology*, July 1993, https://doi.org/10.1002/jso.2930530313; Cho Eujin et al.,"Breast Cancer Cutaneous Metastasis at Core Needle Biopsy Site," *Annals of Dermatology* 22, no.2 (2010): 238-40, https://doi.org/10.5021/ad.2010.22.2.238.

58 K. Shyamala, H.C. Girish, and S. Murgod, "Risk of Tumor Cell Seeding Through Biopsy and Aspiration Cytology," *Journal of the International Society of Preventative and Community Dentistry* 4, no. 1 (January 2014): 5-11, https://doi.org/10.4103/2231-0762.129446.

59 Sebastian R. Nielsen and Michael C. Schmid, "Macrophages As Key Drivers of Cancer Progression and Metastasis," *Mediators of Inflammation* 2017, no. 9624760 (2017), https://doi.org/10.1155/2017/9624760.

60 Thomas N. Seyfried, *Cancer as a Metabolic Disease: On the Origin, Management and Prevention of Cancer*, 133-43.

61 Zhanyu Wang et al., "Metabolic Reprogramming in Triple-negative Breast Cancer," *Cancer Biology & Medicine* 17, no.1 (2020): 44-59, https://doi.org/10.20892/j.issn.2095-3941.2019.0210; Yeon-Kyung Choi and Keun-Gyu Park, "Targeting Glutamine Metabolism for Cancer Treatment," *Biomolecules & Therapeutics* 26,no.1(2018): 9-28, https://doi.org/10.4062/biomolther.2017.178.

62 Thomas N. Seyfried et al., "Consideration of Ketogenic Metabolic Therapy as a Complementary or Alternative Approach for Managing Breast Cancer," *Frontiers in Nutrition* (March 11, 2020), https://doi.org/10.3389/fnut.2020.00021/full.

63 This estimate was developed, using the American College of Surgeons' reported stage I, II, and III breast cancer diagnoses during 2017, as its basis. See: National Cancer Database, American College of Surgeons, "Benchmark Reports", http://oliver.facs.org/BMPub/index.cfm.

64 Kate Pickert, "Why the Women Most Likely to Die of Breast Cancer Have Gotten the Least Attention," *Time*, October 1, 2019, https://time.com/5689570/metastatic-breast-cancer-research-treatment/; Musa Mayer and Susan E. Grober, "Silent Voices: Women with Advanced (Metastatic) Breast Cancer Share Their Needs and Preferences For Information, Support, and Practical Resources," *Living Beyond Breast Cancer*, 2006; https://www.lbbc.org/sites/default/files/LBBCsilentvoices.pdf.

65 Thomas Seyfried, interview with author, Chestnut Hill, MA, February 13, 2017.

66 Thomas N. Seyfried, et al, "Consideration of Ketogenic Metabolic Therapy as a Complementary or Alternative Approach for Managing Breast Cancer," *Frontiers in Nutrition*, March 2020, https://doi.org/10.3389/fnut.2020.00021; Thomas Seyfried, podcast interview with Karl Goldcamp, *Keto Naturopath*, Episodes #42–43, December 18, 2019, https://www.listennotes.com/podcasts/keto-naturopath/episode-42-interview-with-dr-5UqY_o-eFib/ and https://www.listennotes.com/podcasts/keto-naturopath/episode-43-interview-with-dr-2aZUV-zvkIt/.

67 Purna Mukherjee et al., "Therapeutic Benefit of Combining Calorie-restricted Ketogenic Diet and Glutamine Targeting in Late-stage Experimental Glioblastoma," *Communications Biology* 2, no. 200 (May 29, 2019), https://doi.org/10.1038/s42003-019-0455-x; T.N. Seyfried et al., "Press-pulse: A Novel Therapeutic Strategy for the Metabolic Management of Cancer," *Nutrition & Metabolism* 14, no. 19 (2017), https://doi.org/10.1186/s12986-017-0178-2.

68 Matej Mikulic, "Global Metastatic Cancer Treatment Market in 2017 and 2025," October 9, 2019, https://www.statista.com/statistics/940465/metastatic-cancer-treatment-market-worldwide/; Research and Markets, "$40 Billion Breast Cancer Drug Market and Clinical Trial Insights Report, 2020-2025," January 28, 2020, https://www.globenewswire.com/news-release/2020/01/28/1975943/0/en/40-Billion-Breast-Cancer-Drug-Market-Clinical-Trial-Insights-Report-2020-2025.html; Grand View Research, "Breast Cancer Drugs Market Size, Share & Trends Analysis Report By Type (Hormonal Receptors, Mitotic Inhibitors, HER2 Inhibitors, Anti-metabolites, CDK 4/6 Inhibitors), By Region, And Segment Forecasts, 2019 – 2025," February, 2019, https://www.grandviewresearch.com/industry-analysis/breast-cancer-drugs-market.

69 BIS Research, "Global Metastatic Cancer Treatment Market to Reach $98.24 billion by 2025," BIS Research Report, June 28, 2018, https://www.prnewswire.com/news-releases/global-metastatic-cancer-treatment-market-to-reach-9824-billion-by-2025-bis-research-report-686807881.html.

70 Andrew Pollack, "Sloan-Kettering Chief Is Accused of Taking Research," *The New York Times*, February 5, 2012, https://www.nytimes.com/2012/02/06/health/cancer-center-in-lawsuit-says-a-doctor-appropriated-a-discovery.html; Robert Weisman, "Agios Settles Two Lawsuits Over Cancer Research," *Boston Globe*, September 4, 2012, https://www.bostonglobe.com/business/2012/09/04/agios-pharmaceuticals-settles-two-lawsuits-signs-licensing-pact-with-university-pennsylvania/OgeVK4t4wzzoJEUXI4DIVO/story.html; Beth Fand Incollingo, "Considering Cost: What's an Immunotherapy Worth?" *Cancer Updates, Research & Education*, July 16, 2015, https://www.curetoday.com/publications/cure/2015/immunotherapy/considering-cost-whats-an-immunotherapy-worth; "Celgene, Agios, Launch $1B+ Metabolic Immuno-Oncology Alliance," *Genetic Engineering and Biotechnology News*, May 17, 2016, https://www.genengnews.com/topics/omics/celgene-agios-launch-1b-metabolic-immuno-oncology-alliance/81252736/; Bloomberg Business, "BB Biotech Novel Drugs to Battle Cancer on the Verge of Market Launch," June 19, 2017, https://www.bloomberg.com/press-releases/2017-06-19/bb-biotech-ag-novel-drugs-to-battle-cancer-on-the-verge-of-market-launch; Matthew Tontonoz, "License to Build: New Theory of Cancer Puts Metabolism at Center," Memorial Sloan Kettering Cancer Center blog, January 12, 2016, https://www.mskcc.org/blog/license-build-new-theory-cancer-puts-metabolism-center.

71 Craig Thompson, "How Do People Get Cancer/Cancer Awareness," November 20, 2010, https://www.youtube.com/watch?v=WUlE1VHGA40.

72 Bret Stetka, "Fighting Cancer by Putting Tumor Cells on a Diet," National Public Radio, March 5, 2016, https://www.npr.org/sections/health-shots/2016/03/05/468285545/fighting-cancer-by-putting-tumor-cells-on-a-diet.

73 Dr. E. Aubrey Thompson, in Stetka, "Fighting Cancer," 7.

74 Ibid.

75 Anna Wagstaff, "Jim Watson: DNA Revealed the Causes, It May Never Reveal a Cure," *CancerWorld* 56 (September–October 2013), https://cancerworld.net/cover-story/jim-watson-dna-revealed-the-causes-it-may-never-reveal-a-cure/.

76 Sam Apple, "An Old Idea, Revived: Starve Cancer to Death," *The New York Times Magazine*, May 12, 2016, https://www.nytimes.com/2016/05/15/magazine/warburg-effect-an-old-idea-revived-starve-cancer-to-death.html.

77 The Keto Pet Sanctuary is a nonprofit organization in El Segundo, California, that treats rescue dogs, diagnosed with cancer, using metabolic therapies. www.ketopetsanctuary.com. Also see: "The Dog Cancer Series," https://www.youtube.com/channel/UCcBP2Dp1pUnVriNUr_ZqIEg.

78 Ahmed M.A. Elsakka et al., "Management of Glioblastoma Multiforme in a Patient Treated with Ketogenic Metabolic Therapy and Modified Standard of Care: A 24-Month Follow-Up," *Frontiers in Nutrition* 5 (March 2018): 20, https://doi.org/10.3389/fnut.2018.00020; Mehmet Salih Iyikesici et al., "Efficacy of Metabolically Supported Chemotherapy Combined with Ketogenic Diet, Hyperthermia, and Hyperbaric Oxygen Therapy for Stage IV Triple-Negative Breast Cancer," *Cureus* 9, no.7 (July 2017): e1445, https://pubmed.ncbi.nlm.nih.gov/28924531/; Pablo's Journey Through a Brain Tumour, https://www.facebook.com/pablosbrainjourney/; Andrew Scarborough, "My Brain Cancer Story," http://mybraincancerstory.blogspot.com.

79 Thomas Seyfried, "Cancer: A Metabolic Disease," lecture, Annual Cross Fit Health Conference, July 31, 2018, Madison, Wisconsin, https://www.youtube.com/watch?v=KusaU2taxow.

80 Iosif M. Gershteyn interview with Dr. T.N. Seyfried, "Cancer as a Metabolic Disease," *Cognitum*, Episode 9, March 20, 2019; https://www.youtube.com/watch?v=XFcq6Zb4hlg.

81 See Chapter 9.

82 See end note 67 and National Cancer Database, American College of Surgeons, "Benchmark Reports," http://oliver.facs.org/BMPub/index.cfm.

83   Megan Murphy, "Introduction to "#MeToo Movement," *Journal of Feminist Family Therapy* 31, no.3 (2019): 63-65, https://www.tandfonline.com/doi/full/10.1080/08952833.2019.1637088.

84   Sharon Batt, *Patient No More: The Politics of Breast Cancer* (Charlottetown, PEI, Canada: Gynergy Books, 1994), 96.

PART II.
THE FIVE SIMPLE PREVENTION STEPS

2 STEP 1:
Eat Fat to Lose Fat and Keep Mitochondria Healthy

Here's a shocking statistic: About 75 percent of American women are overweight or obese.[1] That's right: In the United States today, it is actually only a small *minority* of women who have a body mass index (BMI) in the "healthy" range. When we consider the role that weight plays in increasing a woman's chance of developing breast cancer, that's a number that should make us sit up and take notice.

The American Cancer Society, the federal Centers for Disease Control (CDC), and the National Institutes for Health (NIH) all report that "being overweight is a risk factor when it comes to breast cancer."[2] Their statements are based on statistics that show us there is an apparent connection between these two epidemics.[3] And it gets worse. The longer a postmenopausal woman remains overweight, the more her risk of developing any and all types of breast cancer increases.[4] Postmenopausal women in the US today face truly astronomical rates of cancer, ranging from 337 to 422 per 100,000, depending on which age subgroupings of older women you examine.[5]

Add stress to the equation, and the news gets even worse! Studies show that when they are overweight or obese, both older and younger women with chronic stress who go on to develop breast cancer are then at higher risk for developing the fast-growing type of disease known as *triple-negative breast cancer.*[6] And if that's not enough to make us all pay more attention to our weight, it turns out that both younger and older overweight women who get diagnosed with breast cancer are *less likely to survive* their diagnosis than their peers who maintain a healthy weight.[7]

Have I gotten your attention? Good. Now let's look at how and why weight plays such a significant role in the development of this dread disease.

The Link Between Obesity and Breast Cancer

As we saw in the last chapter, mainstream oncologists still can't tell a woman why she developed breast cancer when her family members and friends did or did not.[8] That's because mainstream medical schools are still teaching their students the old-fashioned or mainstream *genetic* understanding of cancer; they're not yet teaching their students to understand how cancer is actually a *metabolic* disease that originates in the mitochondria of a cell.[9] If they did, it would be clear to these oncologists why overweight and obese women develop at least 30 percent more breast cancer than their healthy weight peers. Let me explain.

To begin, endocrinologists now realize that a person's excess body fat is actually alive. Known as "biologically active,"[10] this excess fat doesn't just sit there; it *does* something. It generates an enzyme called *aromatase*. This aromatase, in turn, quickly converts itself into a toxic, irritating type of the hormone *estrogen*.[11] Now, estrogens can't enter just any organs in a woman's body; however, estrogens can only enter the cells of a woman's sex organs—and that includes her breasts. Once inside a breast cell, this fat-generated toxic estrogen is able to assault the cells' power batteries (mitochondria), bombarding them nonstop, day in and day out. Interestingly, if a woman's excess fat disappears, these attacks stop—and with that, her risk of developing breast cancer quickly drops.

There's a second connection between excess body fat and breast cancer, as well. This one has to do with the inflammatory enzymes that the adipose (fat) cells generate day after day.[12] These inflammation-producing toxins can enter cells in most of our organs, and that includes the cells in our breasts. Now we have a double whammy: toxic estrogen and inflammatory enzymes both hitting an overweight woman's breast cells at the same time. These are two reasons why overweight and obese postmenopausal women develop 30 percent more breast cancer than their peers.

Age plays a different type of role in this equation for younger women. Studies do not consistently show that obese *younger* women face the same increased risk of developing breast cancer as their older peers.[13] But don't get too comfortable if you are younger. A number of studies have demonstrated that obese younger women are at a higher risk for developing faster-growing triple-negative tumors, right along with their postmenopausal peers, once an obese younger woman is diagnosed with breast cancer.[14] This is a topic we'll return to later on in Chapter 7 and Chapter 8. For now, though, just these few statistics should make it clear that it's worth exploring some lifestyle changes to get ourselves to a healthy weight, no matter our age.

Figure 2.1: Are You Part of Today's Obesity Epidemic?

BODY MASS INDEX

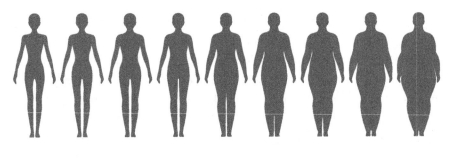

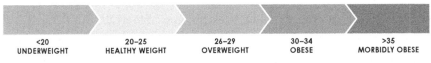

| <20 UNDERWEIGHT | 20–25 HEALTHY WEIGHT | 26–29 OVERWEIGHT | 30–34 OBESE | >35 MORBIDLY OBESE |

Find your body image in the picture above. What is the number under the figure that most looks like you? This is your approximate body mass index (BMI) right now.

Adapted from Best BMI Calculator chart, http://www.bestbmicalculator.com/bmi-chart/women/, Spain.

As Figure 2.1 shows, being *overweight* is defined as having a body mass index (BMI) over 25. Being *obese* is defined as having a BMI over 29. A *healthy* BMI is 20–25.

Being Overweight Is Not Your Fault!

Does this statement surprise you? My research tells me that Americans have been led astray for decades by a variety of so-called "authorities" in the field of nutrition. We've been misled about the best combinations of food, the best types of food, and the best amounts of food to eat each day in order to achieve and maintain our optimal weight—and the health that brings. We've been misled because the US government's Dietary Guidelines for Americans are wrong!

That's right. They're wrong. Nicknamed DGAs, these guidelines are developed and promoted by the US Department of Agriculture (USDA) and the Department of Health and Human Services (HHS), and they're popularized in tools like the "food pyramid" and the more recent *MyPlate* graphic. But as the vast majority of ongoing international metabolic research continues to show, these DGAs go against the best biological-ly-based nutrition research available today. In fact, leading food science experts agree that the types, combinations, and quantities of foods in our DGAs are responsible for today's ever-increasing obesity epidemic.[15]

To understand the scope of the problem facing us as American women trying to stay healthy, it might help to look back and see that it wasn't always this way.

Why Our Ancestors Were Thin: The Way Americans Used to Eat

Our earliest ancestors killed bison and other large game—but only in the fall, when the animals' fat stores were highest. According to histori-ans, humans threw the lean meat to their dogs, and preserved the fattier cuts for themselves. Since natural fat operates as a clean-burning, effi-cient, high-octane fuel, small amounts of these animals' internal organs and fatty meat cuts were able to carry our ancestors through the winter months, even with limited food supplies.[16]

If they were lucky, our Paleolithic ancestors were also able to gather wild fruits in season, along with wild greens, fat-filled nuts, and seeds. They caught fatty fish and small game all through the year. They worked hard to find their food—often eating few (or no) meals for days at a time, depending on the season.[17]

Today, some people mimic the experience of our Paleolithic ancestors by eating diets that are high in natural fats and low in starches/carbs, and even by engaging in periodic water-only fasts that are now the prod-uct of well-informed choice, not necessity. We've learned that inter-mittent fasts of 13–18 hours in a day, with longer water-only fasts last-ing from one to three days at a time, can improve our immune systems, strengthen our cells' mitochondria, and help starve any cancer cells in our bodies.[18] It turns out that eating (and fasting) like our Paleolithic ancestors is actually good for us!

Fast-forward to more recent times. Until the 1970s, high-fat, nutrient-rich eating was the norm throughout US history. Native Americans, African-American slaves, Euro-American immigrants, sharecroppers, laborer groups of all ethnicities, and even the landed gentry—all ate this way. Their diets consisted mainly of high-fat, densely nutritious organ meats, fatty cuts of pork, goat, lamb, and wild animals, along with high-fat poultry, like geese, ducks, turkeys, and chickens. Their diet was rounded out with small fatty fish, lots of green veggies, and lard.[19] History books tell us that our ancestors ate only full-fat dairy products, typically sourced from cows, sheep, and goats. Also, the diet included small amounts of fermented foods, from pickles to sauerkraut. And there were fruits, when they were in season. Because our ancestors ate a diet that was high in fat but low in starches/sugars, their bodies were burning fat—not glucose—most of the time. And as we saw earlier, when your body's operating system is burning fat, you're running your powerful mitochondria on a clean-burning, high-octane fuel. In metabolic terms, you're in a state of *nutritional ketosis*.[20]

No wonder it was easy for most Americans to remain thin before the 1970s! Actually, most people didn't have much choice in the matter. With larger families and less food available, they ate fewer meals. And they ate smaller meals. And the meals they did eat included more greens and more fat, but less starch and sugar. Few homes had electric refrigerators before the 1950s. Prior to that, ice boxes didn't provide nearly as much space or a constant temperature to keep a stash of fresh food. Most families also needed to grow food and store it on their own to have enough year-round.[21] In other words, until the 1980s most people didn't have the opportunity to overeat starchy and sugary carbohydrates and meat. That's why they remained thin—and free of the myriad obesity-related health problems that plague so many Americans today.[22]

One study tells us that back in the 1960s breast cancer was diagnosed in 81 out of every 100,000 women, of all ages, in the United States.[23] Today a national compilation from all state registries tells us that rate is around 71 per 100,000, just for women under 50 years old, and 337 per 100,000 for women 50 years and older.[24] When it comes to breast cancer, the 1960s really were the "good old days."

The Obesity Bullies: The US Congress, Federal Agencies and National Academy of Medicine

So, this is why being fat is not your fault: you've been misled. As near as I can tell, there are three groups, working together for over thirty years now, that have played the most significant roles in coordinating, creating, and maintaining today's obesity and breast cancer epidemics. They are the US Congress and federal government agencies (specifically, the Department of Agriculture and the Department of Health and Human Services). In turn, both branches of government are directed by the processed food industry and the industry's most powerful lobby, the National Academy of Medicine (NAM).

Since you may not be familiar with the last of these organizations, it may be useful to say a word about it. NAM was formerly known as the Institute of Medicine. NAM's president, Dr. Victor Dzau (a longtime PepsiCo board member, until a week before taking leadership of NAM),[25] was recently able to elevate the organization's name to the more prestigious National Academy of Medicine.[26] But where did NAM come from in the first place? Why is this privately funded lobby group, representing the profit interests of the agribusiness, processed food, medical, chemical, and pharmaceutical industries, involved in determining our Dietary Guidelines for Americans?

Back in the early 1970s, NAM was created by a group of physicians. They organized out of concern that the US government might consider adopting a national Medicare or single-payer health insurance system for all Americans. The doctors felt that having a powerful, Washington-based lobby group could help them influence Congress to maintain the country's current private health insurance system. The doctors were not interested in seeing President Lyndon Johnson's new government-run single-payer Medicare program for seniors and the disabled expanded to the entire population.[27] Led by a Midwest physician and medical researcher by the name of Irvine Page, the doctors petitioned the National Academy of Sciences to allow the doctors' lobby to be housed under the Academy, a respected, historic nongovernmental advisory organization.[28]

Soon, the rapidly expanding pharmaceutical, agribusiness, and processed food industries joined the physicians to support the new NAM lobby group. These groups also wanted in on a direct line to those in the government who might be inclined to support industry-backed studies and industry-friendly federal laws.[29] And so, we learn from multiple sources, the contents of our USDA Dietary Guidelines for Americans (DGAs), beginning in the 1980s until today, have always been controlled by the processed food and agribusiness industries.

In the first chapter of her book, *What to Eat: The Ten Things You Really Need to Know to Eat Well and Be Healthy!*, Dr. Luise Light describes her initial experience and conversations in the late 1970s with the Cattlemen's Association, the Grocery Manufacturers, the National Food Processors, the Meat Institute, the Dairy Council and the Egg Board.[30] The meeting was quite unsettling. Dr. Light had recently been hired by the USDA when she was invited to a private dinner with these food industry leaders. Her new government job was to lead the team of nutritionists that was tasked with developing our first comprehensive DGAs. Within a few years, however, Light resigned from her government job. The contents of her team's original food pyramid, containing their well-researched DGAs, had been rejected, replaced by a combination of foods dictated by these leaders of the processed food industry.

Don't take my word for it. Listen to Dr. Light:

> *When the new food guide came back from review by the office of the Secretary of Agriculture, changes had been made to it. The number of servings in the whole grain category has been altered from the original "two to three" to "six to eleven," and the words "whole grains" were nowhere to be found. Dairy was now three or four servings, protein foods had become two to three servings and fats, oils, and sweets to "use moderately," without further explanation. The alterations that were made to the new guide would be disastrous, I told my boss, the agency director. These changes would undermine the nutritional quality of eating patterns and increase the risk for obesity and diabetes, among other disease. At stake here, I told him, was nothing short of the credibility and integrity of the USDA as a source of reliable nutrition information."[31]*

As I later discovered, the wholesale changes made to the guide by the Office of the Secretary of Agriculture, were calculated to win the acceptance of the food industry. My nutritionist group had placed baked goods, made with white flour...at the peak of the pyramid, recommending that they be eaten sparingly. To our alarm, in the 'revised' Food Guide, they were now made part of the Pyramid's base. I vehemently protested that the changes, if followed, could lead to an epidemic of obesity and diabetes—and couldn't be justified on either health or nutritional grounds. To my amazement, I was a lone voice on this issue, as my colleagues appeared to accept the 'policy level' decision. Over my objections, the Food Guide Pyramid was finalized, although it only saw the light of day 12 years later, in 1992. Yet it appears my warning has come to pass.[32]

America's obesity epidemic and breast cancer rates continued to grow hand in hand, once the National Nutrition Monitoring and Related Research Act of 1990 was passed. This first national nutrition law dictated two things: (1) the content and amount of carbohydrates, proteins, and fats to be used in every federally funded food program, and (2) the requirement that every government-funded food program, from day care snacks to subsidized nursing-home fare and Meals on Wheels, must follow these federal guidelines or lose government funding.[33]

In principle, it seems like a good idea that the federal government would offer guidelines on healthy eating to ensure that consumers are informed. One fly in the ointment seems to be the continuing involvement of that powerful lobbying group, NAM; whose funders often have interests other than Americans' health at heart. But how is it that NAM seems to continue to hold such apparent power over our national nutritional guidelines?[34]

The culprit, in my mind, is, in part, a badly written section of the 1990 legislation that established these powerful dietary directives. Section 102 8 (B) of the law mandates that the USDA and HHS contract with "a scientific body *such as* the National Academy of Sciences" to develop the DGAs every two to five years. Are these nebulous words the doorway through which NAM and its multi-million-dollar food and pharma industry funders make their way into the process of determining our food guidelines? Decades later, NAM's power over these DGAs continues on, and every five years we learn that neither our DGAs nor the corresponding food pyramid will see any meaningful change. Both will continue to recommend a high-starch, high-sugar diet, with few ounces of natural fat in sight.[35] But how can I say that NAM's power over our DGAs continues to be controlled by the various elements of the food industry?

Figure 2.2: 1992 USDA Food Pyramid

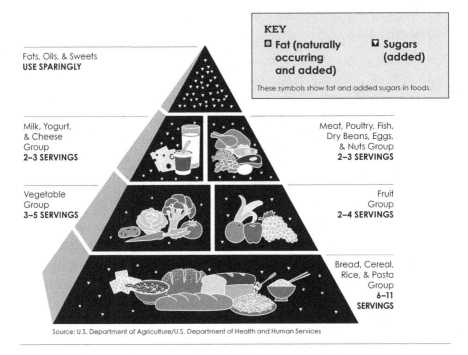

The USDA's original 1992 Food Guide Pyramid recommended that fats be used sparingly; starchy and sugary carbs are to be the mainstay of a person's diet.

Graphic from USDA, https://www.choosemyplate.gov/eathealthy/brief-history-usda-food-guides.

Figure 2.3: The 2005 USDA *"My Pyramid"* and the 2011*"My Plate"*

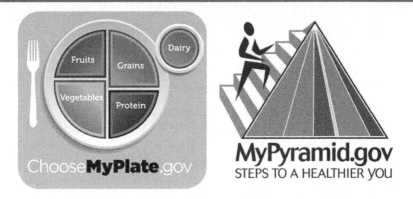

America's current food guides continue to be filled with sugar, starch, fruits and other types of glucose. Natural fats are still hard to find!

Graphic from USDA, https://www.choosemyplate.gov/eathealthy/brief-history-usda-food-guides.

The National Nutrition Monitoring and Research Act of 1990

"Follow the money," as my indomitable Uncle Jack used to tell me. One look at the corporations and those individuals who give literally tens of thousands of dollars each year to the National Academy of Medicine, tells the story. Who are the members of NAM's Catalyst Society (those donating $50,000 or more annually)?[36] Who are those who give NAM million-dollar endowments? In February 2019, NAM was happy to receive such an endowment from Whitney MacMillian, "longtime NAM volunteer" and former chairman of the board and CEO of Cargill.[37] For those who do not recognize this name, Cargill is one of the world's largest companies and a major food supplier to McDonald's, Target, and Stop & Shop. It is active in the deforestation of the Amazon, among its many anti-environmental endeavors. In 2019 Cargill was given the "Worst Company in the World" award by Mighty Earth, the environmental campaign organization chaired by former Congressman Henry Waxman.[38]

The National Nutrition Monitoring and Research Act of 1990

Excerpt from Section 102 8 (B)

The Department of Agriculture and the Department of Health and Human Services will...contract with a scientific body, such as the National Academy of Sciences or the Federation of American Societies for Experimental Biology, to interpret available data analyses, and publish every two years, or more frequently if appropriate, except as provided in subparagraph (B), a report on the dietary, nutritional, and health-related status of the people of the United States and the nutritional quality (including the nutritive and non-nutritive content) of food consumed in the United States. Or (B) if the Secretaries determine that sufficient data analyses are not available to warrant interpretation of such data analyses, inform Congress of such fact at the time a report required in subparagraph (A) would have been published, and publish such report at least once every five years.

(7 USC Ch. 84: NATIONAL NUTRITION MONITORING AND RELATED RESEARCH, From Title 7—AGRICULTURE.) https://uscode.house.gov/view.xhtml?path=/prelim@title7/chapter84&edition=prelim.

And so, our misguided federal food programs continue on. More than 4.8 billion meals, costing $24.3 billion, were given to children under the program in 2018 by the Department of Agriculture's Food and Nutrition Service.[39] These are all meals filled with starchy and sugary carbs, and very little fat—a blueprint for obesity. Additional billions are also spent each year on low-fat, high-starch and sugary carb meals for the disabled, the poor, and the elderly.[40] No wonder our obesity rates continue to rise each year—and our breast cancer rates with them! No wonder the poor, as a population group in the United States, are more obese than the wealthy. In a 2011 *American Diabetes Association Journal* editorial, it was noted that "poverty rates and obesity were reviewed across 3,139 counties in the US. In contrast to international trends, people in America who live in the most poverty-dense counties are those most prone to obesity. Counties with poverty rates of >35% have obesity rates 145% greater than wealthy counties."[41]

Today, the contents of the food pyramid and the *MyPlate* meal guide have changed little from the original plan that caused Luise Light to resign her post as our top government nutritionist in the early 1980s. And so, today, the most vulnerable Americans from cradle to grave continue to be given government-funded meals that are very high in starch and sugar, and very low in natural animal and vegetable fats. Meanwhile, most US physicians continue to blindly counsel patients to follow the popular food pyramid or *MyPlate* chart to achieve optimal health. What a mess.

Agricultural Subsidies: More Support for Our National Obesity Epidemic

Over past decades, the majority of our elected senators and representatives, from both the Democratic and Republican parties, have created a second way of supporting agribusiness and the processed food industry—and our national obesity epidemic, in the process. Each year, Congress continues to give billions of taxpayer dollars in federal kickbacks to huge private agribusiness concerns.[42] These kickbacks, politely known as *food subsidies*, help cover the costs of raising crops, such as GMO soybeans for cheap soybean oil and GMO corn for cheap high-fructose corn syrup, along with GMO wheat, rice, and sorghum (a type of grain used to make ethanol and livestock feed). Wonder why the poor are disproportionately affected by obesity? Many of Americans' cheapest foods today are strange-looking starchy and sugary foodstuffs with stranger-sounding names, like Doritos, Cheetos, Tostitos, and Pepsi.[43]

Can Grassroots Americans Topple MyPyramid and MyPlate?

The US government's key role in creating today's obesity epidemic seems clear. In addition to the firsthand information shared by Luise Light, there are plenty of other books that shed light on the biological—and political—roots of today's cancer-causing obesity epidemic. These include: Ellen Ruppel Shell's *Fat Wars: The Inside Story of the Obesity Industry*;[44] Gary Taub's numerous books on the subject, including, *Why We Get Fat: And What to Do About It*;[45] pediatric endocrinologist Robert Lustig's *The Hacking of the American Mind: The Science Behind the Corporate Takeover of Our Bodies and Brain*;[46] and *The Big Fat Surprise: Why Butter, Meat and Cheese Belong in a Healthy Diet*,[47] by journalist Nina Teicholtz.

Meanwhile, the hard-hitting nonprofit group of investigative journalists, US Right to Know (USRTK),[48] continues its critically important mission of uncovering original documents that establish exactly how the processed food, chemical, pharmaceutical, and agribusiness industries continue to work together to maintain our misguided national nutritional guidelines. USRTK was cofounded in 2014 by the best-selling authors and political activists Stacy Malkin[49] and Greg Palast.[50] USRTK may be the most important fact-finding group we have, when it comes to learning the true history behind our obesity- (and cancer-) creating national food policy.

The Great Sugar Heist

The American public is only beginning to understand exactly how PepsiCo, General Foods and other processed food companies have long been major players in today's national obesity epidemic. One example: In 2016, the *New York Times* reported that researchers had uncovered a deceitful move by sugar industry executives, carried out against the US public in the late 1960s. Apparently, food scientists had been paid to manipulate research to highlight false benefits from sugar, while denigrating the benefits of natural fats.[51] This pro-sugar-industry report, published in 1967 in the *New England Journal of Medicine*, tried to show how natural fat, not sugar, was the culprit in the country's rising heart attack rate.[52]

A second important group was also created in 2014: The Nutrition Coalition, comprised of functional and alternative health practitioners, organic food associations, and interested citizens. With initial funding from the progressive Laura and John Arnold Foundation, the coalition continues its efforts to work with federal legislators to overhaul the American food pyramid and DGAs. The Coalition's goal is to monitor the creation of guidelines that are based on today's best nutritional research, which overwhelmingly supports a person's need to eat lots of natural fat, many fewer starchy and sugary carbs, and lots more greens and non-starchy vegetables to combat obesity and achieve cancer-free, optimal health.[53] Sadly, though, Dr. Dzau's politically powerful

National Academy of Medicine, the Department of Agriculture and possibly other food industry advocates appear to be making it very difficult for the Nutrition Coalition (and, indeed, all other groups bringing objective research to the table) to make headway on changing the American food pyramid.[54] And so, each year, hundreds of billions of taxpayer dollars continue to be spent feeding large segments of the population nothing but low-fat, high-carb meals that worsen our national obesity epidemic—and with it, our breast cancer epidemic, as well.

What About Cholesterol?

Each year my mother would dutifully write out a $10 check to the American Heart Association (AHA) and to the American Cancer Society (ACS). In our household, growing up in the 1950s and 1960s, these groups were akin to motherhood and apple pie. Why? As the iconic writer and cultural change agent, Alice Walker tells us, "Propaganda is amazing. People can be led to believe anything."[55]

Today, mention the word *cholesterol* and most Americans still shudder. Most of us think if our cholesterol number is 200 or above, we're destined for a heart attack or stroke. Most people don't know that our bodies actually need to make large quantities of this important fat (also called a lipid). Most people also don't know that different individuals need different levels of cholesterol to carry out their body's critical daily life functions. Meanwhile, any blood test that measures how much cholesterol is found in your blood right now really has little to do with how many strips of bacon or the number of fried eggs you ate for breakfast this morning. Why are we never told these facts by the American Heart Association?

About 30 pharmaceutical companies each year give the American Heart Association $30 million. This seems to be enough money to carry out their never-ending national pro-statin drug campaign. These cholesterol-lowering drugs continue to reap blockbuster annual global sales, predicted by some analysts to hit $1 trillion by 2020.[56]

In 2015, David Diamond, a statistically savvy neuroscience professor, conducted a stunning study with his team at the University of South Florida. They exposed the pharmaceutical industry's longtime propaganda tactic that continues to push statin drugs on just about everybody.

In a 2015 article describing the study, Diamond had this to say: "We have described the deceptive approach statin advocates have deployed to create the appearance that cholesterol reduction results in an impressive reduction in cardiovascular disease outcomes, through their use of a statistical tool called relative risk reduction (RRR), a method which amplified the trivial beneficial effects of statins."[57]

In the same year that Diamond published this report, for the first time in US history, a group of nutritionists appointed to help develop the 2015 national nutritional guidelines were finally willing to write in their advisory report, *"available evidence shows no appreciable relationship between consumption of dietary cholesterol and serum cholesterol."*[58] In other words, this panel of the nation's top-level nutritionists publicly said, "Guess what? We disagree with the American Medical Society and with the American Heart Association. We believe that today's best research shows that a person's blood cholesterol level has little connection with how much cholesterol (natural fat or lipids) that person eats every day."[59] But never mind. Physicians continue to be told by the AHA and the AMA to prescribe statins to any patient with blood cholesterol levels over 200. And our food pyramid, still controlled by processed food lobbyists within NAM, remains the same. However, that honest top nutritionist, Luise Light, who died in 2010, would have been proud of our 2015 national nutritional team.[60]

Meanwhile, statins continue to be a cash cow for their pharmaceutical industry manufacturers. "Statin products are very high margin. So if a statin generates about 20 percent of a company's sales, it is likely to contribute 30 percent to its profits," according to Dr. Navid Malik, a pharmacologist by training, and a venture capital investor by profession.[61] "Statins have been the fairytale story in the industry. But heart disease is still the number one killer in the western world, so one could argue how much value for money have we really got out of their use?" Malik asks.

Fortunately, more physicians are finally questioning the information they got in medical school, about the importance of keeping blood cholesterol levels below 200. In 2012, Dr. Barbara H. Roberts, director of the Women's Cardiac Center at the Miriam Hospital in Providence, Rhode Island, wrote an entire book about this issue. Here's what she has to say:

Some people can take statins and not develop side effects. But how nec-essary are statins in the first place? Do they really help prevent strokes and heart attacks? Nowadays, doctors are advised to knock down their patients' cholesterol to very low levels with high doses of statins. But cholesterol, far from being the villain it's said to be, is a vital part of every cell in our bodies. This waxy fat, produced primarily by the liver, is absolutely crucial for the normal functioning of muscles, nerve cells, and the brain—and it's also the building block that our bodies use to manufacture many hormones, including the reproductive hormones estrogen and testosterone. How will our muscles, brain cells, and nerves react if they are chronically starved of a chemical that is so necessary for their proper functioning?[62]

Using Statin Drugs Doubles Breast Cancer Rates

Using statins can somehow damage a woman's breast cells' tiny mitochondria. A published, but little-known, 2013 statistical study tells us that *women who have taken statins for more than ten years develop twice as much breast cancer as women who have never taken the drug.* Conducted by epidemiologists at the highly regarded Fred Hutchinson Cancer Research Center in Seattle, the study looked at the long-term statin drug use of about 1,000 women between the ages of 55 and 74, compared to about 900 women who had never taken statins.[63]

Still worried about possible adverse health effects from a high-natu-ral-fat, low-starch, and low-sugar lifestyle? Read Dr. David Perlmut-ter's 2013 best-selling book, *Grain Brain*.[64] This groundbreaking book, revised and updated in 2018, re-educates us on why a diet based on nat-ural fats is best, and why a high-starch and high-sugar diet, especially when overloaded with grains, most fruits, and starchy/sugar-filled vege-tables (think corn, potatoes, peas, beets, and carrots), does not keep the mitochondria in the cells of our brains, hearts, and breasts in top-notch health. Maybe Dr. Perlmutter should have named his best-selling book, *Retraining Your Brain Against Corporate Grain...and Gain!*

Why High-fat Eating Makes It Easy to Lose Excess Body Fat

My son, Anil, is a clever computer tech. When customers ask him to upgrade their old computers, he often installs an inexpensive solid-state hard drive. Suddenly the client's machine starts up in a matter of seconds and can access files, programs, and web browsers faster than ever. That one inexpensive tweak to an old PC rejuvenates the machine's entire operating system and enables wonderful things to happen. Just like that solid-state hard drive, there are at least two reasons why it is fairly easy, and certainly healthy, for most of us to upgrade our body's sugar-burning metabolism to a fat-burning operating system.

As we've already seen, the first good reason is because a fat-burning operating system allows our bodies to lose weight as the liver is able to process our excess body fat into highly efficient and clean-burning ketones, producing high amounts of energy. The second good reason is this: Once our fat-burning system is switched on, two different "I am full" signals can go on in our brains. Switch #1 suddenly makes it incredibly easy to not overeat today. Switch #2 enables us to be a "naturally thin" person for the long term. In other words, this second switch makes it incredibly easy *to not overeat once we hit a healthy body size*. Who knew?

Weight Loss Switch #1: Cholecystokinin (CCK)

When an overweight or obese woman who begins a low-starch/high-natural-fat lifestyle is finally able to keep hunger under control, it's because of a substance called cholecystokinin (CCK). This naturally occurring substance, called a *neuropeptide*, gets turned on in your brain soon after you begin eating any high-fat meal—a meal without any starches or sugars. This CCK, however, stays silent whenever you eat a high-carb/low-fat breakfast of oatmeal and OJ, a bagel, or a fruit smoothie. Sadly, once you eat any starchy or sugary carbs at breakfast, you're sure to be hungry again in a short while. You know the feeling: lunch can't come soon enough![65]

As you're gradually willing to leave those starchy and sugary carbs behind and eat mainly natural fat, some protein, and some low-starch vegetables instead,[66] CCK will arrive to tell your brain and your stomach, "Enough already!" Suddenly, you actually know: "Oh! I'm actually pretty full. In fact, I really can't eat any more." You'll happily stop eating for longer and longer periods of time. Alleluia![67]

CCK

Cholecystokinin (CCK) is a neuropeptide of great benefit to anyone trying to lose weight. CCK is produced by special cells in the intestinal wall in response to a meal that contains some fat. Basically, it causes bile and pancreatic enzymes to be released for fat digestion. Besides helping fat digestion, research has demonstrated that CCK also causes a reduction in food intake in several species, including humans. In other words, it helps you to control your appetite; clearly an advantage if you're trying to eat less and reduce body fat.[68]

Weight Loss Switch #2: Leptin

Ever watch a naturally thin person politely refuse a freshly baked, warm chocolate chip cookie? It can be amazing. But if their body doesn't need to be refueled at that moment, they have an enzyme called *leptin* that switches on. This leptin actually tells that naturally thin person, "You're full. You don't want to eat anything right now." And, until leptin's "I am full" signal turns itself off, naturally thin folks won't touch that cookie.[69]

Since 1984, when the leptin hormone was first discovered, biologists have figured out that leptin can only activate its "Stop eating, you're full" signal in healthy weight people. That signal simply won't turn on if you are overweight. This means that leptin can't help an overweight person stop eating, even when her body has absorbed enough food. Apparently, as scientists are now learning, having excess body fat messes up leptin's normal signaling operation, no matter how much leptin is actually in your body.[70] What a bummer.

But here's some really good news! Once you lose your excess body fat, your body's "I'm full" leptin signal starts to work in your brain. Now you've joined the ranks of naturally thin people! This means that once you've finished eating any type of regular-sized meal, your leptin signal will come on, telling you that you're no longer hungry. Suddenly, you are truly not interested in finishing off that last piece of quiche, or even that warm chocolate chip cookie.

Why Eating Lots of Natural Fats Decreases Your Risk of Breast Cancer

"Ketogenic diets nourish normal cells with healthy fats and proteins and shield them from the damaging effects of excess sugar, starch and protein (all of which can turn into glucose), while simultaneously depriving cancer cells of the fuel they need to grow and spread. There is no other nutritional approach that can do all of these wonderful things."

—Georgia Ede MD

Converting your body's operating system away from a sugar- (or glucose-) burning metabolism and into a fat-burning metabolism helps every woman, of every shape and size, to prevent breast cancer. Why? Here are two biologically based answers.

Reason #1: Your Breast Cells Stop Producing Dirty Exhaust! This Helps Protect Your Cells' Mitochondria.

Eating starchy and sugary carbohydrates provides your body with low-octane, dirty fuel. As we've already seen, using glucose as your body's fuel creates a kind of molecule that I like to describe as dirty diesel exhaust; biologists call it reactive oxygen species (ROS). This ROS molecule, if left in your breast cells, can assault the cells' mitochondria day after day. These assaults, of course, increase the possibility that your mitochondria will become damaged and begin to suffocate. And that suffocation is the first step in the development of a woman's very first breast cancer cells.

Yes, this one simple change can make all the difference in the world: converting your personal operating system (your body's metabolism) to one that's fueled by natural fats. In fact, eating lots of natural fat is similar to filling your car's gas tank with super-octane fuel. A little goes a long way before you need to refuel again.

Reason #2: Fat Does Not Feed Cancer Cells! You're Starving Any Cancer Cells That Form.

As we saw in Chapter 1, all cancer cells love to eat sugar. And these same cancer cells can't process fat-produced ketones. Along with the amino acid called glutamine, sugar is what fuels every cancer cell's growth.[71] This means that if you're only eating natural fats and leafy greens, other low-starch vegetables, no grains, and no fruit, along with a minimal-to-moderate amount of protein, there won't be any glucose available to feed any glucose-loving cancer cells that might decide to form in your breasts.

Eating Natural Fat to Burn Body Fat: An Autobiography

Sometimes it helps to hear other people's stories. So, here's my own tale of switching from a starchy carb, glucose-burning system to my current, clean-running, natural-fat-burning, cancer prevention system. As my body made this switch, I moved from being about 140 pounds (with my BMI around 24 or 25) to my "new normal" of 115–120 pounds (with my BMI around 19–20, instead). Eating lots of natural fat, along with lots of green carbs and other non-starchy vegetables, created a personal metamorphosis. My new fat-burning operating system easily burned off almost 15 percent of my former body weight. Yes, while in my sixties, I evolved back to a shape and weight similar to what I had forty years earlier! This transformation took about eighteen painless months, and it continues to the present day.

Goodbye, Sugar!

Long ago, I stopped eating much sugar. For many people, not only is this the most important step towards ending obesity and high-cancer risk, but it's the hardest step, too. As I began to move further into a keto lifestyle, I tried to give up bread and crackers during my first week. Then I tried to give up rice the next week. Actually, I just gave myself three crackers or half a serving of rice. But at least I was now conscious that I didn't want to eat much bread, crackers, or rice anymore. It was the same with pasta. I still cooked my favorite spaghetti and meatballs; but each time, I got heavier on the meatballs and lighter on the pasta. I still wanted to eat three meals a day, so I did.

My reluctance to just give up the rice and pasta showed me that I actually had a carbohydrate addiction—an issue I had never fully understood or acknowledged. I reasoned that I'd never really been a big-time sugar eater—or even a regular bread eater, for that matter. But once I learned more about "going keto," I realized that my body's new natural-fat-burning operating system didn't know the difference between a scoop of organic brown rice and a scoop of Ben & Jerry's Chocolate Chip Cookie Dough! Both, it turns out, create the same kind of dirty fuel attacking my cells' mitochondria; both break down into glucose.

Hello, Bulletproof Coffee!

My serious fat-burning operation didn't really shift into high gear until I got brave enough to start drinking "bulletproof coffee," named after health food entrepreneur Dave Asprey's line of wellness products and supplements. The concoction is a heady mix of coffee and fat—think heavy cream with an added glob of coconut oil and a chunk of grass-fed butter. Are you still with me?

I bought my jar of unrefined, organic, cold-pressed coconut oil. I was happy to begin cooking with it; hefty chunks went into my scrambled eggs and sautéed asparagus. But put a tablespoon of coconut oil or a glob of unsalted, grass-fed butter into my gorgeous, freshly ground, organic, French-pressed dark roast, with gently heated and frothed organic cream? This was a very hard thing to do.

But after watching a few YouTube videos of hunky young men lauding the hunger-control benefits of drinking a few cups of this so-called "bulletproof" coffee every morning, I found the courage to give it a try.[72] One sip of that bulletproof coffee and I was sold. Talk about a heartwarming, nourishing, and comforting way to start your day! This quickly took the place of eating regular food for breakfast. I was finally on my way towards the keto lifestyle of only one or two meals each day.

Sometimes I change my routine and have bulletproof chaga tea instead of coffee. Chaga is taken from a fungus that grows mainly on the bark of birch trees in cold climates. Chaga is caffeine-free and apparently can reduce cellular inflammation, boost the immune system, enhance liver health, and fight viruses. Other research has found that chaga also has anti-tumor properties which is why it's used by some people to help treat and/or prevent some forms of cancer.[73]

Initially, on mornings when I tried to get by with just a cup of black tea and milk, or merely coffee with half-and-half (instead of heavy cream, butter, or coconut oil), my new fat-focused/low-carb lifestyle went belly-up. Suddenly, I wanted breakfast way before noon. Then I was hungry again at lunchtime, which meant there was no way I could easily keep my daily carb intake below 50 grams. This 50-gram carb limit became my goal during the months I was trying to lose my excess body fat. And when that excess body fat began to disappear, I could say I was reaching that place keto-based nutritionists call *nutritional ketosis*.[74] This is when your body is no longer operating on glucose to fuel your energy. Now the mitochondria in your cells are processing ketones. And those ketones or ketone bodies are being processed from the fat in your cowboy coffee and the fat around your tummy and thighs.

Two Meals a Day
Breakfast at 1 p.m.
My next happy discovery in Keto Land happened when I soon realized I wasn't getting hungry until noon or 1 p.m., having drunk that bulletproof coffee. So, each day, I began eating one or two sausages and an egg or two, scrambled in butter or avocado oil, along with half an avocado, at midday. Fried, scrambled, or poached eggs and bacon (or I might substitute a few boiled eggs and a chunk of salami, if I'm on the run) create a satisfying low-carb/high-fat (or "keto") meal, since these foods don't have more than a speck of carbs in them.[75] I did try to hang onto a half-piece of toast or half a ciabatta roll for a while, with *lots* of grass-fed butter. But after a few weeks of weaning myself off breads and rolls, I was pleasantly surprised to discover that I really didn't miss the bread anymore. And even today, my appetite continues to operate in a really different voice—sometimes so different it's startling.

High-natural fat/green carb dinners
These days, I continue to maintain my BMI of 19–20, and I don't cook rice, pasta, or potatoes for myself at all. I still have some basmati rice in the cupboard, and I'll make it for a dinner party once in a while; but rice,

bulgur, rolls, oatmeal, and potatoes are now gone from my daily life. Instead, I enjoy a high-natural-fat lifestyle, burning ketones more days than I burn glucose. And since I relax by cooking, I've become creative with various dark, fatty poultry and red meats, along with nuts, seeds, cheeses, and all kinds of greens and non-starchy vegetables.

One day, I got up the nerve to cut up, peel, and cook a large knob of celery root (celeriac). This weird, octopus-like, low-starch root vegetable looks a lot like mashed potatoes when it's steamed and mashed, but it has the faint sweet taste of celery. When my son and other mashed-potato-loving men now arrive for a roast lamb dinner, I may throw in one or two small potatoes with the chunks of a peeled, two-pound knob of celery root. No one notices the difference from the mashed potatoes I used to serve before! I think what we really like is simply having different textures, not necessarily starches, on our dinner plate. That mashed celery root, served with piles of sautéed garlicky leafy greens with toasted walnuts and capers, is perfect alongside a small piece of grilled, wild-caught fish or roasted meat. Add a Caesar salad topped with shaved parmesan, and you've got a beautiful meal! I've learned that ripe avocados also provide the same kind of satisfying mashed potato texture, and they go well with just about any meal.

I've never measured or weighed how many green vegetables I'm eating. Since I no longer eat any starchy or sugary carbs, I can just fill up on these healthier greens—things like avocadoes, asparagus, and peppers (or a few tomatoes, if I feel like some more color). This is how I happily transport all my main nutrients—those natural plant and animal fats—into my body, along with a small amount of fatty protein. Today, natural fat fuels my new operating system, while the moderate amount of protein I eat each day (one egg and less than one half-pound of fish or meat) helps me build and maintain muscle.

And even some dessert!
Sometimes, I finish off my high-fat dinners with a square or two of 85% organic dark chocolate, or enjoy a few blueberries atop a good dollop of sour cream—maybe even adding a drop of brandy or rum. It's also fun to make cookies or a loaf cake with the ingredients I've come to love. I use almond flour, coconut flour, almond butter, eggs, butter, coconut oil,

chopped nuts, a few super-dark, semi-sweet chocolate chips, and sunflower seeds. For icing, I'll use a whipped cream, cream cheese, and butter icing, sweetened with a drop of vanilla extract and a drop of maple syrup or stevia, and who knows what else. As you can see, my healthy diet isn't making me suffer!

Food Shopping and Cooking

I now approach the supermarket, fishmonger, and farmers' market with a new set of eyes. Eating this way all the time, I know a good fatty protein when I see one—think duck, chicken thighs, dark wild fish (like sardines, mackerel, sockeye salmon, bluefish, and shellfish), along with those long-forgotten organ meats or offal (like chicken livers, calves' livers, sweetbreads, and beef tongue)—dishes I dimly remember eating in my grandmothers' kitchens.[76]

Being as much a vegetable lover as I am a carnivore, I've also become equally adventurous with my produce selections. In addition to knobs of celery root, I try to buy a new kind of green or low-starch veggie every time I'm at the market—think red and green dandelion greens, broccoli rabe, different kinds of kale, different kinds of chard, radicchio, artichoke, watercress, arugula, collard greens, escarole, brussels sprouts, bok choy, fennel, turnips, and Jerusalem artichokes...to name a few. Hate to prepare fresh veggies? No problem. It's fine to use frozen instead.

According to Dr. Nasha Winters' groundbreaking book with Jess Higgins Kelly, *The Metabolic Approach to Cancer*,[77] Jerusalem artichokes (an unsung hero among veggies), radishes, and leeks are all five-star, low-glycemic/low-sugar vegetables.[78] These are powerhouses for developing a strong biome, that important part of our immune system found in our gut and described further in <u>Chapter 6</u>.[79]

Today, with my BMI happily stuck at 19 or 20, I very rarely need to snack and am usually happy eating just one or two meals a day. It's fun to search through Middle Eastern, Indian, Eastern European, Italian, French, and African American cookbooks, easily finding a wide variety of "naturally keto" recipes to keep my meals interesting. After all, these cultures have always included dishes based on cheap and fatty meat cuts, leafy green vegetables, nuts, olives, and fermented foods.[80] What's not to like about this ketogenic lifestyle?

What About Cocktail Hour?

This was for me, and is for many, the big question: "Can I still drink wine, or have a beer, or a martini, on a fat-focused, low-carb diet?" The answer to this question, in fact, may be the most important part of this chapter—or even a deal-breaker for some.

Wine

As you may know, there are leading scientists and nutritionists in the field of ketogenic lifestyles and type 2 diabetes who have published research demonstrating how a glass or two of wine each day can be stress-reducing, and how, for many, it can improve sleep and longevity.[81] But I've always wondered if some wines are *more good* for me than others. I was delighted to discover a company that offers low-sugar, low-alcohol wine for those of us following a ketogenic lifestyle.

As Todd White, president of Dry Farm Wines, tells potential customers, your fat-burning metabolism will probably come to a halt for a few hours once you have a drink, as your body works hard to burn off the toxic alcohol. But happily, most "fat-adapted folks" will revert back to their fat-burning metabolism just a few hours later.

And what about white wine versus red; which is better? White wine, as a rule, contains more sugar than red wine. Having said this, however, Todd White doesn't entirely disabuse his namesake. Instead, he likes to point out that all American-made wines, white and red, are sweeter than most European wines. American wine makers are appealing to the average American's preference for anything sugary. In order to sell their wines, most US vineyards do not allow the sugar-eating (i.e., fermenting) process to run its full course. The unfermented, leftover sugar found in US wines is absent from most European wines. Here, the sugar has been "disappeared," by allowing the yeast to digest or ferment away all of the sugar in the wine-making vat.[82]

How about martinis and beer?

When it comes to vodka or gin, a martini is much better than a gin and tonic or a vodka and tonic. This is because you're not putting mixers, loaded with sugar or chemical sweeteners, into your body. A lemon peel with your martini is fine, but olives (in fact, *lots* of olives) are a real boon.

They add to your fat intake for the day! On the other hand, drinking beer is drinking pure carbs. Meanwhile, any kind of hard liquor contains lots more alcohol than wine. And as Todd White likes to remind folks, any amount of alcohol is putting poison in your body.

No wonder our body's very clever, fat-fueled operating system quickly shuts down its fat-burning as soon as any spirits go down the throat; it has to turn its attention to processing away that toxic alcohol.[83] Yes, our bodies really do know best. Or, as Hippocrates told us thousands of years ago, "Let food be your medicine and medicine be your food." Unfortunately, alcohol is neither! Meanwhile, now more than ever, I also follow my friend Lorraine's favorite motto: Life is too short to drink cheap wine!

Ketogenic Cookbooks: An Expanding Collection

More and more high-fat/low-carb cookbooks are being published every month. But my favorite remains *The Ketogenic Kitchen*.[84] Actually, this is two cookbooks for the price of one! The first half of the book is filled with low-carb (less than 50 grams a day) recipes for those wanting to stay in nutritional ketosis in order to lose excess body fat, prevent cancer, or block a recurrence of a prior cancer diagnosis. The second half of the book includes recipes that are extremely low-carb (under 20 grams/day). This is best for those currently facing a cancer diagnosis who can use the diet as a medicine to help starve their duplicating cancer cells. These extremely low-carb recipes are also appropriate for women who are obese and focused on rapidly losing a significant amount of weight. *The Ketogenic Kitchen*, with its international and everyday recipes, also contains lively narratives by its two Irish authors, Domini Kemp and Patricia Daly, and it includes a foreword by Dr. Seyfried, the "George Washington" of the new metabolic approach to cancer. Beautifully designed, *The Ketogenic Kitchen* is a critical reference for keto cooks. It also makes a lovely gift.

Maria Emmerich discovered the ketogenic lifestyle many years ago, and used high-fat/low-carb eating to get rid of her excess body fat and then maintain her naturally thin body. Her book, *The 30-Day Ketogenic Cleanse: Reset Your Metabolism with Tasty Whole-Food Recipes & Meal Plans* is a great resource when you're beginning a keto lifestyle.[85] Emmerich's other ketogenic cookbooks, all designed for feeding your entire family, include *Keto Comfort Foods: Family Favorites Made Low-Carb and Healthy,*[86] *Keto Restaurant Favorites,*[87] and *Easy Dairy-Free Ketogenic Recipes.*[88] Each of these books includes beautifully illustrated recipes, along with clearly written basic information about the ketogenic diet that will helpful to anyone beginning this low-carb lifestyle. Finally, Leanne Vogel's *Keto for Women*[89] and Suzanne Ryan of Keto Karma[90] have self-help books, podcasts and other resources, all focusing on women's special issues when utilizing a ketogenic lifestyle for fat loss and optimal health.

Casey Durango, a 60-year-old woman, lost one hundred pounds following a keto lifestyle for a few years. She had carried this extra weight for decades. Now maintaining this lower weight, by continuing to follow this lifestyle, Durango shares her knowledge, philosophy and ongoing experience, by creating informal videos each week for tens of thousands of viewers on her YouTube channel "Go Keto with Casey." A follower of Dr. Eric Westman's work and weight loss protocols at Duke University's Diabetes Clinic, Durango continues to translate the basics and the benefits of a ketogenic diet to women who, like herself, have struggled or continue to struggle with chronic obesity.

Measuring Ketone Levels

How do you know if your body is burning any natural fat instead of your old standard inefficient glucose fuel? One way to answer this question is to measure your body's glucose and ketone blood levels throughout the day, or at least every few days. You can tell if you're in ketosis (burning fat instead of glucose), by using a glucose/ketone meter and the glucose/ketone calculator or GKI formula. This calculation was developed by Dr. Seyfried and a graduate student in 2015 to help guide a brain cancer patient who was using only metabolic therapies to manage her disease. The GKI formula or index measures the ratio of glucose in your blood to the amount of ketones you are producing. You need to have *both* numbers to know if you have hit your body's fat-burning switch![91] By taking her blood glucose reading and her blood ketone reading and calculating the two with the GKI formula, the patient was able to tell if the type and quantity of food she was eating was enabling her to remain in deep ketosis (<1). Cancer patients who are able to keep their GKI index below 1 are able to starve their tumors cells of glucose, slowing or blocking their tumor growth.[92]

You can also use a glucose/ketone meter and the GKI formula to guide you in your fat loss journey. Just keep your GKI number between 3 and 9. This is the place where your body's unique metabolism is able to burn mainly ketones. This means your body can now burn off your excess body fat, and/or the fat you choose to eat today. Any excess ketones you make today will be eliminated in your urine. My favorite way of tracking my glucose/ketone levels is with a simple glucose/ketone meter called the Keto-Mojo.[93] This little device reads both glucose and ketone strips, sourced from the same finger prick. Once you know your two numbers, just use the GKI formula and divide your glucose number by 18; then divide that number by your ketone level. You can do this calculation yourself, or download Keto-Mojo's app, which does the calculation for you! Keto-Mojo will soon offer a glucose-ketone meter that give you your GKI number automatically. Presto! You have your GKI. Again, if your GKI is less than 10, your body is burning ketones. A GKI between 6 and 9 is fine for slow weight loss and maintaining current health. Keto-Mojo's GKI guide can be found on their website and below.[94]

Another way to evaluate the general level of your body's current fat-burning operation is to use a breath analyzer. Two favorites are the Swedish-made Ketonix and the US-made Biosense.[95] All of these keto measurement tools, along with many others, can be found on the website myketokitchen.com.[96] Check it out for yourself.

Order a Complete Blood Panel

Switching to a fat-burning operating system means transitioning your body to a new kind of equilibrium. Women who face thyroid, adrenal, and other types of hormonal or autoimmune conditions, chronic migraines, or obesity, should find a functional health practitioner to help them safely get started on their high-fat/low-carb journey. You can partner with any number of optimal-health or preventive-medicine practitioners or health coaches. Thanks to Skype, Zoom, FaceTime, cell phones, and email, ketogenic-focused health practitioners and coaches can be located near or far. And no matter your health status, it's critical that you or your healthcare professional order a complete blood panel at least twice a year.[97] This panel should include your vitamin D3 level, as well as your C-reactive protein (CRP) level.[98] Your vitamin D3 number, as described in Chapter 3, indicates the current strength of your cell-to-cell communication system, a critically important part of your body's multi-sectional immune system. C-reactive protein (CRP) is a marker for whole-body inflammation, a cause of significant numbers of breast cancer diagnoses.

Figure 2.4: The Glucose Ketone Index

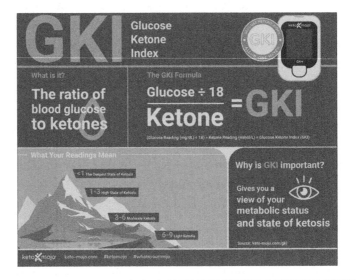

Knowing your GKI helps you experience the most effective ongoing fat loss. Your GKI indicates whether your body is finally burning your own fat and/or the fat you are eating. Likewise, if you eat too much protein, your body will convert it to glucose. A GKI over 9 indicates you are eating too much protein and/or carbs.

keto-mojo.com, *Glucose Ketone Index [GKI]: A biomarker for tracking your metabolic health,* https:// keto-mojo.com/glucose-ketone-index-gki/.

Facing That Loud Voice

As you read through this chapter, do you keep hearing a voice inside your head, screaming, "It's crazy and wrong to eat so much fat every day!" Or is it perhaps telling you, "It's stupid to tell me I shouldn't eat a banana every morning," or, "It's crazy to eat so much fat!" Or, "I have to take that statin drug!" Well, guess what? If you're a woman, that voice you're hearing is actually not your own. That screaming, critical, and commanding voice that keeps yelling at you every day to be cautious, to not make any changes, to not try jumping over that mud puddle—that *other* voice—is really a learned reflex, or a tape from your younger years.

But as women, we each have another voice, as well. This one is located deep within our mind and heart. It's a quieter, more thoughtful voice. This is the one I like to call *myself*, or my *own* inner voice.

In this chapter, I'm asking you and other women to ignore that loud other voice for a while. This chapter has also encouraged you to ignore the US food pyramid, along with the advice of traditional nutritionists and physicians, when it comes to an effective fat-loss lifestyle. Other chapters in this book suggest that you also ignore some other voices of authority—which is, admittedly, hard to do. But you'll see that many policies issued by the National Cancer Institute, by Planned Parenthood, by Susan G. Komen for the Cure, even some policies recommended by your own OB/GYN (not to mention your friends and family members) run counter to the breast cancer prevention steps discussed in this book. But bear in mind that every one of these cancer prevention choices is backed by the best research we have today. Be prepared: You may find it hard to listen to, let alone consider trying, one or more of these effective breast cancer prevention options. Remember, what makes it hard is this *other* voice inside your head, telling you, "No, no, no," even when the best evidence is saying, "Yes, yes, YES!"

For most women, that *other* voice all too often pushes its way in to override the kinder, more intuitive, more personal—and more daring—quiet voice that is our *own*. And so, that *other* voice, with its nagging tone and high volume, often makes it very hard for women to make significant life changes—changes that are often in our own best self-interest; dramatic changes that most men seem to have a much easier time embracing.[99] For women, the internal ranting and raving of that *other* voice can too often block our forward movement, always telling us to do the dishes now, not later; to not waste money on that perfectly gorgeous (fill in the blank); to keep our job security, even if we hate everything about our daily work; to not make drastic changes about how we eat...about anything...at least not now.

That *other* voice loves to utter its harsh, often controlling attack words or phrases, just as we're thinking about doing something revolutionary, something completely new, something we actually would really like to try, just for ourselves. But then that *other* voice starts in: "Keep your mouth shut." "Don't make a fuss." "Be nice." "NO." "Crazy girl." "Stupid woman." "Stop." "You're useless." "That's wrong." "Don't do it." "You can't go there." "That's impossible." "Try to smile." "It won't work." "That's a pathetic idea." "Don't be so gullible." "Who do you think you are, anyway?"

Fortunately, many women are finally becoming able to distinguish between these two voices, the *loud* or *other* one versus their *own*. In fact, this may be why the #MeToo movement continues to strike such a chord. Starting in 2017, women came out in force, shocking ourselves as much as anyone else. Many women, now emboldened, have finally been able to shove that *other* voice out of their way, breaking their silence and daring to publicly decry the countless sexual molestations and harassment that the *other* voice told them to keep silent about—until now.

If that *loud other* voice has been so good at telling us to keep our mouths shut about these horrors for so many years, just imagine what that *other* voice will say when you decide to throw your long-beloved breakfast out the window—your "healthy," organic, steel-cut oatmeal, granola, and banana! "Replace my oatmeal with thick-cut bacon and fried eggs?" And just imagine what that *other* voice might say when you decide that the toast and jam are out the window, but the butter gets to stay!

Where Did That Other Voice Come From in the First Place?

For the past fifty years, psychologists have recognized that girls form a very different, much tighter, bond with our mothers' psyche—and voice—than boys do. That bond develops into an all-critical, loud, internal voice that's hard to separate from, even when women reach far into adulthood. Boys, on the other hand, are usually forced to separate psychologically from their mothers early on. They're first told, and then shown, that they're physically different from Mom; that they are boys. Even as three-year-olds, boys are encouraged to understand that they're more like Daddy than Mommy: "Be a big boy, like Daddy," they're told.[100]

In her short, but very powerful book *Women, Food and God*, Geneen Roth, having lost and gained "over 1,000 pounds" in her own life, has gathered up all this wisdom about women's internal critic and developed a few really important life-knowing and lifesaving guidelines to help herself and other women begin to put ourselves first. Roth calls that *other* voice simply, "The Voice." She then tries to help women learn to ignore The Voice in order reach a healthy weight, regardless of the food they currently eat. Roth's guidelines are all about how we must put that *other* voice in its place—well out of the way of our own good sense. Her guidelines explain what happens when, finally, a woman begins to make her own wise decisions—including decisions about food.[101]

"According to developmental psychologists, The Voice is fully operative in most of us by the time we are four years old, after which it functions as a moral compass, a deterrent to questionable behavior. Instead of being afraid of the disapproval of our parents, we become afraid of the disapproval of The Voice...We become risk aversive. Frightened of change. Depending on our particular parents, this could mean anything from traveling to Asia (all that icky malaria, dysentery, leprosy better stay home) to trusting our own instincts (Trust your instincts? Hello? Have you noticed where that has gotten you?)..."[102]

Neither education nor privilege seems to change the power or the volume of a woman's critical inner monologue very much. Back in the 1970s, the Harvard psychiatrist Dr. Jean Baker Miller, having worked with hundreds of women for decades, wrote, "The sense of pleasing herself has been a very rare experience for most women. When they attain it, it is a newfound joy."[103]

Dr. Baker Miller's Harvard colleague, Carol Gilligan, added to this finding a few years later by eloquently describing how most women are brought up to have a "different voice." Not surprisingly, this "different voice" makes connections with other people seem more important than a woman's own self-determination or her ability to prioritize her own personal wants, needs, and feelings above what other people expect of her.[104]

A decade later, Gilligan and her colleagues studied how girls attending the private Emma Willard School in Troy, New, York started out as feisty ten-year-olds, knowing their own minds. Quickly, though, they lost their sense of self as they become teenagers. They began putting others' wishes ahead their own.[105] As the years and decades go by, with women's own instincts covered over most of the time, it becomes more and more difficult for women to even remember, let alone live each day, without that *other* voice telling us to ignore our own desires for change. Or as the Al-Anon organization tells its members (85 percent of whom are women), "It is unfortunately more common for us to focus on the issues of others, before ourselves."[106]

Having lost sight of our own individual and thoughtful, inquisitive, and daring inner voice, many women find ways to also detach from our physical bodies. And since we've been guided by these voices of "authority" throughout our lives, we're content to be guided and harmed by the authority of today's misguided USDA's food pyramid, even though we thought we were "eating healthy."

Countering the Other Voice with Your Own

Natalie Goldberg, the Zen-inspired writer, teaches us an inexpensive and effective way to get away from that *other* voice for short periods of time. Goldberg's rules for the practice of writing are an easy way to catch a glimpse of our *own*, often distant but nonetheless strong voice, deep inside. Her book *Writing Down the Bones* has sold well over a million copies since it was first published in 1986. Her four simple writing directives enable every woman to break free of that *other* voice, even if just for ten minutes at a time. Her free-writing rules aim at allowing our minds to go jumping and leaping "into witchever whey makes ewe feel less which-like!" Goldberg encourages us to write from our bellies and big toes. And never edit, never cross out—not for "write" now, at least. Using these four writing rules, these "righting ways," can create wonderful moments—even if initially terrifying to some—as women are able to face down and finally put aside that loud, morally superior, controlling inner critic. Goldberg calls that *other* voice our "Monkey Mind."[107]

Meanwhile, Anne Lamott, a writer as funny as she is wise, calls that *other* voice "Radio Station KFKD."[108] According to Lamott, "Less lyrical people (like Sigmund Freud) call it the superego, the internalized parent, the inner critic." The teacher and writer Byron Katie has a compassionate and effective method of managing that *other* voice. She says, "I love my thoughts. I'm just not tempted to believe them."[109]

The fat-loss author and coach Geneen Roth also tells us, "So long as we cannot control that *other* voice in our minds, we cannot listen to our *own* voice telling us which foods to eat, how much food we should have, and when. No wonder it's so hard for so many women to change the way we eat. Even if our lives depend on it. Which they do."

When beginning to follow a ketogenic lifestyle, then, it's totally natural to feel guilty. But then it becomes deliciously exciting, sautéing that red chard, spinach, or watercress in tablespoons of olive oil...adding in some toasted pine nuts or walnuts...topping it off with olives, capers, lemon, and chunks of feta...and guiltlessly devouring it all with a thick, fatty pork chop and a glass of very dry red wine alongside.

This chapter has included some of the most important information in the entire book. By taking charge of your body with a high-fat/low-carb lifestyle, you really can switch your body's operating system from one that burns cancer-creating and -feeding sugar to one that burns natural fat instead. And doing so will have both fat-loss and breast cancer prevention benefits. What more motivation do you need? Following this high-fat ketogenic lifestyle, you'll lose your excess body fat and maintain a healthy body size. You'll eliminate dirty, glucose-driven ROS molecules from your breast cells (and other body cells), pumping in lots of life-giving oxygen to keep your mitochondria clean and healthy. There's no question about it: eliminating all your excess body fat, and keeping your body in a fat-burning mode, is one of the most important breast cancer prevention steps on the planet!

Along with sharing this important lifestyle information in this chapter, we also confronted the biggest obstacle to making a life-saving change: that loud, nagging, *other* voice in our heads. But if we can find ways to stand up to that voice, we can not only change our food...we can change our lives!

Beyond diet, there are other concrete changes we can make to take charge of our health. The next chapter describes another simple, inexpensive, and healthy step all woman can take to help keep breast cancer out of our bodies. Keeping your vitamin D3 blood level over 60 ng/ml year-round is a highly effective second line of defense, should a cancer cell ever begin to develop in your breast. Let's learn more!

2 CHAPTER ENDNOTES

1   National Institutes for Health, "Overweight and Obesity Statistics," https://www.niddk.nih.gov/health-information/health-statistics/overweight-obesity.

2   Stacey Simon, "How Your Weight May Affect Your Risk of Breast Cancer," October 4, 2018, https://www.cancer.org/latest-news/how-your-weight-affects-your-risk-of-breast-cancer.html;"Cancers Associated with Overweight and Obesity Make Up 40 Percent of Cancers Diagnosed in the United States," (October 3, 2017), https://www.cdc.gov/media/releases/2017/p1003-vs-cancer-obesity.html; Shawna B. Matthews and Henry J. Thompson, "The Obesity-Breast Cancer Conundrum: An Analysis of the Issues," *International Journal of Molecular Sciences* 1, no. 6 (June 22, 2016): 989, https://www.mdpi.com/1422-0067/17/6/989.

3   Marian L. Neuhouser et al., "Overweight, Obesity, and Postmenopausal Invasive Breast Cancer Risk: A Secondary Analysis of the Women's Health Initiative Randomized Clinical Trials," *JAMA Oncology* 1, no. 5 (2015): 611–21, https://doi.org/10.1001/jamaoncol.2015.1546.

4   Melina Arnold, "Duration of Adulthood Overweight, Obesity, and Cancer Risk in the Women's Health Initiative: A Longitudinal Study from the United States," *PLOS Medicine* (August 16, 2016), https://doi.org/10.1371/journal.pmed.1002081; Aiko Sueta et al., "Differential Impact of Body Mass Index and its Change on the Risk of Breast Cancer by Molecular Subtype: A Case-control Study in Japanese Women," *SpringerPlus* 1, no. 1 (2012): 39, https://doi.org/10.1186/2193-1801-1-39.

5   North American Association of Central Cancer Registries, "NAACCR Age-Adjusted Incidence Rates and 95% Confidence Intervals; 2000 US Standard Population By Age at Diagnosis; Female Breast, All Races, Female, U.S. Combined 2012-2016," NAACR.org. See Chapter 9 for discussion of US cancer statistics.

6   Andrew G. Renehan, et al., "Adiposity and Cancer Risk: New Mechanistic Insights from Epidemiology," *Nature Reviews Cancer* 15 (2015):484–98, https://doi.org/10.1038/nrc3967; Masaaki Kawai et al., "Height, Body Mass Index (BMI), BMI Change, and the Risk of Estrogen Receptor-positive, HER2-positive, and Triple-negative Breast Cancer among Women Ages 20 to 44 Years," *Cancer* 120, no.10 (2014): 548–56, https://acsjournals.onlinelibrary.wiley.com/doi/full/10.1002/cncr.28601; Heng Sun et al. "Triple-Negative Breast Cancer and its Association with Obesity," *Molecular and Clinical Oncology* 7, no. 6 (2017): 935–42, https://pubmed.ncbi.nlm.nih.gov/29285353/; Linda Vona-Davis, et al., "Triple-negative Breast Cancer and Obesity in a Rural Appalachian Population," *Cancer Epidemiology, Biomarkers & Prevention* 17, no. 12 (2008): 3319–24, https://doi.org/10.1158/1055-9965.EPI-08-0544.

7   Manual Picon-Ruiz et al., "Obesity and Adverse Breast Cancer Risk and Outcome: Mechanistic Insights and Strategies for Intervention," *CA: A Cancer Journal for Clinicians* 67, no.5 (2017): 378–97, https://doi.org/10.3322/caac.21405.

8   Ana M. Soto and Carlos Sonnenschein, "The Somatic Mutation Theory of Cancer: Growing Problems with the Paradigm?", *Bio Essays* 20 (September 2004): 1097–1107, https://doi.org/10.1002/bies.20087.

9   T.N. Seyfried, *Cancer As A Metabolic Disease; On the Origin, Management and Prevention of Cancer*, (Hoboken, Wiley, 2012).

10 M. Coelho, T. Oliveira, and R. Fernandes, "Biochemistry of Adipose Tissue: An Endocrine Organ," *Archives of Medical Science* 9, no.2 (2013): 191–200, https://doi.org/10.5114/aoms.2013.33181.

11 There are different types of estrogens, and there are substances that mimic estrogens. All are able to enter breast cells. Some naturally-produced estrogens, including plant based estrogens, are important for women's development and ongoing health; most other estrogens are toxic and can harm breast cells' mitochondria.

12 Kassem Makki et al., "Adipose Tissue in Obesity-related Inflammation and Insulin Resistance: Cells, Cytokines, and Chemokines," *ISRN Inflammation* 139239, (December 22, 2013), https://doi.org/10.1155/2013/139239.

13 Aiko Sueta et al., "Differential Impact of Body Mass Index and Its Change on The Risk of Breast Cancer by Molecular Subtype: A Case-Control Study in Japanese Women," *SpringerPlus* 1,no.1 (2012): 39. doi:10.1186/2193-1801-1-39.

14 Picon-Ruiz et al., "Obesity and Adverse Breast Cancer Risk and Outcome" (2017), https://doi.org/10.3322/caac.21405.

15 Marion Nestle, *Unsavory Truth: How Food Companies Skew the Science of What We Eat*, (New York: Hachette Book Group, 2018).

16 Steven Phinney and Jeffry Volek, *The Art and Science of Low Carbohydrate Living: An Expert Guide to Making the Life-Saving Benefits of Carbohydrate Restriction Sustainable and Enjoyable*, (Phoenix, AZ: Beyond Obesity, LLC, 2011).

17 Ibid.; see also Colin Barras, "Ancient Leftovers Show the Real Paleo Diet was a Veggie Feast," *New Scientist*, December 6, 2015, https://www.newscientist.com/article/2115127-ancient-leftovers-show-the-real-paleo-diet-was-a-veggie-feast/.

18 Ruth E. Patterson et al., "Intermittent Fasting and Human Metabolic Health," *Journal of the Academy of Nutrition and Dietetics* 115, no.8 (2015):1203–12, https://pubmed.ncbi.nlm.nih.gov/25857868/; Seyfried, 2012.

19 Adrian Miller,"The Surprising History of African-American Mashup Cuisine," September 10, 2015, https://firstwefeast.com/eat/2015/09/the-surprising-history-of-african-american-mashup-cuisine; African American Registry AAREG, "Soul Food: A Brief History," https://aaregistry.org/story/soul-food-a-brief-history/.

20 Joseph Mercola, *Fat for Fuel* (New York: Hay House, 2017); Joseph Mercola, *KetoFast: Rejuvenate Your Health with a Step-by-Step Guide to Timing Your Ketogenic Meals* (New York: Hay House, 2019).

21 Howard Zinn, the American historian, civil rights leader, and son of immigrant Russian Jewish parents, describes his family's normal state of hunger growing up in NYC in the 1920s in his autobiographical book, *You Can't Be Neutral on a Moving Train: A Personal History of Our Times* (Boston: Beacon Press, 2002).

22 Cheryl D. Fryar et al., "Prevalence of Overweight, Obesity, and Extreme Obesity Among Adults: United States, Trends 1960–1962 Through 2009–2010," CDC.gov, http://creativecatsolutions.com/uploads/1/0/6/4/10642571/prevalence_of_overweight_obesity_and_extreme_obesity_among_adults.pdf.

23 Andrew G. Glass, James V. Lacey Jr. and Robert N. Hoover, "The Rise in Breast Cancer Incidence, 1960-2003, is Largely Confined to ER+ Tumors", *Epidemiology 9: Descriptive Epidemiology and Methodology*, 46, no. 9 (2005) Supplement, https://cancerres.aacrjournals.org/content/65/9_Supplement/953.4.

24 North American Association of Central Cancer Registries, "Age-Adjusted Incidence Rates 2012-2016," NAACCR.org, https://faststats.naaccr.org/selections.php?series=cancer.

25 Larry Forbes, "Victor Dzau Leaving Duke to Head the Institute of Medicine," Feb 2, 2014, Forbes.com, https://www.forbes.com/sites/larryhusten/2014/02/19/victor-dzau-leaving-duke-to-head-the-institute-of-medicine/#101a332b2e4b; Roy M. Poses, "Incoming President of IOM Outed as Member of Boards of Alnylam Pharmaceuticals, Medtronic and PepsiCo," *Health Care Renewal*, (February 24, 2014), http://hcrenewal.blogspot.com/2014/02/incoming-president-of-iom-outed-as.html; David Armstrong, "PepsiCo Director Quitting to Lead Health Institute That Touted Soda Tax," *Bloomberg Business Week*, (February 21, 2014), https://www.bloomberg.com/news/articles/2014-02-21/victor-dzau-leaving-pepsicos-board-to-lead-institute-of-medicine.

26 National Academies, "Institute of Medicine to Become National Academy of Medicine," press release, April 28, 2015, https://www8.nationalacademies.org/onpinews/newsitem.aspx?RecordID=04282015.

27   Edward D. Berkowitz, *To Improve Human Health: A History of the Institute of Medicine* (Washington, DC: National Academies Press, 1998); Lawrence K. Altman, "Dr. Irvine Page is Dead at 90: Pioneered Hypertension Research," *The New York Times*, June 12, 1991. Accessed March 10, 2019, https://www.nytimes.com/1991/06/12/obituaries/dr-irvine-h-page-is-dead-at-90-pioneered-hypertension-research.html.

28   The National Academies of Sciences, Engineering, and Medicine, "History of the National Academies," nationalacademies.org, http://www.nationalacademies.org/about/history/index.html, accessed March 10, 2019.

29   National Academies of Science, Engineering, and Medicine, "New Report Identifies Five Breakthroughs to Address Urgent Challenges and Advance Food and Agricultural Sciences by 2030," July 18, 2018, nationalacademies.org, 2018, https://www.nationalacademies.org/news/2018/07/new-report-identifies-five-breakthroughs-to-address-urgent-challenges-and-advance-food-and-agricultural-sciences-by-2030.

30   Luise Light, *What to Eat: The Ten Things You Really Need to Know to Eat Well and Be Healthy!* (New York: McGraw Hill, 2006), 14.

31   Ibid.

32   Luise Light, "A Fatally Flawed Food Guide," 2004, http://www.whale.to/a/american_food_pyramid.html; Also see: Luise Light, *What to Eat: The Ten Things You Really Need to Know to Eat Well and Be Healthy!*, 14.

33   H.R.1608–National Nutrition Monitoring and Related Research Act of 1990, 101st Congress (1989-1990), www.congress.gov/bill/101st-congress/house-bill/1608.

34   National Academies of Sciences, Engineering, and Medicine, "Review of the Process to Update the Dietary Guidelines for America," http://www.nationalacademies.org/hmd/Activities/Nutrition/DietaryGuidelinesforAmericans.aspx.

35   David Lazarus, "A Former Corn-syrup Lobbyist is Drafting New Federal Dietary Rules (Seriously)," *Los Angeles Times*, May 7, 2019, https://www.latimes.com/business/lazarus/la-fi-lazarus-food-industry-shapes-dietary-guidelines-20190507-story.html.

36   National Academies, "Giving to the National Academies," https://sites.nationalacademies.org/Giving/givingsocieties/index.htm; "Support the National Academy of Medicine," https://nam.edu/support-the-nam/.

37   National Academies, "Whitney and Betty MacMillan: A Gift for a Better Future," https://www.nationalacademies.org/giving/whitney-and-betty-macmillan.

38   Mighty Earth, "Cargill Named 'Worst Company in the World,' "(July 11, 2019), https://www.mightyearth.org/cargillreport.

39   EveryCRSReport, "U.S. Domestic Food Assistance Programs," December 11, 2018, https://www.everycrsreport.com/reports/R45433.html#_Toc532546877.

40   Food and Nutrition Service, "National School Lunch Program," https://www.fns.usda.gov/nslp.

41   James A. Levine, "Poverty and Obesity in the U.S," *Diabetes* 60, no.11 (November 2011): 2667–68, https://doi.org/10.2337/db11-1118.

42   Adam Andrzejewski, "Mapping the U.S. Farm Subsidy $1M Club," *Forbes*, August 14, 2018, https://www.forbes.com/sites/adamandrzejewski/2018/08/14/mapping-the-u-s-farm-subsidy-1-million-club/#45913c6d3efc.

43   These are all food products produced by PepsiCo. NAM's president, Victor Dzau received more than $7 million dollars from annual compensation and stocks from membership on PepsiCo and various pharmaceutical companies' boards of directors during his lengthy tenure with PepsiCo and the other boards, resigning most positions in 2014, weeks before accepting the position of

NAM's chief executive. See: Larry Husten, "Newly Elected President of Institute of Medicine is on the PepsiCo Board of Directors," *Forbes*, February 19, 2014, https://www.forbes.com/sites/larryhusten/2014/02/19/newly-elected-president-of-institute-of-medicine-is-on-the-pepsico-board-of-directors/#58d69a3e258c.

44   Ellen Ruppel Shell, *Fat Wars: The Inside Story of the Obesity Industry* (New York: Atlantic Books, 2003).

45   Gary Taub, *Why We Get Fat: And What to Do About It* (New York: Anchor, 2011).

46   Robert Lustig, *The Hacking of the American Mind: The Science Behind the Corporate Takeover of Our Bodies and Brains* (New York: Avery, 2017).

47   Nina Teicholtz. *The Big Fat Surprise: Why Butter, Meat and Cheese Belong in a Healthy Diet* (New York: Simon and Schuster, 2014).

48   Common Dreams, "Monsanto Internal Documents Reveal Campaign Against U.S. Right to Know," August 8, 2019, https://www.commondreams.org/newswire/2019/08/08/monsanto-internal-documents-reveal-campaign-against-us-right-know.

49   Stacy Malkin, *Not Just a Pretty Face: The Ugly Side of the Beauty Industry* (New York: Harmony, 2009).

50   Greg Palast, "Stacey Abrams Hires Palast Investigations Team for Massive Federal Suit to Restore Voting Rights," November 24, 2019, https://www.gregpalast.com/stacey-abrams-hires-palast-investigations-team-for-massive-federal-suit-to-restore-voting-rights/.

51   Stacey Malkin, "USRTK Research Director Carey Gillam Receives SEJ Award for Reporting," https://usrtk.org/news-releases/u-s-right-to-know-research-director-carey-gillam-receives-prestigious-sej-book-award/.

52   Anahed O'Connor, "How the Sugar Industry Shifted Blame to Fat," *The New York Times*, September 13, 2016, https://www.nytimes.com/2016/09/13/well/eat/how-the-sugar-industry-shifted-blame-to-fat.html; Cristin E. Kearns, "Sugar Industry and Coronary Heart Disease Research: A Historical Analysis of Internal Industry Documents," *JAMA Internal Medicine* 176, no.11 (2016): 1680–85, https://pubmed.ncbi.nlm.nih.gov/27617709/. R.B. McGandy et al., "Dietary Fats, Carbohydrates and Atherosclerotic Vascular Disease," *New England Journal of Medicine* 277, no.4 (July 27, 1967): 186–92 contd. https://doi.org/10.1056/NEJM196707272770405; R.B. McGandy et al. "Dietary Fats, Carbohydrates and Atherosclerotic Vascular Disease," *New England Journal of Medicine* 277, no. 5 (August 3, 1967): 245–47 concl. https://nature.berkeley.edu/garbelottoat/wp-content/uploads/Mcgandy-1967-part-1-1.pdf.

53   J.M.W. Wong et al., "Effects of a Low Carbohydrate Diet on Energy Expenditure During Weight Loss Maintenance: Randomized Trial," *BMJ* 363 (November 2018), https://doi.org/10.1136/bmj.k4583; Joseph Mercola, *Fat for Fuel* 2017.

54   Nina Teicholtz, "2020 Dietary Guidelines Repeating Past Mistakes, Lacks Scientific Rigor," October 31, 2019, https://www.nutritioncoalition.us/news/2020-dietary-guidelines-repeating-past-mistakes.

55   Alice Walker, *We Are the Ones We Have Been Waiting For: Inner Light In a Time of Darkness* (New York: The New Press, 2006).

56   Gordon H. Sun, "Statins: The Good, the Bad, and the Unknown, Clinicians Are Talking About Statins," Medscape.com, October 10, 2014, https://www.medscape.com/viewarticle/832841.

57   David M. Diamond and Uffe Ravnskov, "How Statistical Deception Created the Appearance that Statins Are Safe and Effective in Primary and Secondary Prevention of Cardiovascular Disease," *Expert Review of Clinical Pharmacology* 8 no. 2 (2015) 201-10, https://doi.org/10.1586/17512433.2015.1012494.

58   "Scientific Advisory Report on 2015 Dietary Guidelines," Health.gov (February; 2015), https://health.gov/dietaryguidelines/2015-scientific-report.

59 N.G. Puaschitz et al., "Dietary Intake of Saturated Fat is Not Associated with Risk of Coronary Events or Mortality in Patients with Established Coronary Artery Disease," *Journal of Nutrition* (February 2015): 299-305, https://doi.org/10.3945/jn.114.203505. Epub 2014 Dec 10.

60 "Luise Light Obituary," *Brattleboro (VT) Reformer*, April 20, 2010, https://www.legacy.com/obituaries/brattleboro/obituary.aspx?n=luise-light&pid=142028322.

61 Rachel Cooper, "Statin: The Drug Firms' Goldmine," *The Daily Telegraph*, London, (January 19, 2011), https://www.telegraph.co.uk/news/health/news/8267876/Statins-the-drug-firms-goldmine.html.

62 Barbara H. Roberts, *The Truth About Statins* (New York: Pocket Books/Simon & Schuster, 2012).

63 Jean A. McDougall et al., "Long-term Statin Use and Risk of Ductal and Lobular Breast Cancer Among Women, 55 to 74 Years of Age," *Cancer, Epidemiology, Biomarkers and Prevention* 22, no. 9 (September 2013):1529-37, https://doi.org/10.1158/1055-9965.EPI-13-0414.

64 David Perlmutter, Grain Brain: *The Surprising Truth About Wheat, Carbs, and Sugar: Your Brain's Silent Killers*, revised 2018 (New York: Little Brown, 2013).

65 Richard C. Rogers and Gerlinda E. Hermann, "Mechanisms of Action of CCK to Activate Central Vagal Afferent Terminals," *Peptides* 29, no.10 (October 2008): 716-25.

66 Comprehensive Diabetes Center, "Non-Starchy Vegetables/Protein/Fat," University of Michigan, http://www.med.umich.edu/1libr/MEND/Diabetes-NonCarbFoods.pdf.

67 A.A. Gibson, et al., "Do Ketogenic Diets Really Suppress Appetite? A Systematic Review and Mega-analysis," *Obesity Reviews* 16, no.1 (January 2015): 64-76, https://pubmed.ncbi.nlm.nih.gov/25402637/; Jens F. Rehfeld, "Cholecystokinin: From Local Gut Hormone to Ubiquitous Messenger," *Frontiers in Endocrinology* 8, no. 47 (April 13, 2017), https://doi.org/10.3389/fendo.2017.00047.

68 Gene Bruno, Huntington College of Health Science; also see: B. Perry and Y. Wang, "Appetite Regulation and Weight Control: The Role of Gut Hormones," *Nutrition & Diabetes* 2, no. e26 (2012), https://doi.org/10.1038/nutd.2011.21.

69 Josh Axe, "How to Turn on Your Fat Burning Switch, Leptin: Your 'Starvation Hormone," drxe.com, https://draxe.com/health/leptin/; also see: Ellen Ruppel Shell, *The Hungry Gene: The Inside Story of the Obesity Industry* (New York: Grove Press, 2003).

70 Martin G. Myers Jr. et al., "Obesity and Leptin Resistance: Distinguishing Cause from Effect," *Trends in Endocrinology and Metabolism* 21, no.11 (November 2010): 643-5, https://doi.org/10.1016/j.tem.2010.08.002; Vajiheh Izadi, Sahar Saraf-Bank, and Leila Azadbakht, "Dietary Intakes and Leptin Concentrations, Review Article," *Atherosclerosis ARYA* 10, no. 5 (September 2014): 266-72, http://docplayer.net/48965056-Dietary-intakes-and-leptin-concentrations-vajiheh-izadi-1-sahar-saraf-bank-1-leila-azadbakht-1-review-article.html.

71 Purna Mukherjee et al., "Therapeutic Benefit of Combining Calorie-restricted Ketogenic Diet and Glutamine Targeting in Late-stage Experimental Glioblastoma," *Communications Biology*, 2, no. 1 (2019), https://doi.org/10.1038/s42003-019-0455-x.

72 Dave Asprey, "How to Make Bulletproof Coffee...And Make Your Morning Bulletproof," bulletproof.com; Food News, "The History of Bulletproof Coffee," https://news.yummyeveryday.com/2018/11/17/the-history-of-bulletproof-coffee/.

73 Satoru Arata et al., "Continuous Intake of the Chaga Mushroom (Inonotus obliquus) Aqueous Extract Suppresses Cancer Progression and Maintains Body Temperature in Mice," *Heliyon* 2, no. 5, (May 12, 2016), https://doi.org/10.1016/j.heliyon.2016.e00111; Joseph Mercola, "Chaga Tea: Benefits of This Unusual But Health-Boosting Beverage", https://articles.mercola.com/teas/chaga-tea.aspx.

74 Vincent J Miller, Frederick A. Villamena, and Jeff S. Volek, "Nutritional Ketosis and Mitohormesis: Potential Implications for Mitochondrial Function and Human Health," *Journal of Nutrition and Metabolism* (February 2018), 1, https://doi.org/10.1155/2018/5157645.

75 Amanda Missimer et al., "Consuming Two Eggs per Day, as Compared to an Oatmeal Breakfast, Decreases Plasma Ghrelin While Maintaining the HDL/LDL Ratio," *Nutrients* 9, no. 2 (January 2017): 89, https://doi.org/10.3390/nu9020089.

76 Robert Sietsema, "The Offal-Eaters Handbook: Untangling the Myths of Organ Meats," Eater. com, June 16, 2015, https://www.eater.com/2015/6/16/8786663/offal-organ-meat-handbook-cuts-sweetbreads-tripe-gizzard; Katie Parla and Kristina Gill, *Tasting Rome: Fresh Flavors and Forgotten Recipes from an Ancient City*, (New York: Clarkson Potter, 2016).

77 Nasha Winters and Jess Higgins Kelley, *The Metabolic Approach to Cancer: Integrating Deep Nutrition, the Ketogenic Diet*, and *Nontoxic Bio-Individualized Therapies* (White River Junction, VT: Chelsea Green Press, 2017), 135–38.

78 *Johns Hopkins Medical Newsletter*, "The Truth about Low Glycemic Diets," Hopkinsmedicine. org, https://www.hopkinsmedicine.org/health/wellness-and-prevention/the-truth-about-lowglycemic-diets.

79 Winters and Higgins Kelley, 2017; NIH Human Microbiome Project, "About the Human Microbiome," hmpdacc.org.

80 Nassib Bezerra Bueno et al., "Very-low-carbohydrate Ketogenic Diet v. Low-fat Diet for Long-term Weight Loss: A Meta-analysis of Randomized Controlled Trials," *British Journal of Nutrition*, 110, No. 7 (October 14, 2013): 1178-87, https://doi.org/10.1017/S0007114513000548.

81 Y. Gepner et al., "Effects of Initiating Moderate Alcohol Intake on Cardiometabolic Risk in Adults With Type 2 Diabetes: A 2-Year Randomized, Controlled Trial," *Annals Internal Medicine* 163, no. 8(2015;):569-79, https://doi.org/10.7326/M14-1650; R. Paul Robertson, "Red Wine and Diabetes Health: Getting Skin in the Game," *Diabetes* 63 (2014): 31–38, https://doi.org/10.2337/db13-1318.

82 Interview with Todd White, Keto f(x) Summit, February 2018; Todd White, Dry Farm Wines, dryfarmwines.com.

83 Arthur I. Cederbaum, "Alcohol Metabolism," *Clinics in Liver Disease* 16, no. 4 (2012): 667–85, https://doi.org/10.1016/j.cld.2012.08.002.

84 Domini Kemp and Patricia Daly, *The Ketogenic Kitchen: Low Carb, High Fat. Extraordinary Health*, (White River Junction, VT: Chelsea Green, 2016).

85 Maria Emmerich, *The 30-Day Ketogenic Cleanse: Reset Your Metabolism with Tasty Whole-food Recipes & Meal Plans* (Las Vegas: Victory Belt, 2016).

86 Maria Emmerich, *Keto Comfort Foods, Family Favorite Recipes Made Low Carb and Healthy* (Las Vegas: Victory Belt, 2016).

87 Maria Emmerich, *Keto Restaurant Favorites: More Than 175 Tasty Classic Recipes Made Fast, Fresh, and Healthy* (Las Vegas: Victory Belt, 2017).

88 Maria Emmerich, *Easy Dairy-Free Ketogenic Family Favorites Made Low-Carb and Healthy* (Las Vegas: Victory Belt, 2018).

89 Leanne Vogel, healthfulpursuit.com, https://www.healthfulpursuit.com.

90 Suzanne Ryan, ketokarma.com, https://ketokarma.com.

91 See The GKI Formula, Figure 2.4 below.

92 Joshua Meidenbauer, Purna Mukherjee, and Thomas Seyfried, "The Glucose Ketone Index Calculator: A Simple Tool to Monitor Therapeutic Efficacy for Metabolic Management of Brain Cancer," *Nutrition & Metabolism* 12, no. 12 (March 11, 2015), https://doi.org/10.1186/s12986-015-0009-2.

93 https://keto-mojo.com

94 Keto-mojo.com, "Glucose Ketone Testing," https://cdn.keto-mojo.com/wp-content/uploads/2020/01/GKI/.

95 https://www.ketonix.com; Mybiosense.com.

96 See myketokitchen.com.

97 Andreas Eenfeldt et al., "Monitoring Patients on Low Carb: Lab Tests," dietdoctor.com, https://www.dietdoctor.com/low-carb/for-doctors/monitoring-lab-tests.

98 Lanwei Guo et al., "C-reactive Protein and Risk of Breast Cancer: A Systematic Review and Meta-analysis," *Scientific Reports* 5, no.10508, (May.22, 2015) https://doi.org/10.1038/srep10508.

99 Penelope Green, "Carefully Smash the Patriarchy," The New York Times, March 18. 2019, https://www.nytimes.com/2019/03/18/style/carol-gilligan.html.

100 Nancy Chodorow, *The Reproduction of Motherhood*, (Berkeley, CA: University of California Press, 1978); Francine Prose, "Confident at 11, Confused at 16," *The New York Times Magazine*, January 7, 1990, https://www.nytimes.com/1990/01/07/magazine/confident-at-11-confused-at-16.html; Mary Belenky et al., *Women's Ways of Knowing: The Development of Self, Voice and Mind* (New York, Basic Books, 1986); Jean Baker Miller, *Toward a New Psychology of Women* (Boston: Beacon Press,1976).

101 Geneen Roth, *Women, Food and God: An Unexpected Path to Almost Everything* (New York: Scribner, 2010), 127-141.

102 Geneen Roth, *Women, Food and God: An Unexpected Path to Almost Everything* (New York: Scribner, 2010), 128.

103 Jean Baker Miller, *Toward a New Psychology of Women*, (Boston:Beacon Press, 2nd edition: 1986) 110.

104 Carol Gilligan, *In a Different Voice*, (Cambridge: Harvard University Press, 1982); Sujat Massey, *The Widows of Malabar Hill* (New York: Soho Press, 2018), a novel that looks at "The Voice" across religions and in twentieth-century East Indian history.

105 Carol Gilligan, *Making Connections: The Relational World of Adolescent Girls at Emma Willard School*, (Cambridge: Harvard University Press, 1990).

106 Al-Anon, an international group formed to help family and friends of alcoholics, is comprised of 85 percent women. See https://al-anon.org/.

107 Natalie Goldberg, *Writing Down the Bones: Freeing the Writer Within* (Boulder, CO: Shambhala, 1986).

108 Anne Lamott, *Operating Instructions: A Journal of my Son's First Year* (New York: Pantheon, 1993).

109 Byron Katie, *Loving What Is: Four Questions That Can Change Your Life* (New York: Harmony, 2003), as cited in Roth, *Women, Food and God*, 135.

STEP 2:
Keep Your Vitamin D3 Blood Level Above 60

The Good News for Women

What if I told you that there was one change that American women could make that would reduce breast cancer diagnoses in the United States by as much as 80 percent? Well, pay attention, because there is! Leading researchers estimate that as the majority of women in the United States raise their vitamin D3 blood levels above 60 nanograms/milliliter (ng/ml), we could see at least 80 percent fewer breast cancer diagnoses each year.[1] Let that sink in. Instead of the three hundred thousand women now being diagnosed in the US with breast cancer each year, about a quarter million fewer women would get this horrifying news. What an incredible moment, as hundreds of thousands of women in the US take a single simple step that literally blocks most breast cancer tumors from unnecessarily taking root in our bodies!

The Bad News for Investors

What is good news for women, though, is bad news for investors. As we saw earlier, market research firms all tell us that the US breast cancer treatment market "accounted for (the) largest share of industry revenues in 2018 and is expected to grow 9.1% annually over the forecast period" (2018–2025). Worldwide, the breast cancer market (radiation, drugs, surgeries, tests, physicians' and hospitals' fees, etc.) will "surpass $30 billion by 2025."[2] Any significant decrease in the number of women developing breast cancer each year, especially in the US, would significantly hurt industry investors' currently anticipated jump in income. Yes, once individual women are able to learn how to keep themselves well, the breast cancer business will suffer.

What can happen when any industry feels threatened by the discovery of a better product? Often, the threatened industry will find ways to sabotage its competition. Do you remember the quick demise of that precious little electric car, the EV-1, in 2003? It was billed as "an electric automobile that requires no gas, oil, muffler or brake changes and is, seemingly, the world's first perfect car. Yet six years later, GM recalls and destroys the EV-1 fleet."[3] The documentary film *Who Killed the Electric Car?* examines the birth and death of this revolutionary vehicle. The film points the finger at the oil industry and car companies. Both allegedly feared lower long-term profits once huge chunks of the population switched to electric cars. But now, less than two decades later, all seems to have changed. Amidst increasing existential fears of global warming, along with other shifting economic and political dynamics, dozens of electric car models are now available on the US market. Sales are soaring, led by the luxury electric carmaker, Tesla.[4]

In the eyes of the cancer industry, it seems that vitamin D3 could, today, be the EV-1 of the early twenty-first century. This "sunshine vitamin" is possibly the most effective way for most women to keep breast cancer out of our bodies. As one pharmacology researcher tells us, "this vitamin may be used for the prevention of cancer and included as an adjuvant in combination [with] chemotherapy for the treatment of cancer."[5]

At a mere $5-$10 per bottle for a month's supply, depending on the strength or IUs of each capsule, vitamin D3 has become a major political football in the United States. Every few years, Big Pharma, using their Disinformation Playbook to discredit vitamin D3,[6] produces an industry-funded study by the Institute of Medicine or the National Cancer Institute that carries an anti-D3 headline, such as: "Vitamin D Supplements Don't Reduce Cancer Incidence, New Trial Shows."[7] Often broadcast for weeks on end, this kind of misinformation by today's corporate media about D3's cancer prevention abilities has the purpose and the net effect of confusing the American public.[8]

But before we go further into the politics and economics of this subject, it's important to understand vitamin D3's *proven* ability to stop breast cancer cells from forming. Having adequate levels of vitamin D3 streaming through your blood actually powers up your body's immune system, preventing the majority of today's breast cancer tumors from developing.[9] So, let's look at the biology of how vitamin D3 activates our immune system cells. And then let's look at how we can easily and inexpensively maintain high levels of this protective vitamin (actually considered a hormone)[10] in our bodies throughout the year.

Here is a quick summary of the most current research on vitamin D3 and breast cancer prevention, taken from dozens of peer-reviewed scholarly journals, written by epidemiologists, biochemists, clinicians, and physiologists. Many of these leading researchers, working on D3 studies in their respective institutions around the globe for decades, have more recently been loosely organized and promoted by the nonprofit San Diego-based group GrassrootsHealth.[11] This unique nonprofit education and research entity, created by breast cancer survivor and retired marketing maven Carole Baggerly, recommends women raise their D3 levels above 60 ng/ml in order to maintain optimal health, including the prevention of breast cancer.[12] Unlike the National Cancer Institute, the Centers for Disease Control, and the National Academy of Medicine, GrassrootsHealth does not seek or accept pharmaceutical industry funding, as we will see below.

What's the Right Level of D3?

When we are able to keep at least 30 ng/ml of D3 in our blood all throughout the year, the D3 hormone improves our muscle strength and immune function, and it reduces many inflammatory processes within our bodies.[13] This minimal level of vitamin D3 also promotes the absorption of calcium from the gastrointestinal tract, and it helps maintain adequate blood levels of calcium and phosphate, needed for bone formation, mineralization, growth, and repair.[14]

If we are able to double that D3 level, and keep 60 ng/ml in our blood throughout the year, research indicates that the hormone is able to block the development of breast cancer cells as they form.[15] This amount of D3 switches on the body's "internal Wi-Fi," our cell-to-cell communication system, to its highest level. Then, when a breast cell becomes damaged because its mitochondria begin to suffocate, our healthy breast cells are able to work together to call in our immune system's killer T-cells. The T-cells help the suffocating breast cell(s) to self-destruct. Biologists call this clever operation *apoptosis*.[16]

There is one more substance involved when the D3 in our blood activates our internal Wi-Fi: a protein called *E-cadherin*. This sticky E-cadherin literally helps our breast cells stick together. But it's important to know this: "E-cadherin is activated or switched on only when there is a sufficient amount of vitamin D3 circulating in our blood."[17]

Going back to our Wi-Fi analogy, I like to think of a "sufficient" amount of vitamin D3 as being similar to the amount of electricity needed to power up our Wi-Fi. That sticky E-cadherin acts as the Wi-Fi's modem. In other words, without enough electricity (Vitamin D3), our modem (E-cadherin), won't work. But when we have enough Vitamin D3 in our blood, the E-cadherin switches on and takes charge. Communication among our breast cells and our immune system's killer T-cells now happens, enabling our body to stop those first cancer cells from fully developing. And the more D3 we have circulating in our blood, the faster our Wi-Fi operates!

No wonder studies of breast cancer patients consistently show that most women diagnosed with invasive breast cancer *never* have a vitamin D3 blood level above 60 ng/ml.[18] In fact, most studies indicate that women diagnosed with invasive breast cancer have an average D3 blood level of only 17 ng/ml.[19] So, *what is your D3 blood level right now?* This could be the most important biomarker for you to track.

The Cancer Industry Tries to Dismiss Vitamin D3

In Chapter 2, we saw the role that the American "food pyramid," controlled by the National Academy of Medicine (NAM), plays in today's obesity epidemic. And we saw how this obesity epidemic, in turn, feeds our current breast cancer epidemic. That led us to the realization that women have to speak up and question the authorities who benefit from the status quo. In this chapter, we'll see that it's also important to question these same authorities when they talk about vitamin D3 and its relationship to breast cancer prevention.

Behind its role of having final control over the contents of the American food pyramid, NAM enjoys another government-delegated power: the ability to establish our federal Dietary Reference Intakes (DRIs).[20] DRIs are those numbers found on the labels of every bottle of vitamins and minerals we buy. Each DRI is the government's recommended daily dosage for a particular vitamin, required to maintain optimal health. The food pyramid is supposed to be based on these DRIs.[21]

The Food and Nutrition Board within the NAM continues to tell the American public that "there is no connection between vitamin D3 blood levels and breast cancer prevention."[22] In 2019, however, The Office of Dietary Supplements with the National Institutes of Health, finally ignored NAM's D3 and breast cancer guidance and acknowledged that research existed illustrating that vitamin D3 could be helpful in breast cancer prevention.[23] Here is what NIH's "Fact Sheet on Vitamin D3" tells us: "Laboratory and animal evidence as well as epidemiological data suggests that vitamin D status could affect cancer risk. Strong biological and mechanistic bases indicate that vitamin D plays a role in the prevention of colon, prostate, and breast cancers."[24] Alleluia.

A second industry lobby group also likes to talk down the importance of vitamin D3. Just like NAM, this private group also operates under the guise of an official-sounding name: It's called the US Preventive Services Task Force (USPSTF). More on this group later.

If you receive your nightly news from national TV or most radio stations (including National Public Radio), or from billionaire-owned newspapers (such as the *Washington Post*, the *Wall Street Journal*, *The Boston Globe*, or *The New York Times*), you're no longer getting "all the news fit to print."[25] Sadly, that's especially true when it comes to vitamin D3 and breast cancer. Instead, you're likely to hear that one or another major national report on vitamin D3 has just been published, showing "there is no connection between vitamin D3 and cancer prevention,"[26] or "it is not necessary to have an annual or twice-a-year D3 blood test as part of your regular physical check-up."[27] And, you may be shocked to discover that none of corporate media's news represents the most recent findings of the world's most respected researchers. The nonprofit group GrassrootsHealth's website, however, continues to update and share the best international research on breast cancer prevention and Vitamin D3.[28]

Meanwhile, the National Cancer Institute's most recent (2013) stance, on vitamin D3 and breast cancer prevention, sadly remains the same: "In summary, daily high-dose vitamin D supplementation for 5 years...did not reduce incidence of cancer ..."[29] In contrast, that same year, the Centers for Disease Control (CDC), the federal agency responsible for tracking the prevalence of various diseases, actually published a promising statement about vitamin D3. Following numerous statistical and laboratory assessments, the CDC reported that 41.6 percent of Americans were "deficient" in vitamin D3.[30] This statement was based on an independent national study estimating that almost half of the US population had less than 20 ng/ml of D3 in their blood during this time. Today, however, the CDC's recommendations regarding vitamin D3 continue to defer to the National Academy of Medicine's 2011 vitamin D3 report, dismissing the existence of a national D3 deficiency epidemic.[31] Is it any wonder that women's breast cancer rates have continued to rise throughout all age groups in the US during this past decade?[32]

Keeping women's D3 blood levels low pays off for the breast cancer industry. Breast cancer treatment is about a $30 billion a year industry in the United States today.[33] In 2017, the average cost of an American woman's first year of treatment after her initial diagnosis was:

stage 0 (DCIS): $60,637

stages I and II: $82,121

stage III: $129,387

stage IV: $134,682[34]

Any massive reduction in the disease represents a big chunk of change that the breast cancer industry could lose.

Some Personal Questions and Important Facts About Vitamin D3

Is your personal D3-powered Wi-Fi system "online" right now? Do you even know your current vitamin D3 blood level? And do you know why a woman's D3 blood level is *especially* important when it comes to preventing breast cancer, compared to other types of cancer? Here are some important facts to consider.

Fact #1: The VDR Gene

We each have a specific gene whose job is to provide instructions for making a protein called vitamin D receptor (VDR). This protein allows the body to utilize vitamin D properly.[35] Women born with a mutated or damaged VDR gene sometimes have an incredibly hard time maintaining D3 levels over 60 ng/ml.[36] (We'll return to this topic in Chapter 7, in conjunction with our discussion of triple-negative breast cancer, and again in Chapter 8, in conjunction with the tumor watchdog genes BRCA1 and BRCA2.)

Fact #2: Most Breast Cancer Tumors Appear to Grow Quickly

Researchers have long realized that some breast cancer cells duplicate much faster than cancerous cells in other organs of the body. Many independent vitamin D3 studies show that maintaining D3 blood levels around 40 ng/ml may be sufficient protection against these slower-growing cancer cells.[37] But "slow-growing" is not how many women, especially premenopausal women, often describe their invasive breast tumors.

How often have you heard this story? "I had a mammogram in July, and it showed no trace of any tumor. But in September, when my boyfriend and I were playing around, bam! He feels a lump in my right breast. This just doesn't make any sense! I thought it took cancerous tumors a long time to grow."

For a long time, we've known that breast cancer tumors can grow and become palpable in a matter of five years in older (or postmenopausal) women. Case in point: Twenty years ago, thousands of postmenopausal women who participated in the National Health Initiative's Prempro Study developed 26 percent more breast tumors than women not given this progestin-based hormone replacement therapy (HRT) drug.[38] We will never know for sure, but given Americans' longstanding D3 deficiency epidemic, we can assume that about half of the women in that national Prempro study had less than 20 ng/ml of vitamin D3 in their blood during this period of time.[39] This means their internal Wi-Fi systems were not working very well, offering them virtually no immune system protection against the growth of their Prempro-initiated or progestin-accelerated invasive breast tumors.[40]

Here is more evidence that breast tumors can grow much faster than other types of cancerous tumors. Bill Grant is the NASA physicist who, in retirement, founded the Sunlight, Nutrition and Health Research Center (SUNARC), an internationally respected vitamin D3 think tank. Grant recently questioned why clinicians, along with the American Cancer

Society, all recommend annual or biannual mammograms for women 40 years and older, compared to the Society's recommendation that those over 50 have a colonoscopy every ten years.[41] "Does the American Cancer Society also believe that breast cancer tumors grow much faster than, say, colon cancer tumors?" Grant writes, "Results: I provide evidence that 25(OH)D (60ng/ml) concentration values are only useful for short follow-up times for breast cancer since it develops rapidly."[42]

Fact #3: More Sun = Less Cancer

During the 1970s, two young epidemiologists, Doctors Cedric and Frank Garland began their lifelong study of vitamin D3 and its connection to the development of cancer. The brothers were the first to report that men living in northern latitudes within the United States developed about twenty percent more colon cancer than individuals in southern states.[43] This study documented a landmark finding about vitamin D3 and cancer. More than two decades later it was republished in its original form in the same journal.[44]

In a 1997 study, another vitamin D3 and sun-related phenomena appeared. This research showed that most women in the northern low-sunshine regions, including the Netherlands and Scandinavia, are diagnosed with breast tumors in the fall and spring, rather than in the summer and winter.[45] But why?

Biologists today believe this interesting seasonal growth pattern for breast tumor development happens because our bodies make more immune-strengthening vitamin D3 in sunnier months, and more melatonin (another immune-boosting hormone) in the darker winter months.[46] That's right: Researchers believe this natural hormonal duet of D3 and melatonin apparently slows the growth of some breast tumors during the winter and summer months in northern geographical areas! Who knew?

In a more recent epidemiological study, using data from a National Cancer Institute SEER database, "US women who were diagnosed with invasive breast cancer during the summer months had better outcomes (i.e. longer survival times) than women similarly diagnosed during the fall, winter or spring.[47] "These observations contribute to the mounting evidence that vitamin D3 may affect the progression of cancer.

Since the 1970s, the Garland brothers, along with hundreds, if not thousands of other researchers have continued to substantiate the Garlands' original D3 research, initially connecting sunshine to colon cancer protection.[48] Today, it is also statistically certain that women in the US who live year-round in high-sunshine areas have at least 20 percent fewer breast cancer diagnoses than women who live in more northern, less sunny regions. Just look at the list of US states where women continue to enjoy the lowest rates of breast cancer: New Mexico, Texas, Nevada, Utah, Florida, and West Virginia.[49]

Now, look at five states where women continue to have the highest breast-cancer rates: New Hampshire, Massachusetts, and Connecticut, followed by North Dakota and Rhode Island. In these northern American regions, the only way many women can keep their D3 blood levels above the optimal 60 ng/ml mark year-round is by combining sufficient levels (IUs) of vitamin D3 supplements with safe indoor and outdoor tanning.[50]

As a side note: Hawai'i is the only southern state included in this CDC list of states with the highest breast cancer rates.[51] Hawai'i currently leads other states in their mammography rates. In 2018, 87% of women 40 and over in Hawai'i, chose to have a regular screening mammogram. This is a far cry from today's average national mammogram rate of 72%. As described in Chapter 5, mammograms are leading tens of thousands of US women each year to be overdiagnosed and overtreated, possibly contributing to Hawai'i's above-average breast cancer rate.[52]

African American and Other Darker-Skinned Women

African American women and others who have darker skin tones (especially those living in northern regions across the United States) have a much harder time absorbing sufficient vitamin D3 merely from sunshine.[53] This is because their skin contains lots of sun-protecting melanin. Meanwhile, people native to northern regions like Scandinavia and northern Asia have very light skin, containing almost no melanin. This lack of sun-blocking melanin allows them to efficiently absorb what few UVB rays do occur, living so far away from the equator.[54]

The statistical research is also clear. Women who are born with darker skin tones and who live in northern latitudes have lower average vitamin D3 blood levels than those with less melanin in their skin. Doctors Marc Sorenson's and William B. Grant's treatise, *Embrace the Sun: Are You Dying in the Dark?*, helps us understand the many benefits of absorbing as much of our vitamin D3 from sunshine, as possible, instead of just taking D3 supplements.[55]

D3 Blood Tests

But how can you find out your D3 blood level? Ask your health practitioner to order a D3 blood test, called *25-hydroxy*, twice a year. One test should happen in the summer and one in the winter. This way you can see how much your D3 blood level may fluctuate between the sunnier summer months and the darker winter months each year. For those without adequate health insurance, the nonprofit research organization GrassrootsHealth and the vitamin company Life Extension both offer affordable at-home D3 testing.[56]

Can I Overdose on Vitamin D3?

Fortunately, it appears to be very difficult for healthy individuals to get too much vitamin D3 from supplements and/or safe tanning sessions. According to one recent study conducted by leading D3 researcher Dr. Michael Holick, a person can take up to 15,000 international units (IUs) of D3 daily for more than six months without having any adverse effects.[57]

Overweight Women Need More Sunlight, More Indoor Tanning, More Supplements

Biologists currently know at least three things about obesity and vitamin D3. First, if you are overweight, you probably have a low vitamin D3 blood level, especially if:

- you do not live in a sunny climate
- you have not been taking enough D3 supplementation, and/or
- you do not practice safe year-round tanning.[58]

Why is it much harder for a woman with excess body fat to reach and maintain adequate D3 blood levels? It turns out that a larger size body requires more D3 production in order to reach higher blood levels of the hormone.[59] Excess body fat will absorb much of the D3 gained from safe tanning and from supplements. This D3 hormone, now housed within your body's excess fat cells, is not available to power up your body's internal Wi-Fi immune system and help destroy that first breast cancer cell, should one form.[60]

But there is some good news about fat-stored vitamin D3. Although it's not able to raise your D3 blood levels, fat-stored vitamin D3 can help lower the amount of inflammation being produced by your excess fat.[61] This is helpful to know, since (as we saw in Chapter 1) whole-body inflammation remains the cause behind most breast cancer diagnoses among obese women today.[62]

Researchers at the Fred Hutchinson Cancer Institute in Seattle tell us that most vitamin D3 stored in excess body fat will literally "let go" and surge into your blood once you lose 15 percent or more of your original body weight. At this point in your fat-burning/fat-loss journey, some researchers suggest you can stop taking vitamin D3 supplements for a while, if you are already maintaining a D3 blood level above 60.[63]

Finally, when taking vitamin D3 (as well as calcium, magnesium, and vitamin K supplements), it is important to do so with the largest meal of the day. This appears to increase whatever absorption can happen, no matter your current body size.[64]

Older Women and D3

As we age, vitamin D3 absorption becomes more difficult. Is this another reason breast-cancer rates increase during and after menopause, as age increases, and weight gain can begin to happen much too easily? There is no doubt, that with all of these factors connecting low vitamin D3 blood levels to higher breast cancer rates, postmenopausal women must use a variety of ways to keep their D3 blood levels above 60 ng/ml year-round.[65]

Add Calcium, Vitamin K2 and Magnesium

Alongside vitamin D3 supplements, many researchers and functional medicine clinicians recommend taking a small amount of calcium (1000 IUs), vitamin K2 (90–150 mcg), and magnesium with your D3 supplements. Supplementing with magnesium, which activates the D3, should be considered as an important aspect of vitamin D therapy.[66] Also, vitamin K2, taken with calcium, helps put the calcium in the bones and not into soft tissue such as blood vessels.

Dr. Joseph Mercola, a company called New Chapter, and others have created supplements that combine these various immune-boosting and bone-building vitamins and minerals into a single vitamin capsule.[67] But remember: When purchasing D3 supplements, one size, or one amount of IUs in each capsule, does not fit all. GrassrootsHealth offers a free, online D3 supplement calculator that can get you started on how many IUs of vitamin D3 your body may need each day to push your D3 blood levels past 60 ng/ml and maintain this optimal breast cancer prevention level.[68]

Sunscreen and Breast Cancer

We all know that most people (both children and adults) are spending much more time indoors than we did just a generation ago. Blame it on TV, computers, urban crime, commuter traffic—the reason doesn't matter so much as the result: much less sunshine touches our skin. But even the time we spend outdoors often doesn't manage to raise our vitamin D3 levels the way it should. Did you know that overuse of high-SPF sunscreen also contributes to our vitamin D3 deficiency? And North Americans—mainly women—use about *one third* of all sunscreen products sold globally by this expanding $15-billion-a-year industry.[69]

Why do we need sunscreen in the first place? And how safe are the chemicals in most lotions? Fifty or sixty years ago, sunscreen lotions were not available. Back then, the incidence of malignant melanoma skin cancer (the big killer among all types of skin growths) was much lower than it is today—and so was the incidence of breast cancer.[70] Back then, nobody thought the sun was out to hurt us. Back then, the sun was strengthening our D3-powered immune system in ways we don't allow it to do today.

The sun actually helps *prevent* any number of potentially lethal tumors from developing. I know this sounds illogical, but listen up! Over the past fifty years, national melanoma rates have more than doubled for women and quadrupled for men.[71] Why? Aren't today's highly advertised and dermatologist-recommended, high-SPF sunscreens supposed to make these melanoma statistics run in the other direction? Since when did you believe in "truth in US advertising"?

Figure 3.1: Increasing Melanoma Rates: 1975–2014

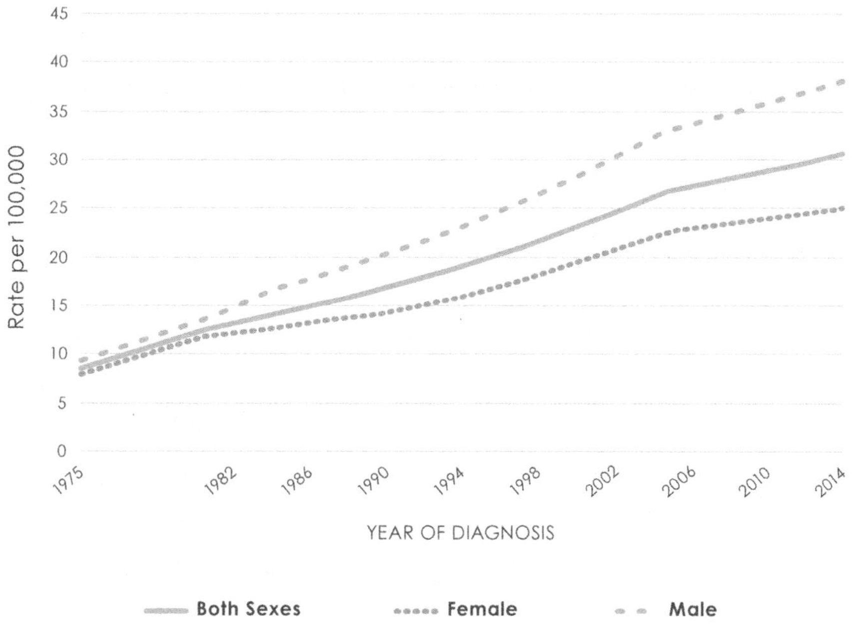

The National Cancer Institute calculated the annual rate of melanoma for men and women between 1975 and 2014. Their national data estimates that melanoma rates have continued to significantly increase during this time.

National Cancer Institute, "Melanoma of the Skin, Long Term Trends in SEER Incidence Rates, 1975– 2014," SEER, *cancer.gov*.

The charts in Figure 3.1 and 3.2 illustrate the steep rise in US melanoma cases over the last two generations, as first sunscreen and then high-SPF sunscreen products were introduced to the American public. These statistics ought to make us question the usefulness of high-SPF sunscreens in preventing melanoma. Given the historical statistical data in these graphs, one from the National Cancer Institute and the other from the Connecticut Tumor Registry, why don't we ever see ads telling us how UVB rays from the sun can improve our immune system and actually *lower* our melanoma risk?

Figure 3.2 should really give avid sunscreen users some pause. This graph, using data from the Connecticut Tumor Registry, illustrates how melanoma rates have continued to soar ever *since* the chemical industry introduced their high-SPF sunscreen to the US public! Astounding. Isn't it time to ask whether high-SPF sunscreen does more harm than good?[72]

Figure 3.2: Introduction of high-SPF sunscreen lotion has resulted in increasing melanoma rates

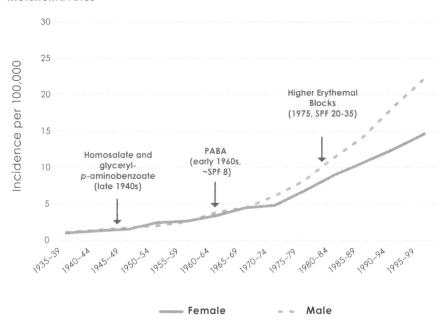

This chart shows that in Connecticut between 1935–1999, melanoma rates increased each time higher SPF lotions were brought to the market.

Data source: Connecticut Tumor Registry; https://www.grassrootshealth.net/blog/skin-cancer-vs-sunscreen-dilemma/.

And here is a final concern about sunscreen: A recent study by US Food and Drug Administration researchers indicates that specific chemicals from high-SPF sunscreen lotions can be carcinogenic for those who chronically use the lotion in large amounts.[73] From the metabolic perspective, this is probably because these SPF chemicals assault melanin cells' mitochondria, helping suffocate these skin cells and thus causing the development of that first cancer cell.[74]

The History of Sunscreen and Sunblock

As a young teen in the mid-1960s, I would see a dermatologist for sunlamp treatments for the acne on my back. We also had a sunlamp at home, so I could treat my erupting teenage skin and gently develop a protective base tan before waitressing at the Jersey Shore each summer.[75] At some point during the late 1970s, however, a new product arrived on the scene: protective "suntan" lotion. Instead of putting on a t-shirt or finding some shade when you had absorbed enough sun, as evidenced by the reddish tinge on your skin, this new sun lotion was advertised as something that could allow you to remain in the sun longer, while still avoiding a bad sunburn. Of course, these high-SPF lotions also blocked *healthy* UVB rays from being absorbed by your skin, which meant blocking an important source of vitamin D3.

So, where did the idea of sunscreen come from? Benjamin Green, an airman and pharmacist during World War II, was trying to protect himself and other soldiers from severe open-cockpit, high-altitude sunburns. He invented Green's Lotion—a greasy, unpleasant substance that created a physical barrier between the skin and the sun.[76] After the war, Green tweaked his recipe, adding cocoa butter and coconut oil. This combination soon became Coppertone lotion. Almost two decades later, sun protection factor (SPF), a clear chemical compound, was developed by a Swiss national, Hans Greiter. Its role was to protect mountain climbers when they were at altitudes above 10,000 feet.[77]

In the mid-1980s, when we heard that the earth's protective ozone layer over the Antarctic had begun to come undone, high-SPF sunscreen sales really took off in the United States. This normally thin layer of ozone, miles above the planet, had always protected people around the globe from overexposure to damaging UVA and UVB rays—and it still does. In 1985, the journal *Nature* reported that small, seasonal holes were developing over the Antarctic during the fall months. Light-skinned, northern European immigrant populations in Australia and New Zealand (countries closest to Antarctica) began experiencing higher levels of sunburns and increased levels of all types of skin growths.[78] Most of these skin growths, however, once noticed, are easily removed. These basal and squamous cell growths are considered so prevalent and insignificant that they aren't even registered by state tumor and cancer boards.[79] It is usually only the rare type of skin growth, cutaneous malignant melanoma, that can prove lethal.

Cutaneous Malignant Melanoma

Cutaneous malignant melanoma accounts for 3 to 5 percent of all skin cancers and is responsible for approximately 75 percent of all deaths from skin cancer. Persons with an increased number of moles, dysplastic (also called atypical) nevi, or a family history of the disease are at increased risk for this type of skin cancer, compared with the general population.[80]

The Montreal Protocol

That 1985 *Nature* article also told us that that a specific type of manmade chemicals, called ozone-depleting substances (ODS), contained chlorine and bromines and were rising up into the upper stratospheres, from aerosol sprays. This was causing increasing damage to the southern hemisphere's fragile ozone layer.[81] Major countries of the world took action. First coming together in Vienna in 1985,[82] these nations signed an agreement two years later in Montreal to ban the production and continued use of these chemicals.[83] Today, more than thirty years later, China, the US, Russia, the European Union, and other signatories to the Montreal Protocol have continued to support the International Ozone Commission. This independent international group continues to monitor these seasonal ozone holes over Antarctica, and other sections of the world.[84]

But despite any positive news around the Montreal Protocol or those seasonal ozone holes that occur only over Australia and New Zealand, the sunscreen and personal care industries continue promoting their successful anti-sunshine scare tactics. Today, the global sunscreen market is valued at $15.8 billion—and expected to rise to $24.9 billion by the end of 2024. North American women remain the largest consumers of SPF lotions.[85] Is this just one more reason why women in the United States currently experience some of the highest breast-cancer rates in the world?[86]

The D3 Good Guys and the D3 Bad Guys

Have you ever asked your physician for a vitamin D3 test, only to be told such tests are "unnecessary," "too expensive," or "not worth it"? Or has your physician told you to just take 1,000 IUs of vitamin D3 every day, without first ordering a vitamin D3 blood test to check your current D3 blood level? This could mean your primary care physician is contributing (intentionally or not) to today's anti-D3 forces.

These same doctors and nurse practitioners are actually well-meaning healthcare workers. But they are being fed misinformation about D3 supplementation from pharmaceutical, chemical, and medical industry-funded groups, including the American Cancer Society, the NAM, the American Medical Association, the NCI, and others. Before discussing these anti-D3 messengers, though, let me introduce you to the leaders of a group I have named "the D3 Good Guys." These are laboratory, clinical, and statistical researchers, optimal health activists, and community health professionals who are teaching the public about the life-saving, biologically-based, and clinically proven benefits of keeping an adequate level of D3 in your bloodstream, year-round.

The D3 Good Guys

These pro-D3 forces are grounded in the ongoing D3 research of Dr. Cedric Garland, the late Dr. Frank Garland, and Dr. Michael Holick, whom we met earlier in this chapter. During the past decade or so, these D3 icons have been joined by the D3 educator Carole Baggerly, founder of GrassrootsHealth; Dr. Azzie Young at the American Public Health Association; Dr. John Cannell, founder of the Vitamin D Council; Dr. Marc Sorenson, with his Sunlight Institute; Dr William W Grant's studies within his Sunlight, Nutrition, and Health Research Center (SUNARC); and by D3 Wiki founder, Henry Lappen. Add to this group the dozens of

pharmacologists, biologists, epidemiologists, clinicians, and health educators whose peer-reviewed, published studies are cited throughout this
book. Today, in fact, there are thousands of D3 researchers who have
continued to build on the Drs. Garland's and Holick's early vitamin D3
findings, showing how adequate levels of vitamin D3 are critical, in dozens of ways, for maintaining a person's optimal health.

Michael Holick, PhD, MD, MPH

*"If you expose your skin to a limited amount of UVB rays from either
sunshine or indoor tanning on a regular basis, you have a much lower
risk of developing breast and many other types of cancers."*[87]

In the 1970s, Michael Holick was a graduate student in biochemistry at the University of Wisconsin when he became the first person to
identify and isolate the major circulating form of vitamin D3, called
"25-hydroxycholecalciferol." This is the marker still used by medical
labs today to assess a person's vitamin-D3 blood levels.[88]

Dr. Holick is a dermatologist, endocrinologist, medical researcher, and
medical school professor, with an MD, an MPH, and a PhD in biochemistry. He has always recommended using natural sunshine or a sunlamp
to expose the skin to short periods of ultraviolet (UVB) light, as a safe
and excellent healing method for many skin conditions. Since the 1990s,
Dr. Holick, unlike most of his dermatologist peers, has continued to
recommend this same sensible tanning option, along with sufficient
amounts of daily vitamin D3 supplements, to help prevent and mitigate
cancer.[89] Thanks to Dr. Holick's ability to first isolate that 25-hydroxy in
human blood, epidemiologists and clinicians have since been able to figure out the optimal vitamin D3 blood levels needed to prevent breast
cancer in specific groups of women, depending on one's age, race, and
body mass index.

Cedric Garland, DPH

*"There is no compelling reason to wait for further studies to incorporate
vitamin D supplements into standard care regimens, since a safe dose
of vitamin D needed to achieve high serum levels above 30 nanograms/
milliliter, has already been established."*[90]

Dr. Cedric Garland, an epidemiologist at the University of California, San Diego (UCSD), and adjunct professor at the UCSD Medical School, has dedicated the past forty-plus years of his life to understanding how, and by how much, vitamin D3 works to help prevent and treat breast cancer, along with many other diseases. As we've already seen, it was back in the 1970s that Dr. Garland and his brother Frank were the first to organize data illustrating how women in northern regions of the United States developed twenty percent more breast cancer than women living in southern regions of the country. Their landmark 1980 statistical study on colon cancer showed this same phenomenon, and it became the first peer-reviewed published study to link higher invasive cancer levels and subsequent mortality with low exposure to sunshine. This single study has now been cited by over 900 peer-reviewed published academic studies.[91] Today, Dr. Garland and his associates at UCSD, and in partnership with GrassrootsHealth, continue to be a leading worldwide force in helping women understand the best ongoing D3 blood levels for the prevention and the treatment of invasive breast cancer.[92]

Azzie Young, PhD and the American Public Health Association

"Four populations in the US are at risk of vitamin D deficiency: women of childbearing age; breastfed infants not receiving D3 supplements; people with dark or brown skin type, including a large portion of African American and Mexican American adolescents and adults; elderly people. Besides adequate exposure to sunlight and eating food rich in vitamin D, dietary supplements provide another source of intake as noted earlier for populations at highest risk for vitamin D deficiency and insufficiency."[93]

The American Public Health Association (APHA) was probably the first major national health organization to recognize our nationwide vitamin D3 deficiency epidemic. Back in 2005, Dr. Azzie Young, a veteran APHA member, was the longtime president and executive officer of the Mattapan Community Health Center, serving Boston's largest Haitian American population. Once Dr. Young learned about the benefits of adequate vitamin D3, she discovered that her own muscular, neurological, and autoimmune concerns soon vanished when she raised her D3 blood level from less than 10 to above 30 ng/ml, simply using D3 and calcium supplements.

Dr. Young quickly formed a national Vitamin D3 Task Force within the mammoth APHA, with its membership of 25,000 community health practitioners and educators. In 2008, Dr. Young's task force published APHA's first Vitamin D3 Policy Statement, calling for education and research into our national epidemic of vitamin D3 deficiency.[94] The APHA's national network of 9,200 rural and urban community health clinics continues to serve large populations of impoverished Hispanic, African American, Euro-American, and Native American communities, including the elderly.[95]

Figure 3.3: Vitamin D Supplementation World Market Size, by Region, 2015–2020 ($Million)

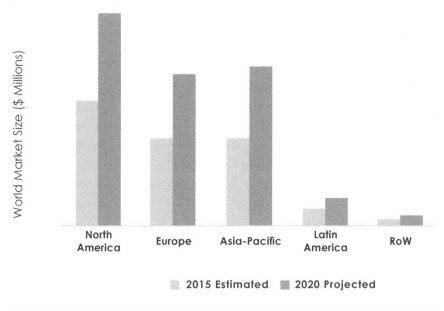

Adapted from a chart by Markets and Markets, press release: 2015, https://www.marketsandmarkets.com/Market-Reports/vitamin-d-market-22034298.html.

Carol Baggerly and GrassrootsHealth

In 2007, Carole Baggerly was a recent breast cancer patient and a newly retired corporate marketing manager. With a wide-ranging background in project management, sales, marketing, and organizational change within the aerospace and electronics industries, Baggerly attended a meeting of vitamin D3 experts in San Diego. This was the first time she had heard the good news: When you have enough of the "sunshine vitamin" in your blood, your body is able to prevent all types of cancer, autoimmune diseases, and other chronic muscular and bone conditions from developing.[96]

"But," Baggerly quietly asked the gathering of experts, "who is teaching healthcare practitioners about this old and new research? Who is teaching the public about the health benefits of having sufficient vitamin D3 blood levels?" She was met with blank stares.

Baggerly immediately understood that, despite four decades of developing hard data on vitamin D3's various health benefits, our federal health agencies, along with the American Medical Association, remained silent about the benefits of vitamin D3. She decided it was important to share this lifesaving D3 information with the public. Yes, it was finally time to begin to help end this unnecessary modern-day national (and international) weakened immune system epidemic.[97]

In 2007, Baggerly formed GrassrootsHealth. This nonprofit group's outstanding work continues to effectively counter the medical industry's media attacks against our best vitamin D3 research.[98] Baggerly's mantra, the foundation of her effective D3 work, has always been *testing*— specifically, the importance of each person knowing her current vitamin D3 blood level. "Measurement is the key to action. It provides every individual with the information needed to make a logical, informed decision about their health. It puts you in charge. We all need measurement to keep our bodies in a disease-fighting state."[99] Since 2007, Carole Baggerly's incredibly effective work with GrassrootsHealth has:

- Brought together many of the leading vitamin D3 researchers from around the world to work cooperatively;[100]

- Produced and publicized large-scale, cutting-edge research on all aspects of effective D3 supplementation research, including work on breast cancer prevention;[101]

- Substantially increased the number of individuals in this country and elsewhere who now have annual vitamin-D3 blood-level tests;[102]

- Helped fuel consumer sales of vitamin D3 from a $50 million market in 2005 to an estimated $550 million in 2010, to an expected $2.5 billion by 2020 (the North American market is growing the fastest, at least doubling in the half decade from 2015–2020[103]); and

- Compiled fact sheets summarizing the most significant international research studies on vitamin D3 and breast cancer prevention.[104]

Other Vitamin D3 Resources

Sunlight Nutrition and Health Research Center (SUNARC)

As mentioned earlier, SUNARC advocates the importance of using natural sunlight in the prevention and treatment of cancer, as well as infectious diseases. The center, let by former NASA physicist, Dr William B. Grant, also publishes papers that synthesize and summarize the vitamin D3 field from a highly scholarly perspective, while advising government and healthcare leaders around the world on vitamin-D3-based disease prevention.[105]

Vitamindwiki.com

This website contains a catalogue of thousands of published research papers on vitamin D3's connection to a variety of health issues. Created by a retired engineer, Henry Lahore, the website is constantly updated. It contains a listing of more than 200 peer-review papers on the single subject, "Vitamin D3 and breast cancer prevention and treatment."[106]

The D3 Bad Guys

As mentioned several times already, the National Academy of Medicine (NAM) (formerly the Institute of Medicine) is the group that continues to control the contents of the American food pyramid. This is the group that consequently, may be most responsible for today's national obesity and breast cancer epidemics. A well-financed and highly effective lobby group that receives substantial funding from a number of industries, including the pharmaceutical and medical industries, NAM also continues to tell the US public that low vitamin D3 blood levels and breast cancer, have nothing to do with each other. Here is a summary of the conclusions from NAM's most recent study on this topic: "There are no known connections between vitamin D3 and breast cancer prevention or treatment."[107] And here is the NAM study's full list of jaw-dropping recommendations regarding vitamin D3 and breast cancer prevention:

1. Calcium and vitamin D3 are only useful in regard to bone health; there is not enough research to indicate vitamin D3 is helpful in preventing or treating any other diseases or health conditions.

2. Individuals should avoid sunshine, because of the risk of developing skin cancer.

3. Most individuals should not take more than 600 ng/ml of vitamin D3 each day, while those over 71 years old should take 800 ng/ml.

4. Each person should take 1000 IU of calcium each day, in order to absorb the D3.

5. There are no benefits, in fact there might be harm, in taking higher doses.

"Most of the other "bad guys," unfortunately are heavily influenced by NAM's policy statement on Vitamin D3."

Who Funds the NAM?

As interesting as this question is, it's not easy to answer. More importantly, why do NAM's funders, given the information described in this chapter thus far, appear interested in ignoring the best international research linking high D3 blood levels to effective breast cancer prevention?

A large part of this private lobby's hundreds of millions of dollars in annual funding appears to come through government agencies. But did you know that government agencies are now allowed to accept millions of dollars each year from private companies? Subsequently, today, as described below, pharmaceutical companies can ask the NCI to conduct specific research and then publish the sought results in the name of the NCI or NAM, creating a report that can be adopted or seen as "official government policy."[108]

CRADAs and the CDC Foundation

Today, the NCI, the CDC, the American Cancer Society, and most national breast cancer organizations appear to be heavily funded by the cancer treatment industry. All of these groups also continue to ignore the best biological, clinical, and statistical research on D3, usually telling us there is no connection between breast-cancer prevention and one's vitamin-D3 blood level. Why are these institutions and agencies promoting these false statements? It probably has something to do with money.

In 1986, President Ronald Reagan signed the *Federal Technology Transfer Act*. This law allowed private industry to give direct grants to federal government agencies for specific corporate-directed projects. As a result, it became (and remains) quite easy for corporations and industry associations to make very large grants in order to have government agencies do industry-backed studies. These so-called "government studies" are then published under the name of the National Cancer Institute, or another federal agency.

The National Institutes of Health tells us, "Cooperative Research and Development Agreements [*CRADAs*] provide an exciting opportunity for National Institutes of Health investigators to join with their colleagues from industry and academia in the joint pursuit of common research goals."[109] In other words, CRADAs enable the medical, pharmaceutical, chemical, and food-processing industries to add millions of dollars each year to the National Cancer Institute's and other federal agencies' budgets.[110] Specifically, with regard to our present topic, it is possible these funds can be handed over by a federal agency to NAM to conduct studies on vitamin D3, obesity, or other topics, on behalf of the government.

The Centers for Disease Control has its own special way of receiving private industry money. They use something called the CDC Foundation. This is an independent nonprofit organization that receives money from corporations within the chemical, medical, pharmaceutical, and other industries, to do jointly developed drug research. In return, the CDC can lend its name and approval to these industry-funded reports.[111] However, don't think that means the profits from these joint taxpayer–private company endeavors are shared. No. Future profits from drugs and inventions produced through this research usually go to the funding corporation.[112]

Here is how the CDC likes to describe this extra money it receives from the drug industry:

The CDC Foundation partnerships help CDC launch new programs and expand existing programs. In each partnership, this external support gives CDC the flexibility to quickly and effectively connect with other experts, information and technology needed to address a public health challenge. Some partnership programs are initiated by the CDC...Other times, a private-sector organization has specific public health interests that are also of interest to CDC as part of its public health agenda.[113]

Not surprisingly, as a consequence of these cozy partnerships, ranking government officials appear to be further rewarded, sometimes receiving highly lucrative positions once they leave government service. One possible example is Dr. Julie Gerberding, CDC chief under President George W. Bush. Her government responsibilities included overseeing the public's need, use, and the safety of vaccines. Just days after leaving this position, Gerberding was given the multimillion-dollar-a-year job as president of Merck Pharmaceutical's Vaccine Division.[114]

Put another way, thanks to CRADAs and the CDC Foundation, the US public no longer enjoys that assurance of unbiased, independent government research directed towards the health interests of our citizens— and that certainly includes the vital areas of vitamin D3 and breast cancer research. Instead, we now allow two industry lobby groups, the US Preventive Services Task Force (USPSTF) *organization* (not the task force itself) and the NAM, to determine federal policies—policies that continue to significantly contribute to at least three preventable current US epidemics: obesity, vitamin D3 deficiency, and breast cancer.

NAM's Fundraising Program

It is publicly reported that the NAM receives about half of its annual funding as tax-deductible contributions from individual donors and private business interests.[115] Those individuals and organizations that give the NAM more than $100,000 over the course of a lifetime become members of the NAM's prestigious Einstein Society. Those whose cumulative giving reaches $20,000 to $99,999 become members of the NAM Society, and those individuals and companies that give between $1,000 and $10,000 annually receive other types of recognitions.[116] But if we're patting all these generous donors on the back, we should also be concerned. Our nation's harmful nutritional and dietary guidelines, including the DRIs for vitamin D3, is being largely controlled by these wealthy individuals and by private, for-profit corporations, as they also receive huge tax-deductible contributions each year. Who's looking out for the *US public's* health??

The US Preventive Services Task Force

As mentioned above, a second industry-directed and industry-financed lobby, the US Preventive Services Task Force (USPSTF) organization, also continues to issue its own propaganda against the D3 Good Guys' research. Created and directed by the American Medical Association and other medical groups, the USPSTF's name gives the impression that it's an official government agency. It's not.

The USPSTF structure appears to include an innocent "front man" in the form of a task force. This is an unpaid, all-volunteer group of respected, well-meaning, healthcare professionals from various sectors of the medical, diagnostic testing, family medicine, and preventive services arms of the US healthcare industry. Each member is nominated or volunteers for a three-year term. Each year, the USPSTF organization's permanent officials, representing private health insurance companies and medical association interests (who refer to themselves as "partners"[117]) ask their temporary task force volunteers to review specific information about preventive health topics. Subjects include how often a woman should have a routine mammogram, and whether it's necessary for a person's annual physical exam to include a vitamin D3 blood test.[118] The volunteer task force members are then asked to use the information they're given by the USPSTF officials, to develop a consensus statement on the specific question being posed. This is where the trouble often starts.

Recent history tells us it doesn't seem to matter what these objective task force volunteers actually report, once they've reviewed the selected information on whatever subject they have been asked by the organization's officials to study. That's because USPSTF officials or partners have the ability to write up the press releases, describing the task force's recent conclusions. These press releases often fit the organization's political, economic, and public relations needs and blatantly ignored the task force's actual findings.

For example, in 2011, when asked to come up with a consensus statement about vitamin D3 supplementation and cancer prevention, based on the information studied, the honest task force volunteers said in their final recommendations that there is, "insufficient information on vitamin D3 and cancer prevention to make any recommendations. Evidence is not sufficiently robust to draw conclusions regarding the **benefits or harms** of vitamin D supplementation for the prevention of cancer."[119]

But guess what? The USPSTF organization appeared to ignore their volunteer task force's actual statement regarding "insufficient evidence." Instead, according to *The New York Times'* subsequent headline and article, the organization apparently issued a misleading press release. "The institute's expert committee, which included bone specialists, concluded that most people don't need supplements of these critical nutrients and warned of serious health risks from the high doses some now take—including kidney stones and heart disease linked to calcium supplements, and the very falls and fractures that vitamin D is meant to protect against,"[120] *The New York Times* article said, that next day. Go figure!

Five years later, a new crop of volunteer task force members was asked to review additional selected D3 research presented to them by the USPSTF officials. This time, the new task force was asked to decide if annual vitamin D3 testing is appropriate for the general public. This new volunteer group again issued an "insufficient evidence" statement, similar to their predecessors: "The USPSTF concludes that the current evidence is insufficient to assess the balance of benefits and harms of screening for vitamin D deficiency in asymptomatic adults."[121]

But once more, here are some headlines from the American press that appeared after USPSTF officials sent out yet another of their apparently misleading press releases on behalf of their volunteer task force:

- *Vitamin D Testing Not Recommended for Most People*
  Julie Corliss, Executive Editor, *Harvard Heart Letter* November 26, 2014[122]

- *Vitamin D Screening Not Backed by Expert Panel*
  Anahad O'Connor, *The New York Times* June 23, 2014[123]

- *USPSTF: No Evidence for Routine Vitamin D Screening*
  Nancy A Melville, *Medscape.com* November 24, 2014[124]

Once again, the USPSTF apparently chose to ignore its volunteer task force's "insufficient evidence" statement and instead substituted a statement that supported the organization's interests. Once again, the American public awoke to more fictitious headlines announcing that "a major national study" had dismissed the importance of vitamin D3 testing—of even knowing one's vitamin D3 blood level! You can't make this stuff up!

The American Cancer Society

Our largest national cancer foundation, the billion-dollar American Cancer Society,[125] receive tens of millions of dollars each year from corporations, especially from radiology and cancer drug companies that soundly benefit from today's $7.8 billion US mammography industry.[126] Corporate contributions help maintain the organization's salaries, which amounted to almost half-a-billion dollars in 2017 for the ACS's 6,000 employees, along with its growing endowment of $1.6 billion in 2017, which produced $28 million in annual income that same year.[127]

In February 2019, the American Cancer Society's website, citing NAM's and USPSTF's reports on vitamin D3, offered this guidance to women regarding the importance of vitamin D3 in effective breast cancer prevention: "So far, no study has shown that taking vitamins or other supplements reduces the risk of breast cancer (or any other cancer)."[128] Hopefully, the majority of women will soon realize that, like the NAM and USPSTF, the American Cancer Society is not always a reliable, objective, or unbiased authority when it comes to the best ways to keep breast cancer out of our bodies.

Where Do We Go from Here?

This chapter has shown how safe outdoor and indoor tanning, along with taking enough vitamin D3 supplements, can be a highly effective breast cancer prevention step. In the process, we've seen once again why women have to make their own decisions about effective breast cancer prevention steps and once again must consider questioning the recommendations of the federal government, the American Cancer Society, the NAM, the USPSTF, and possibly one's own unaware primary care physician or oncologist. This is especially true regarding the all-important role of vitamin D3 in breast cancer prevention. Proper attention to keeping our vitamin D3 blood levels above 60 ng/ml, could, by itself, drop breast cancer rates in the United States by as much as 80 percent!

But important as it is, vitamin D3 is only part of the answer. In <u>Chapter 4</u>, we'll now turn our attention to progestin. This chemical, found in all birth control drugs, has now been traced to the development and acceleration of breast tumors in large numbers of premenopausal women. Beware: to my mind, this next chapter contains some of the most upsetting information you'll find in this entire book.

CHAPTER ENDNOTES

1   S.L. McDonnell et al., "Breast Cancer Risk Markedly Lower With Serum25-Hydroxyvitamin D Concentrations >60 vs >20 ng/ml (150 vs 50 nmol/L): Pooled Analysis of Two Randomized Trials and a Prospective Cohort," *PLoS One*, 2 (June 15, 2018):e0199265, doi:10.1371/journal.pone.0199265. GrassrootsHealth, "Studies on Vitamin D and Breast Cancer: Key Findings from Last Ten Years," 2017, https://www.grassrootshealth.net/project/breast-cancer-prevention/.

2   Global Market Insights, "Breast Cancer Therapeutics Market to Hit $30,637.7 Million by 2025," press release, March 14, 2019, https://www.globenewswire.com/news-release/2019/03/14/1752945/0/en/Breast-Cancer-Therapeutics-Market-to-hit-30-637-7-million-by-2025-Global-Market-Insights-Inc.html.

3   Top Documentary Films, *Who Killed the Electric Car?* Directed by Chris Paine (2006), https://topdocumentaryfilms.com/who-killed-the-electric-car.

4   Julia Pyper, "U.S. Electric Vehicle Sales Increased by 81% in 2018," January 7, 2019, GreenTech Media, https://www.greentechmedia.com/articles/read/us-electric-vehicle-sales-increase-by-81-in-2018.

5   Chandra Kanti Chakraborti, "Vitamin D as a Promising Anticancer Agent," *Indian Journal of Pharmacology* 43, no. 2 (April 2011): 11320, https://www.ncbi.nlm.nih.gov/pmc/articles/PMC3081446/, https://doi.org/10.4103/0253-7613.77335.

6   William B Grant, "Vitamin D Acceptance Delayed by Big Pharma Following the Disinformation Playbook," *Orthomolecular Medicine News Service*, October 1, 2018, http://orthomolecular.org/resources/omns/v14n22.shtml.

7   National Cancer Institute, "Vitamin D Supplements Don't Reduce Cancer Incidence, Trial Shows," December 13, 2018, cancer.gov, https://www.cancer.gov/news-events/cancer-currents-blog/2018/vitamin-d-supplement-cancer-prevention; Institute of Medicine; "Report Brief: Dietary Reference Intakes for Calcium and Vitamin D," November 2010 http://www.nationalacademies.org, https://www.nap.edu/catalog/13050/dietary-reference-intakes-for-calcium-and-vitamin-d.

8   Nicolas Rapp and Aric Jenkins, "Chart: These 6 Companies Control Much of U.S. Media," Fortune.com, July 24, 2018, https://fortune.com/longform/media-company-ownership-consolidation/.

9   Sharon L. McDonnell et al., "Breast Cancer Risk Markedly Lower with Serum 25-hydroxyvitamin D Concentrations ≥60 vs <20 ng/ml (150 vs 50 nmol/L): Pooled Analysis of Two Randomized Trials and a Prospective Cohort," *PLOS One* (June 15, 2018), https://doi.org/10.1371/journal.pone.0199265.

10 The Endocrine Society, "Vitamin D3," youandyourhormones.com, https://www.yourhormones.info/hormones/vitamin-d/.

11 "International Scientists Panel," GrassrootsHealth Nutrient Research Institute, https://grassrootshealth.net/project/our-scientists/.

12 "Scientists' Call to D* Action," www.grassrootshealth.net, https://grassrootshealth.net/wp-content/uploads/2017/12/scientists_call-to-daction_121817.pdf.

13 W. Liu et al., "The Anti-Inflammatory Effects of Vitamin D in Tumorigenesis," *International Journal of Molecular Science* 19, no. 9 (September 13, 2018):2736, https://doi.org/10.3390/ijms19092736; A. Mousa et al., "Effect of Vitamin D Supplementation on Inflammation: Protocol for a Systematic Review," *BMJ Open* 6, no. 4 (2016), http://dx.doi.org/10.1136/bmjopen-2015-010804.

14 Daniel D. Bikle, "Vitamin D and Bone," *Current Osteoporosis Reports* 10, no. 2 (2012): 151–59, https://doi.org/10.1007/s11914-012-0098-z.

15 Sharon L. McDonnell et al., "Breast Cancer Risk Markedly Lower," *PLOS One* (June 15, 2018).

16 James C. Fleet et al., "Vitamin D and Cancer: A Review of Molecular Mechanisms," *The Biochemical Journal* 441, no.1 (Jan 1, 2012): 61–76, https://doi.org/10.1042/BJ20110744; Chakraborti, "Vitamin D as a Promising Anticancer Agent," 14-15.

17 Y. Xin et al., "E-cadherin Mediates the Preventive Effect of Vitamin D3 in Colitis-associated Carcinogenesis," *Inflammatory Bowel Disease* 23, no.9, (Sept 23, 2017):1535–43; https://doi.org/10.1097/MIB.0000000000001209; Rajeev Singhai et al., "E-Cadherin as a Diagnostic Biomarker in Breast Cancer," *North American Journal of Medical Sciences* 3, no. 5 (May 2011): 227–33, https://www.ncbi.nlm.nih.gov/pmc/articles/PMC3337742/, https://doi.org/10.4297/najms.2011.3227; Sharif Mohr, "What is the Dose-Response Relationship between Vitamin D and Cancer Risk?" *Nutrition Review* 65, no. 8 (2007): S91–S93, https://www.academia.edu/4267204/What_is_the_Dose-Response_Relationship_between_Vitamin_D_and_Cancer_Risk; Nives Pecina-Slaus, "Tumor Suppressor Gene E-Cadherin and its Role in Normal and Malignant Cells," *Cancer Cell International* 3, no. 17 (October 2003), accessed March 12, 2019, https://cancerci.biomedcentral.com/articles/10.1186/1475-2867-3-17.

18 Sherif B. Mohr et al, "Meta-analysis of Vitamin D Sufficiency for Improving Survival of Patients with Breast Cancer," *Anticancer Research* 34 (2014): 1163–66, https://pubmed.ncbi.nlm.nih.gov/24596354/.

19 Cedric F. Garland, et al., "Greater Levels of Vitamin D Associated with Decreasing Risk of Breast Cancer," University of California- San Diego, *Medical Express.com*, https://medicalxpress.com/news/2018-06-greater-vitamin-d-decreasing-breast.html; Cara Nicole Inglese, "The Role of Vitamin D Signaling in the Interaction between Mesenchymal Mammary Tumor Cells and Macrophages," (MS thesis, Queen's University Kingston, Ontario, Canada) 2016, https://search.proquest.com/openview/b877423f8ed5452c7843e7fad4799e5f/1.pdf?pq-origsite=gscholar&cbl=18750&diss=y.

20 Nutrient Recommendations, National Institutes of Health, https://ods.od.nih.gov/Health Information/Dietary_Reference_Intakes.aspx.

21 S. P. Murphy et al., "History of Nutrition: The Long Road Leading to the Dietary Reference Intakes for the United States and Canada," Reviews from ASN EB 2015 Symposia, American Society for Nutrition, 7, (2016): 157–68, https://doi.org/10.3945/an.115.010322; For a coherent understanding of the food industry's long-standing involvement in lobbying Congress and various governmental food agencies regarding DRIs and DGAs, see Marion Nestle, *Food Politics: How the Food Industry Influences Nutrition and Health* (10th Anniversary Edition), (Berkeley: University of California, 2013).

22 "Committee to Review Dietary Reference Intakes for Vitamin D and Calcium," A. Catharine Ross et al., editors, in *Dietary Reference Intakes for Calcium and Vitamin D.* (Washington, DC: National Academies Press; 2011). Available from: https://www.ncbi.nlm.nih.gov/books/NBK56069/.

23 Institute of Medicine. *Dietary Reference Intakes for Calcium and Vitamin D.* (Washington, DC: The National Academies Press, 2011), https://doi.org/10.17226/13050.

24 NIH, "Vitamin D Fact Sheet for Health Professionals," March 24, 2020, https://ods.od.nih.gov/factsheets/VitaminD-HealthProfessional/.

25 Kate Vinton, "These 15 Billionaires Own America's News Media Companies," *Forbes*, June 1, 2016, https://www.forbes.com/sites/katevinton/2016/06/01/these-15-billionaires-own-americas-news-media-companies/#54b733bf660a.

26 Julie Corliss, "Vitamin D Testing Not Recommended for Most People," *Harvard Heart Letter*, November 26, 2014, https://www.health.harvard.edu/blog/vitamin-d-testing-recommended-people-201411267547.

27 Gina Kolata, "Why Are So Many People Popping Vitamin D3?" *The New York Times*, April 10, 2017, https://www.nytimes.com/2017/04/10/health/vitamin-d-deficiency-supplements.html.

28 GrassrootsHealth, "D*Action Breast Cancer Prevention Society, Show Me the Research," https://www.grassrootshealth.net/?post_projects=breast-cancer-prevention.

29 J.E. Manson, et al., "Vitamin D Supplements and Prevention of Cancer and Cardiovascular Disease,"*New England Journal of Medicine* 380, no.1(2019): 33-44, doi:10.1056/NEJMoa1809944.

30 "National Health and Nutrition Examination Survey: Analytic Guidelines, 1999–2010," *Vital and Health Statistics, Series 10, Data from the National Health Survey*, No. 161 (September 2013), CDC. gov, accessed March 12, 2019, https://stacks.cdc.gov/view/cdc/21305; Kimberly Y.Z. Forrest and W.I. Stuhldreher, "Prevalence and Correlates of Vitamin D Deficiency in U.S. Adults," *Nutrition Research* 31, No.1 (January 2011): 48–54, https://doi.org/10.1016/j.nutres.2010.12.001; See Chapter 9 for data on rising breast cancer rates.

31 Institute of Medicine, (US) Committee to Review Dietary Reference Intakes for Vitamin D and Calcium; A. C. Ross, C.L. Taylor, A.L. Yaktine et al., editors. "Dietary Reference Intakes for Calcium and Vitamin D, (Washington, DC: National Academies Press, 2011). Available from: https://doi.org/10.17226/13050.

32 Tyler Scott, "Annual Report to the Nation on Status of Cancer, Focus on Younger Adults," North American Association of Central Cancer Registries, July 11, 2019, https://www.naaccr.org/11457-2/; Elaine Schattner, "Breast Cancers Are Rising in Younger and in Older Women: Reasons for Concern," *Forbes*, June 16, 2015, https://www.forbes.com/sites/elaineschattner/2015/06/16/nci-investigators-report-breast-cancers-are-rising-in-younger-and-older-women-reasons-for-concern/#b9fbe98582fb.

33 Kim Farina, "The Economics of Cancer Care in the United States," *American Journal of Managed Care* 18, no. 1, (2012) https://www.ajmc.com/journals/evidence-based-oncology/2012/2012-2-vol18-n1/the-economics-of-cancer-care-in-the-united-states-how-much-do-we-spend-and-how-can-we-spend-it-better.

34 Courtney Elder, "How Much Does Breast Cancer Treatment Cost in the U.S?" November 21, 2017, blog post on singlecare.com, https://www.singlecare.com/blog/breast-cancer-treatment-cost-u-s/; H. Blumen, K. Fitch and V. Polkus, "Comparison of Treatment Costs for Breast Cancer, by Tumor Stage and Type of Service," *American Health & Drug Benefits* 9, no. 1 (2016):23–32, PMCID: PMC4822976.

35 National Institutes of Health, "VDR Gene: Vitamin D Receptor: Genetics Home Reference," https://ghr.nlm.nih.gov/gene/VDR.

36 Meis Moukayed and William B. Grant, "Review: Molecular Link between Vitamin D and Cancer Prevention," *Nutrients* 5 (September 30, 2013): 3993–4021, https://doi.org/10.3390/nu5103993.

37 Sang-Min Jeon and Eun-Ae Shin, "Exploring Vitamin D Metabolism and Function in Cancer," *Experimental and Molecular Medicine* 50, no. 20, (April 2018), https://doi.org/10.1038/s12276-018-0038-9.

38 NIH, "Clinical Alert: NHLBI Stops Trial of Estrogen Plus Progestin Due to Increased Breast Cancer Risk, Lack of Overall Benefit," National Heart, Lung, and Blood Institute (NHLBI), July 9, 2002, nih.gov.

39 See Chapter 4 for more on the National Prempro Study.

40 Kimberly Y. Forrest and Wendy L. Stuhldreher, "Prevalence and Correlates of Vitamin D Deficiency in U.S. Adults," *Nutrition Research* 31, no. 1 (January 2011): 48-54. https://doi.org/10.1016/j.nutres.2010.12.001.

41 William B Grant, "25, Hydroxyvitamin D and Breast Cancer, Colorectal Cancer, and Colorectal Adenomas: Case-Control Versus Nester Case-Control Studies," *Anticancer Research* 35 (2015): 1153–60; Alexander Ho et al., "Seasonality Pattern of Breast, Colorectal, and Prostate Cancer is Dependent on Latitude," *Medical Science Monitor* 20 (May 19, 2014): 818–24, https://pubmed.ncbi.nlm.nih.gov/24835144/.

42 William B. Grant, "25, Hydroxyvitamin D and Breast Cancer…", 1.

43 Cedric F. Garland and Frank C. Garland, "Do Sunlight and Vitamin D Reduce the Likelihood of Colon Cancer?" *International Journal of Epidemiology* 9 (1980): 227-31, https://doi.org/10.1093/ije/9.3.227.

44 Cedric F. Garland and Frank C. Garland, "Do Sunlight and Vitamin D Reduce the Likelihood of Colon Cancer?, (republished in *International Journal of Epidemiology* 35, no. 2 (April 2006): 217-20, https://doi.org/10.1093/ije/dyi229.

45 Alexander Ho et al., "Seasonality Pattern of Breast, Colorectal, and Prostate Cancer is Dependent on Latitude," *Medical Science Monitor: International Medical Journal of Experimental and Clinical Research* 20, (May 19, 2014): 818-24, https://doi.org/10.12659/MSM.890062.

46 Thomas Wehr, "Melatonin and Seasonal Rhythms," *Journal of Biological Rhythms* 12, no. 6 (December 12, 1997): 518-27, https://doi.org/10.1203/00006450-200101000-00015.

47 Alexander Ho et al., "Seasonality Pattern of Breast, Colorectal, and Prostate Cancer…" *Medical Science Monitor*, 818.

48 Cedric F. Garland et al. "The Role of Vitamin D in Cancer Prevention," *American Journal of Public Health*. 96, no.2, (2006): 252-61, https://doi.org/10.2105/AJPH.2004.045260.

49 Centers for Disease Control "Female Breast, All Ages, All Races/Ethnicities, Female Rate per 100,000 Women," *Leading Cancer Cases and Deaths, Female*, 2016, https://gis.cdc.gov/Cancer/USCS/DataViz.html.

50 M. F. Holick, "Vitamin D Deficiency," *New England Journal of Medicine* 7, no. 357 (2007): 266–81, https://doi.org/10.1056/NEJMra070553.

51 Hawai'i Heath Matters, "Mammogram History: Ages 50-74," http://www.hawaiihealthmatters.org/indicators/index/view?indicatorId=2333&localeId=14.

52 G. Maskarinec, L. Wilkens and L. Meng, "Mammography Screening and the Increase in Breast Cancer Incidence in Hawaii," *Cancer Epidemiol Biomarkers Preview* 6, no.3, (March 1, 1997): 201-08, https://cebp.aacrjournals.org/content/6/3/201.long; also see: Chapter 5.

53 Yanyuan Wu et al., "Association of Vitamin D3 Level with Breast Cancer Risk and Prognosis in African-American and Hispanic Women," *Cancers* 9, no.10 (October 2017): 144, https://doi.org/10.3390/cancers9100144.

54 Nina G. Jablonski and George Chaplin, "Colloquium Paper: Human Skin Pigmentation as an Adaptation to UV Radiation," *Proceedings of the National Academy of Sciences of the United States of America* 107, no. Suppl 2 (2010): 8962-8, https://doi.org/10.1073/pnas.0914628107.

55 Marc B. Sorenson and William B. Grant, *Embrace the Sun: Are You Dying in the Dark?* (Salt Lake City, UT: Marc Sorenson, 2018).

56 GrassrootsHealth, "Do You Know Your Vitamin D Level?" https://www.grassrootshealth.net/project/daction/; Life Extension, "Vitamin D, 25-Hydroxy Blood Test". https://www.lifeextension.com/lab-testing/itemlc081950/vitamin-d-25-hydroxy-blood-test.

57 S. M. Kimball, N. Mirhosseini, and M. F. Holick, "Evaluation of Vitamin D3 Intakes up to 15,000 International Units/day and Serum 25-hydroxyvitamin D Concentrations up to 300 nmol/L on Calcium Metabolism in a Community Setting," *Dermato-endocrinology* 9, no.1 (April 2017): e1300213, https://doi.org/10.1080/19381980.2017.1300213.

58 For scholarly information on the importance of practicing safe year-round tanning, see: SUNARC.org; sunlightinstitute.org and European Sunlight Association, "Updated Scientific Overview," http://europeansunlight.eu/cms/wp-content/uploads/2019/07/Updated-scientific-overview.pdf.

59 A.T. Drincic et al, "Volumetric Dilution, Rather Than Sequestration Best Explains the Low Vitamin D Status of Obesity," *Obesity* 20, no.7, (July 2012):1444-8, https://doi.org/10.1038/oby.2011.404.

60   Angela Carrelli et al., "Vitamin D Storage in Adipose Tissue of Obese and Normal Weight Women," *Journal of Bone and Mineral Research* 32, no. 2 (2017): 237-242, https://doi.org/10.1002/jbmr.2979.

61   Shivaprakash J. Mutt et al., "Vitamin D and Adipose Tissue: More than Storage," *Frontiers in Physiology* 5, no. 228 (June 2104), https://doi.org/10.3389/fphys.2014.00228.

62   Adriana Villaseñor et al., "Postdiagnosis C-Reactive Protein and Breast Cancer Survivorship: Findings from the WHEL Study," *Cancer Epidemiology and Prevention* 23, no. 1 (January 2014), https://doi.org/10.1158/1055-9965.EPI-13-0852.

63   Caitlin Mason et al., "Effects of Weight Loss on Serum Vitamin D in Postmenopausal Women," *The American Journal of Clinical Nutrition* 94, no. 1 (2011): 95-103, https://doi.org/10.3945/ajcn.111.015552.

64   G.B. Mulligan and A. Licata, "Taking Vitamin D with the Largest Meal Improves Absorption and Results in Higher Serum Levels of 25-Hydroxyvitamin D," *Journal of Bone Mineral Research* 25, no.4 (April 2010): 928–30, https://doi.org/10.1002/jbmr.67

65   Barbara Boucher, "The Problem of Vitamin D Insufficiency in Older People," *Aging and Disease* 3, no. 4 (August 2012): 313–29, PMCID: PMC3501367.

66   P. Reddy and L.R. Edwards, "Magnesium Supplementation in Vitamin D Deficiency," *American Journal of Therapy*, 2019;26(1):e124-e132, https://doi.org/10.1097/MJT.0000000000000538; Anna Marie Uwifonza and Mohammad Razzaque, "Role of Magnesium in Vitamin D Activation and Function," *The Journal of the American Osteopathic Association* 118 (March 2018): 181–89, https://doi.org/10.7556/jaoa.2018.037.

67   Joseph Mercola, "What are the Health Benefits of Vitamin K2?", https://articles.mercola.com/sites/articles/archive/2019/03/04/health-benefits-of-vitamin-k2.aspx, mercola.com and newchapter.com; New Chapter, "Calcium, Magnesium and Other Minerals," https://www.newchapter.com/products/calcium/.

68   GrassrootsHealth "Vitamin D* Calculator," https://www.grassrootshealth.net/project/dcalculator/

69   Global Sun Care Market, "Rising Awareness about Adverse Effects of Solar Radiation Ensures Steady Growth in Demand," *Transparency Market Research*, November 14, 2016, 2, https://www.transparencymarketresearch.com/pressrelease/global-sun-care-market.htm.

70   Centers for Disease Control, "Rates of New Melanomas—Deadly Skin Cancers—Have Doubled Over Last Three Decades," June 2, 2015, https://www.cdc.gov/media/releases/2015/p0602-melanoma-cancer.html.

71   Alan C. Geller et al., "Melanoma Epidemic: An Analysis of Six Decades of Data from the Connecticut Tumor Registry," *Journal of Clinical Oncology* 31, no.33 (November 20, 2013):4172-4178, https://doi.org/10.1200/JCO.2012.47.3728.

72   Michael Castleman, "Think Sunscreen Protects Against Cancer? Think Again," *Mother Jones*, May/June 1998, https://www.motherjones.com/politics/1998/05/sunscam/; Terry Tillaart, "Sunscreen Not Sunshine Causes Cancer- Proof," July 24, 2016, https://www.terrytillaart.com/single-post/2016/07/24/Sunscreen-Not-Sunshine-Causes-Cancer-Proof.

73   Theresa Michele et al., "Effect of Sunscreen, Application Under Maximal Use Conditions on Plasma Concentration of Sunscreen Active Ingredients A Randomized Clinical Trial," *Journal of the American Medical Association* 321, no. 21(June 4, 2019): 2082–2091, https://doi.org/10.1001/jama.2019.5586.

74   See Chapter 1.

75   Kyle P. Radack et al., "A Review of the Use of Tanning Beds as a Dermatological Treatment," *Dermatology and Therapy* 5, no. 1 (2015): 37–51, https://doi.org/10.1007/s13555-015-0071-8.

76 *The New York Times*, "Sunscreen: A History," June 23, 2010, https://www.nytimes.com/2010/06/24/fashion/24skinside.html.

77 Ibid

78 J. C. Farman, B. G. Gardiner and J. Shanklin, "Large Losses of Total Ozone in Antarctica Reveal Seasonal ClOx/NOx Interaction," *Nature* 315, no. 6016 (May 16, 1985): 207–10, https://doi.org/10.1038/315207a0; also see: TheOzoneHole.com for updated information on this topic. This website is sponsored by a number of international environmental groups, unaffiliated with the chemical and sunscreen industries.

79 NCI, "Reportable List: SEER Training Modules," cancer.gov, https://training.seer.cancer.gov/operations/management/list.html.

80 Donald W. Shenenberger, "Cutaneous Malignant Melanoma: A Primary Care Perspective," *American Family Physician* 85, no.2 (January 2012):161–68, PMID: 22335216.

81 Farman et al., *Nature*, 315, no. 6016, May 16, 1985, p. 207

82 US Environmental Protection Agency, "Basic Ozone Layer Science," https://www.epa.gov/ozone-layer-protection/basic-ozone-layer-science.

83 US Department of State, "The Montreal Protocol on Substances that Deplete the Ozone Layer," https://www.state.gov/key-topics-office-of-environmental-quality-and-transboundary-issues/the-montreal-protocol-on-substances-that-deplete-the-ozone-layer/.

84 International Ozone Commission, "The International Ozone Commission, on the 30th anniversary of the Montreal Protocol, Reports Signs of Healing of the Ozone Hole in Antarctica," press release, September 15, 2016, International Association of Meteorology and Atmospheric Science (IAMAS), http://www.io3c.org/sites/io3c.org/files/upload/documents/io3c_press_release_2016.pdf; 30th Anniversary of the Discovery of the Ozone Hole, Cambridge Centre for Climate Science, May 14, 2015, https://www.climatescience.cam.ac.uk/news/30th-anniversary-of-the-discovery-of-ozone-hole.

85 ReportLinker, "Global Sun Care Products Industry", *March 11*, 2020, https://www.globenewswire.com/news-release/2020/03/11/1998542/0/en/Global-Sun-Care-Products-Industry.html?pr; Statista.com, "Sun Care Industry- Statistics & Facts," March 15, 2018, https://www.statista.com/topics/1990/sun-care-industry/.

86 See Chapter 9.

87 Michael F. Holick, "Cancer, Sunlight and Vitamin D3," *Journal of Clinical and Translational Endocrinology* 1, no. 4 (2014): 179–86, https://doi.org/10.1016/j.jcte.2014.10.001.

88 Michael F. Holick, H. F. Deluca and L. V. Avioli, "Isolation and Identification of 25-hydroxycholecalciferol from Human Plasma," *Archives of Internal Medicine* 129, no. 1 (1972): 56–61, https://doi.org/10.1001/archinte.1972.00320010060005.

89 Michael F. Holick et al., "Vitamin D and Brain Health: The Need for Vitamin D Supplementation and Sensible Sun Exposure," *Journal of Internal Medicine* 277, no. 1 (January 2015): 90–93, https://doi.org/10.1111/joim.12308.

90 S.B. Mohr et al., "Meta-analysis of Vitamin D Sufficiency for Improving Survival of Patients with Breast Cancer, *Anti-Cancer Research* 34, no. 3 (March 2014): 1163-66, accessed March 13, 2019, https://www.ncbi.nlm.nih.gov/pubmed/24596354, PMID: 24596354

91 Frank Garland and Cedric F. Garland, "Do Sunlight and Vitamin D Reduce the Likelihood of Colon Cancer?", 1

92 GrassrootsHealth, "Scientists Call to D*action for Public Health," https://www.grassrootshealth.net/project/our-scientists/.

93 American Public Health Association, "Call for Education and Research into Vitamin D Deficiency/ Insufficiency," Policy Number: 20081 (Oct 28, 2008), accessed March 13, 2019, https://www.apha. org/policies-and-advocacy/public-health-policy-statements/policy-database/2014/07/07/18/10/ call-for-education-and-research-into-vitamin-d-deficiency-insufficiency.

94 Ibid.

95 Azzie Young and Michael F. Holick, "Health Disparities and the Vitamin D Connection: Local and Global Health Concerns," APHA Annual Meeting, Boston, MA, November 2013, https://apha. confex.com/apha/141am/webprogram/Paper285890.html.

96 GrassrootsHealth, "About Us," https://www.grassrootshealth.net/project/about-us/.

97 Yangshen Lhamo et al., "Epidemic of Vitamin D Deficiency and Its Management: Awareness among Indian Medical Undergraduates," *Journal of Environmental and Public Health* (2017): 2517207, https://doi.org/10.1155/2017/2517207.

98 Joseph Mercola, "Gamechanger of the Year," August 7, 2018, mercola.com; Gina Kolata, "Why Are So Many People Popping Vitamin D?" *The New York Times*, April 10, 2017, accessed March 13, 2019, https://www.nytimes.com/2017/04/10/health/vitamin-d-deficiency-supplements.html.

99 Carole Baggerly, "Letter from the Director," www.grassrootshealth.net. http://archive. constantcontact.com/fs187/1102722411090/archive/1119367034884.html.

100 Carole Baggerly, "Scientists' Call to D* Action: The Vitamin D Deficiency Epidemic," grassrootshealth.net/project/our-scientists/, accessed March 13, 2019, https://grassrootshealth. net/project/our-scientists/.

101 GrassrootsHealth, "Last Ten Years," 2017.

102 Colata, "Why Are So Many People..." 2017.

103 Market Research Report, "Vitamin D Market by Analog (Vitamin D2, Vitamin D3), Form (Dry, Liquid), Application (Functional Food & Beverage, Pharma, Feed, and Personal Care), End User (Children, Adult, and Pregnant Women), Iu Strength and Region–Global Forecast to 2025," Press Release, May 2019, https://www.marketsandmarkets.com/Market-Reports/vitamin-d-market-22034298.html.

104 GrassrootsHealth, "D*Action Breast Cancer Prevention Society, Show Me the Research," https:// www.grassrootshealth.net/?post_projects=breast-cancer-prevention.

105 William B. Grant, www.sunarc.org.

106 Henry LaHore, "Vitamindwiki.com," https://vitamindwiki.com/Cancer+-+Breast, https:// vitamindwiki.com/VitaminDWiki.

107 Catharine A Ross et al., "The 2011 Report on Dietary Reference intakes for Calcium and Vitamin D from the Institute of Medicine: What Clinicians Need to Know," *The Journal of Clinical Endocrinology and Metabolism* 96, no. 1 (2011): 53-8, https://doi.org/10.1210/jc.2010-2704.

108 It is beyond the scope of this book to identify specific breast cancer studies that have been initiated and directed by industry and published as objective national studies by the NCI or CDC. The independent nonprofit group, US Right to Know, however, continues to publish original source documents that identify some of the ways industry continues to influence the work of federal food and medical agencies. Some examples are found in Stacy Malkin, "10 Revelations from U.S. Right to Know Investigations," September 19, 2019, https://usrtk.org/ our-investigations/10-revelations-usrtk.

109 National Institutes of Health, "CRADAs, Overview," Office of Intramural Research, Office of Technology Transfer, https://www.ott.nih.gov/policy/cradas.

110 Tom Stackhouse, "An Industry Guide to Partnering with the National Cancer Institute," December 9, 2003, Technology Transfer Branch, National Cancer Institute, Washington, D.C.

https://tier7.us/wp-content/uploads/2013/09/NCI_An_Industry_Guide_to_Partnering1.pdf;
Percy Ivy, "NCI Cooperative Research and Development Agreements, Review Article," December
1, 2000, https://pdfs.semanticscholar.org/539c/9b728d7ab57513027408618bf76085db7b39.pdf;
Cancer Network.com, "Special Sources of Funds: CRADAs," https://www.cancer.gov/about-nci/
budget/fact-book/data/special-sources.

111 Matt Richtel and Andrew Pollack, "Harnessing the U.S. Taxpayer to Fight Cancer and Make
Profits," *The New York Times*, December 18, 2016, https://www.nytimes.com/2016/12/19/health/
harnessing-the-us-taxpayer-to-fight-cancer-and-make-profits.html.

112 Samuel Epstein, *The Politics of Cancer Revisited*, indexed edition (Hankins, NY: East Ridge Press,
1998).

113 CDC Foundation, "Our Story," www.cdcfoundation.org/our-story.

114 Reuters, "Former CDC Head Lands Vaccine Job at Merck," December 21, 2009, https://www.
reuters.com/article/us-merck-gerberding/former-cdc-head-lands-vaccine-job-at-merck-
idUSTRE5BK2K520091221; For additional examples, see Samuel Epstein, *National Cancer
Institute and American Cancer Society: Criminal Indifference to Cancer Prevention and Conflicts of
Interest*, (Bloomington, IN: Xlibris, 2011).

115 National Academy of Medicine, "National Academy of Medicine 2018 Annual Report," https://nam.
edu/wp-content/uploads/2019/05/National-Academy-of-Medicine-2018-Annual-Report.pdf.

116 National Academy of Medicine, "Philanthropic Societies, National Academy of Medicine,"
Accessed March 15, 2019, https://nam.edu/support-the-nam/philanthropic-societies/.

117 US Preventive Services Task Force, "Our Partners," https://www.uspreventiveservicestaskforce.
org/uspstf/about-uspstf/our-partners.

118 Michael McBureney, Sonia Hartunian-Sowa, and Nathan V. Matusheski, "Implications of U.S.
Nutrition Facts Label Changes on Micronutrient Density of Fortified Foods and Supplements,"
The Journal of Nutrition: Issues and Opinions 147, no. 6 (June 2017): 1025–30, https://doi.
org/10.3945/jn.117.247585.

119 Mei Chung et al., "Vitamin D With or Without Calcium Supplementation for Prevention of Cancer
and Fractures: An Updated Meta-Analysis for the U.S. Preventive Services Task Force," December
2011, https://doi.org/10.7326/0003-4819-155-12-201112200-00005.

120 Jane Brody, "Long and Short of Calcium and Vitamin D," *The New York Times*, January 24, 2011,
https://www.nytimes.com/2011/01/25/health/25brody.html.

121 USPSTF, "Vitamin D, Calcium, or Combined Supplementation for the Primary Prevention
of Fractures in Community-Dwelling Adults: Preventive Medication," USPSTF.
org, April 2018, https://www.uspreventiveservicestaskforce.org/Page/Document/
RecommendationStatementFinal/vitamin-d-calcium-or-combined-supplementation-for-the-
primary-prevention-of-fractures-in-adults-preventive-medication.

122 Julie Corliss, "Vitamin D Testing Not Recommended for Most People," *Harvard
Heart Letter*, November 26, 2014, https://www.health.harvard.edu/blog/
vitamin-d-testing-recommended-people-201411267547.

123 Anahad O'Connor, "Vitamin D Screening Not Backed by Expert Panel," *The
New York Times*, June 23, 2014, https://well.blogs.nytimes.com/2014/06/23/
vitamin-d-screening-not-backed-by-expert-panel/.

124 Nancy A Melville, "USPSTF: No Evidence for Routine Vitamin D Screening," MedScape.com,
November 24, 2014, https://www.medscape.com/viewarticle/835369.

125 American Cancer Society, "ACS, Inc. Form 2017 990: For Fiscal Year Ended December 31, 2017,"
https://www.cancer.org/about-us/financial-governance-information/irs-form-990s.html.

126 See Chapter 5.

127 American Cancer Society 2017 Annual Report, https://www.cancer.org/content/dam/cancer-org/online-documents/en/pdf/forms/american-cancer-society-inc_990_PIC_2017-final.pdf.

128 American Cancer Society, "Can I Lower My Risk of Breast Cancer?" Accessed March 15, 2019, https://www.cancer.org/cancer/breast-cancer/risk-and-prevention/can-i-lower-my-risk.html.

STEP 3:
Avoid All Birth Control Drugs and Choose Hormone-Free Options Instead

Helen's Story

"I always used to say to my doctor, 'Are you really sure these pills aren't going to hurt me? I've been on these things for decades,'" an exasperated Helen told me as we walked the beach in our hometown of Manchester, Massachusetts.

Helen, 48, an airline attendant for the past twenty-five years, had been diagnosed days earlier with invasive breast cancer. As she settled into a comfortable position on her couch to read one evening, relaxed and bra-free, Helen's fingers touched something rock-hard in her left breast. Like most women, Helen had found her tumor herself.

"So, after the oncologist called and gave me the bad news about the tumor, I went in for my next appointment and they shrieked at me," Helen said. "'What?! You haven't stopped taking your birth control pills yet? Stop those things immediately!' the nurse told me."

"How was I supposed to know?" a frustrated Helen asked. "Why has my regular doctor always told me, 'Oh, those contraceptive drugs are fine, don't worry.' I never wanted to have kids; I've been on those damn pills nonstop for over twenty-five years."

Yes, the medical profession knows. Helen's doctor and other oncologists have their personal patient profiles; they have the evidence of a connection between birth control drug use and breast cancer, right before their eyes. Still, the cat is not yet out of the bag when it comes to the general public. But finally, at least, one paw is sticking out. It's only a matter of time until most women refuse to use today's popular birth control drugs, choosing hormone-free alternatives instead. That's never been more true than it is right now.

For decades we have had the statistical proof comparing progestin drug users with those who "just say no" (those who choose progestin-free options instead).[1] Today we finally have documented, award-winning, published proof that spells out the biology of what exactly is happening to breast cells in women who develop breast cancer while using progestin drugs and progestin-laced IUDs. The first piece of this research, published in 2010 in the journal Nature, begins to explain how healthy breast cells are transformed into cancer cells, and how tumor growth from existing breast cancer cells can become accelerated when progestin is introduced into breast cells.[2] Additional research, published in 2012, describes exactly how the mitochondria in breast duct cells can suffocate from such toxic chemical or toxic hormone attacks, and revert back to their prehistoric, mindlessly duplicating state, becoming modern-day cancer cells, now growing within a woman's breast.[3] Merging these two discoveries together, we can finally understand why Helen (and thousands of other women) develop breast cancer while using progestin-based birth control options and progestin-based menopausal relief drugs.

American women turn too easily to these progestin drugs, both for birth control and for fast relief from menopausal symptoms. As we will also see later in this chapter, there are other, much safer options women can choose today, options that offer effective birth control, hormonal balancing, and menopausal relief.

In September 2010, a study published in the influential academic journal *Nature* revealed that an international team of medical researchers had finally traced some of the biological links between a man-made chemical, *progestin*, and breast cancer. This eight-member research team was headed up by the Austrian biologist Josef Penninger, and included the current President and CEO of Boston's Dana Farber Cancer Institute, Dr. Laurie Glimcher. Together, this blue-ribbon international group succeeded in their ten-year quest to identify and validate the steps that take place when the chemical, progestin, enters a woman's breast cells.[4] Significantly, this chemical is found in all types of birth control drugs, in some IUDs, and in all combination hormone replacement therapy (HRT) drugs (for menopausal relief).

Through their work with laboratory mice, the researchers were finally able to witness the horrible trajectory the progestin takes as it activates a specific protein called RANKL,[5] which in turn apparently assaults the mitochondria within breast cells. These attacks can cause significant damage to those tiny power batteries in our breast cells. And as we've already seen, once healthy, oxygen-processing mitochondria suffocate, these damaged organelles are able to connect with their cell's nucleus, initiating the formation of a breast cancer cell. The research team also described how these progestin-induced RANKL attacks can exponentially accelerate the ability of new and existing breast cancer cells to duplicate. The faster a cancer cell duplicates, of course, the more quickly breast tumors can form and grow.

Here are excerpts from the press release in which Dr. Penninger's Vienna-based Institute of Molecular Biotechnology (IMBA) announced their findings to the world. Their press release cautions the public about the clear and present danger of using birth control drugs and progestin-based HRT drugs. Curiously, the online news digest *Science Daily* appears to be the only US media outlet that carried this life-saving news.[6]

How HRT and the Pill Can Lead to Breast Cancer

Medical scientists have uncovered how hormone replacement therapy can increase the risk of breast cancer,...the link is a protein molecule RANKL, which is essential to regulate bone mass, and which is also involved in milk production. The...researchers have shown that a synthetic progesterone, frequently used in HRT and hormonal contraception, can switch on the activity of RANKL within breast cells, causing them to divide and multiply and preventing them from dying when they should. Moreover, stem cells in the breast become able to renew themselves, ultimately resulting in breast cancer.

Breast cancer is one of the most common cancers, affecting up to one in eight women during their lives in Europe, the UK and USA. Large population studies such as the Women's Health Initiative and the Million Women Study have shown that synthetic sex hormones called progestins used in hormone replacement therapy, HRT, and in contraceptives can increase the risk of breast cancers...

> Now medical researchers...have identified a key mechanism which allows these synthetic sex hormones to directly affect mammary cells...
>
> "Ten years ago, we formulated the hypothesis that RANKL might be involved in breast cancer and it took us a long time to develop systems to prove this idea," says Prof. Josef Penninger. "I have to admit it completely surprised me just how massive the effects of the system were. Millions of women take progesterone derivatives in contraceptives and for hormonal replacement therapy."
>
> This work was an international collaboration between lead researchers at IMBA and scientists at the Medical University of Vienna; the Garvan Institute of Medical Research, Sydney, Australia; the Ontario Cancer Institute, University of Toronto, Toronto, Canada; Harvard School of Public Health, Harvard Medical School and the Ragon Institute of MGH/MIT and Harvard, Boston, USA; the Institute for Genetics, Centre for Molecular Medicine (CMMC), and Cologne Excellence Cluster (CECAD), University of Cologne, Germany; University College London, UK; and the University of Erlangen-Nuremberg, Germany.
>
> *IMBA Press Release, October 1, 2010*

Progestin: A Required Ingredient in All Birth Control Drugs

All birth-control drugs contain a chemical hormone called *progestin*. This chemical mimics a pregnant woman's high progesterone level. Progestin is able to stop new eggs from dropping into the uterus, protecting a woman from an unwanted pregnancy. In progestin-laced IUDs, the chemical changes the chemistry of the mucous in a woman's cervix. The progestin stops live sperm from entering the uterus.[7]

Many women feel funny when they start using some form of progestin birth control—whether in the form of a pill, a vaginal ring, an implant, an injection, or a progestin-laced IUD.[8] Complaints include weight gain, depression, lack of libido, insomnia, hair loss, a weakened immune system, and increased body hair.[9] This is probably because a woman quickly stops making her own natural progesterone once she begins using a progestin birth control drug. This is too bad since our natural hormone, progesterone, has any number of important health functions. When using the chemical progestin instead, a woman is robbing her body of:

- Better sleep, due to normal melatonin levels[10]
- A stronger immune system[11]
- Normal serotonin levels that prevent or minimize depression[12]
- A solid libido[13]

What about the *estrogen* in contraceptive drugs? What kind of estrogen is used in birth control drugs today? Is this estrogen also a manmade chemical, or is it natural? During the 1960s, when "the Pill" (as it was then called) was first developed, birth control drugs all contained high amounts of estrogen derived from the urine of pregnant mares (hence the brand name, Premarin: *pregnant mare's urine*). Most of today's contraceptive drugs still contain Premarin, but at significantly lower levels than before. And now, with the 2010 publication of the Penninger/Glimcher team's laboratory study, we can see clearly that the progestin chemical used in these drugs, has always been, and continues to be a significant instigator and accelerator of breast cancer in many women while using these drugs.[14]

For readers with some background in cell biology, here is how the team describes their historic discovery of this progestin–breast cancer link:

> *"…synthetic progesterone derivatives (progestins) such as medroxy-progesterone acetate (MPA), used in millions of women for hormone replacement therapy and contraceptives, markedly increase the risk of developing breast cancer. Here we show the **in vivo**[15] administration of MPA triggers massive induction of the key osteoclast differentiation factor RANKL (receptor activator of NF-KB ligand)[16] in mammary-gland epithelial cells…These data show that the RANKL/RANK system controls the incidence and onset of progestin-driven breast cancer."[17]*

Translated once more into everyday English, and framed within the context of the metabolic understanding of cancer,[18] the Penninger-Glimcher team found that progestin activates a protein called RANKL. This protein then apparently mounts massive assaults on healthy, oxygen-processing mitochondria within breast cells. At some point, these cumulative assaults cause the mitochondria in women's healthy breast cells to suffocate. As described in Chapter 1, those mitochondria can then transform themselves into sugar-loving, fermenting, duplicating breast cancer cells. If these cells are not destroyed by a woman's immune system,[19] that single breast cancer cell can go on to replicate itself endlessly—forming more cells that eventually become invasive breast tumors.[20]

Progestin Discovery Wins $7.4 Million Award

This 2010 research by the Penninger-Glimcher team was apparently a huge deal among those working in the breast cancer drug industry. It was such a monumental discovery that two years later, the highly selective congressionally-funded Breast Cancer Research Program (BCRP) awarded Dr. Penninger its coveted $7.4 million annual *Innovator Award*. The award was given to help the Austrian scientist test if an existing osteoporosis drug, Amgen's denosumab (XGEVA), that slows RANKL's activity in bones, could also be used as a breast cancer prevention drug in women who are born with a genetic mutation that gives them an increased breast cancer risk.[21]

The National Breast Cancer Research Program (NBCRP) is a small government agency that prides itself on funding unique projects that can create a tangible impact on the prevention and treatment of breast cancer throughout the US. However, this agency has not yet taken the opportunity to announce the Penninger-Glimcher Team's findings to the US public. Nor has the breast cancer research group yet taken the opportunity to fund the design of an obvious effective intervention into our rising national breast cancer rates, now facing premenopausal women. One way the NBCRP might intervene, is to fund a public information and education campaign to help premenopausal women calmly switch from using progestin-based birth control drugs and progestin IUDs to equally effective progestin-free contraceptive options. (see Chapter 10)

Today, almost a decade after this direct link between birth control drugs and increasing breast cancer in our premenopausal women was published, the American public and our primary care providers still remain unaware that younger women are unnecessarily increasing their risk of developing breast cancer as each day they continue to use birth control drugs or continue to keep a progestin-laced IUD in their bodies. Today premenopausal women in the US are experiencing an all-time high breast cancer incidence with about 72 out of every 100,000 women of child-bearing age developing breast cancer each year.[22] This is a higher incidence than breast cancer rates facing women of all ages living in Eastern European countries today!

Epidemiologists also tell us that 20,000 deaths were averted within a five-year period among postmenopausal women in 2002, once the public had been informed by the National Institutes of Health of the connection between using progestin HRT drugs and developing breast cancer. Three million women in the US quickly stopped filling their progestin prescriptions, knocking down breast cancer incidence and subsequent deaths among this older population within just the next few years.[23] How many more deaths can now be averted in the next five years once we begin helping young women switch off of their progestin-based contraceptive IUDs and pills? It is time to help women choose equally effective hormone-free contraceptive options instead.

To his credit, Dr. Penninger has twice now tried to share this important news with women, worldwide. Here are excerpts from his second press release, where he again mentions the dangerous connection between contraceptive drugs and breast cancer risk. This 2012 release, also issued by his Vienna-based institute, is announcing the scientist's $7.4 million research award from the U.S. Breast Cancer Research Program. This 2012 press release was distributed to many thousands of media outlets on every continent.[24] Once again, the online journal *Science Daily* appears to be the only American media outlet to publish this piece of news.[25]

In 2012, when I first discovered both of these press releases from Dr. Penninger's research institute, I published a notice on my *Busting Breast Cancer* blog, and published a short e-book: *Learn the Terrible Truth: Birth Control Drugs and Breast Cancer*.[26] I had long believed there had to be a biological connection between progestin and the development of breast cancer. Why else had I run into the same story over and over again? In dozens of statistical studies, conducted by a wide variety of epidemiologists and published in numerous scholarly journals over the past few decades, the results were always the same: *Using all types of birth control drugs which contain progestin, and progestin-based HRT drugs, increases a woman's risk of breast cancer.*[27]

To follow up this new knowledge with data, a Busting Breast Cancer study compared estimated annual breast cancer incidence for US premenopausal women under 45 years old, for the five year period between 2007 and 2011. Using breast cancer incidence data published by the American Cancer Society in their biennial booklets, "Breast Cancer Facts and Figures,"[28] our calculations show that this group of premenopausal women suffered nearly a twelve percent increase in invasive breast cancer incidence over these five years. No other age groups, according to the Cancer Society's data, experienced anything close to this increase in breast cancer. In fact, the data showed that the next group of women, those between the ages of 45 and 64, faced a less-than-one-percent increase in breast cancer incidence over this same time period.[29] Was this because most women within this menopausal and postmenopausal age group of 45-64 stopped taking progestin HRT drugs during the fall of 2002, once the huge National Health Initiative study publicly announced a significant connection between progestin HRT and breast cancer?[30]

Breast Cancer Advance Wins $7.4m US for Austrian Research Institute[25]

22-Oct-2012 5:50AM EDT, by Institute of Molecular Biotechnology

A new approach to possible future prevention of breast cancer and slowing the spread of tumors has won Austrian researcher Josef Penninger, director of the Institute of Molecular Biotechnology of the Austrian Academy of Sciences (IMBA) in Vienna, a $7.4 million innovator's award to continue his research, from the USA's Congressionally Directed Medical Research Program.

Newswise—The innovator's award recognizes Josef Penninger's work in identifying a key molecular pathway how hormone replacement therapies and contraceptive pills can lead to breast cancer. His team provided the first genetic proof that a protein called RANKL is the master regulator of bone loss, which has contributed to the development of a novel drug already approved for the treatment of osteoporosis and skeletal related events in multiple cancers. He was also the first to discover that RANKL not only regulates bone loss but is absolutely essential to enable sex hormone driven lactation in pregnant females, a finding that could explain further the connection between sex hormones and bone loss. Based on these groundbreaking findings, Penninger's group went on to show that RANKL is indeed a missing link between sex hormones, in particular the sex hormone progesterone, and breast cancer, leading to the hypothesis that RANKL is a key driver of breast cancer initiation.

...Supported by the $7.4 million award, Josef Penninger intends to further use this knowledge to develop a new diagnostic method that helps in making predictions concerning the chances that any patient will develop breast cancer. At risk patients will then be able to start preventative treatment using the existing RANK ligand-blocking medicines. Josef Penninger adds: "If our experimental data could be extrapolated to humans, which is what we strongly believe, then we might have an entirely novel way of early breast cancer detection and, since RANKL inhibition is already used in patients, we even would have a medicine within immediate reach that could be used to possibly prevent the disease in those women at high risk."

Institute of Molecular Biotechnology, "Breast Cancer Advance Wins $7.4m US for Austrian Research Institute," newswire.com, Oct 22, 2012.

Behind the Historic Discovery of the Progestin–Breast Cancer Link

Here is some background on two researchers who have played key roles, among many, in discovering this critically important biological link between progestin-based drugs and breast cancer.

Dr. Josef Penninger had already been called the most brilliant scientist of the twenty-first century.[31] Even before his international team's

2010 discovery of the link between progestin and breast cancer, Dr. Penninger had been the first to show how the bone disease, osteoporosis, is also connected to this same RANKL/RANK protein combo. As a principal investigator at the Amgen Institute in Toronto from 1995-2002, Dr. Penninger had used his RANKL/RANK discovery to enable Amgen to develop numerous bone protection drugs still on the market today.[32] A press release by Amgen in April of 2010,[33] announcing the breast cancer link, was further described in the Penninger-Glimcher Team's *Nature* article in October of that year, along with a related article in the same issue, by current Amgen researchers.[34] Penninger's 2012 award of $7.4 million from American taxpayers was apparently given to test Amgen's existing osteoporosis drug, denosumab, as a breast cancer prevention or treatment drug. This was the same drug that Dr. Penninger had developed years earlier, when employed by Amgen Institute.[35]

Dr. Laurie Glimcher, another high-profile member of Penninger's all-star team, was professor of immunology at the Harvard School of Public Health and professor of medicine at Harvard Medical School when she joined this progestin research group more than a decade ago. She later became dean of the Medical College at Weil Cornell Medicine in New York City, until she was named president and CEO of Dana Farber Cancer Institute in Boston in 2016.

From 1997 until 2017, Dr. Glimcher was also a board member of Bristol-Myers Squibb Pharmaceutical Company, for which she received $90,000, annually, plus company shares.[36] Bristol-Myers Squibb is now developing a male contraceptive drug that also uses progestin.[37]

In the summer of 2017, Dr. Glimcher announced she was giving up her board position with Bristol-Myers Squibb and jumped ship. She then joined the board of the British pharmaceutical company GlaxoSmithKline, almost doubling her annual board member compensation set at $160,000. Announcing her appointment to their board in July of 2017, GSK chairman Philip Hampton said that Dr. Glimcher had agreed to offer her "wealth of expertise in scientific and medical innovation and public health, which will be invaluable to GSK."[38]

Dr. Glimcher also continues to sit on the board of the Waters Corporation, where the annual median pay for directors has more than doubled over the past eight years to $336,360.[39] Waters offers cost-reduction manufacturing processes for progestin and other types of generic drugs.[40] Meanwhile, Dr. Glimcher has received millions of dollars in research funding over the years from Merck and Co., a worldwide leader in the birth control drug market.[41]

As Dana Farber's CEO, one of Glimcher's many responsibilities today is the cancer center's "Young and Strong Program for Young Women with Breast Cancer." The program was established in 2005 in response to the increasing numbers of young premenopausal women, those in their early forties and younger, who are now being diagnosed with invasive breast cancer.[42] According to a Dana Farber brochure, "The Young and Strong Program for Young Women with Breast Cancer offers young women with breast cancer (diagnosed at age 44 or younger) a personalized blend of clinical expertise, research discoveries, support, and education within a world-class cancer center." By 2018, Dana Farber's "Young and Strong Program" reported it had treated more than 4,500 premenopausal breast-cancer patients.[43]

To put a sour cherry on this bitter, progestin-filled cake, US treatment costs for young women under forty, during their first year after a breast cancer diagnosis, now averages $97,500—significantly more than first-year treatment costs for a postmenopausal woman with a similar diagnosis.[44] Meanwhile, as the silence about these progestin drugs continues, women of all ages, year after year, continue to stand in line each month, waiting to collect their supply of progestin-based birth control and progestin HRT drugs, still ignorant of the fact that these drugs are assaulting their breast cells' fragile mitochondria, day after day after day. American women are still unaware that these progestin-based drugs are increasing their risk of developing breast cancer by anywhere from 26 to 200 percent.[45]

Forty Years of Government Censorship and Orchestrated Confusion About Progestin

To be fair, the Breast Cancer Research Program, along with Dana Farber's CEO and the rest of the Penninger-Glimcher team, are only a few of the many people and organizations within government, academia and the entire breast cancer industry who have yet to share this life-saving information with the American public. Meanwhile, the *Physicians' Desk Reference (PDR)*, considered the physicians' bible, continues to ignore the existence of progestin as a unique chemical. Instead, both the *PDR* and the FDA websites make no distinction between natural *progesterone* and the various formulations of the carcinogenic chemical *progestin*. *Therefore, researchers and clinicians are able to overtly or in ignorance use these two terms interchangeably when discussing these two very different substances. Go figure!*[46]

This is not the first time this misleading situation has been discussed. In the many and ever-popular books jointly written by Dr. John Lee, Dr. David Zava, and Virginia Hopkins, the authors describe a woman's life-long need for natural progesterone, and the need to avoid the progestin chemical.[47] Their warnings have also been joined for decades by many functional health practitioners including Dr. Sherrill Sellman[48] and numerous grassroots women's health advocates.[49] All have repeatedly questioned this medically enforced or apparently orchestrated confusion around the two terms, *progesterone* and *progestin*.

Progestin-Based Hormone Replacement Drugs

Many older women have known since 2002 that some hormone replacement (HRT) drugs can increase breast cancer risk. Studies show that postmenopausal women who use a progestin-based hormone replacement drug face a 26 percent increased risk of invasive breast tumors. This double-digit breast cancer risk became widely known in the fall of 2002. That's when the National Institutes of Health announced it had just shut down its 16,000-woman Prempro study.[50] This study had made up one section of the NIH's $700-million, multifaceted National Health Initiative (NHI), which looked at multiple health benefits and liabilities surrounding postmenopausal women's use of two types of hormone replacement therapy (HRT) drugs. Project directors found that, among the thousands of women studied, 26 percent more of those being given the drug containing progestin were being diagnosed with palpable breast tumors, compared with those women taking a no-progestin placebo. Prempro study directors quickly sent letters to those taking the progestin-based medication, telling them to *stop taking this progestin/ estrogen drug.* Meanwhile, other women participating in a similar study, but using the estrogen-only drug known as Premarin, did not experience increased breast cancer diagnoses. This part of the NHI study continued.

Once the NIH put out a press release announcing the early cessation of their Prempro study, Wyeth Pharmaceutical saw its stock price drop 24 percent overnight. By the following month, half of the six million post-menopausal women in the United States who had been using Wyeth's Prempro stopped filling their monthly prescriptions.[51]

By the following year, US breast cancer rates for postmenopausal women decreased by 15 percent.[52] Women were elated. But Wyeth's investors weren't happy. The swift financial fallout from the aborted national study continued to hit Wyeth, as millions of older women refused to fill their Prempro prescriptions and physicians stopped prescribing the drug. Once they've got the facts, women and their physicians are not stupid enough to ignore them!

Decrease in Breast Cancer Rates Related to Reduction in Use of Hormone Replacement Therapy

Led by senior investigator Donald Berry, PhD, of the University of Texas M.D. Anderson Cancer Center, Houston, Texas, the research team showed that the decrease in breast cancer incidence began in mid-2002 and leveled off after 2003. Comparing rates from 2001 and 2004 showed a decrease in annual age-adjusted incidence of 8.6 percent. The decrease occurred only in women over the age of 50...*The speed at which breast cancer rates declined after the WHI announcements may indicate that extremely small ER-positive breast cancers may have stopped progressing, or even regressed, after HRT was stopped...*[53] [Emphasis added.]

"By the end of 2003, the use of hormone-replacement therapy had decreased by 38% in the U.S., with approx. 20 million fewer Prempro prescriptions written in 2003 than in 2002."[54]

Women who had developed breast cancer while taking Prempro sued. In 2009, the flailing Wyeth was acquired by the pharmaceutical giant Pfizer.[55] By 2012, Wyeth and Pfizer had jointly paid out $1.2 billion in court-related settlements from the harm caused to women by their progestin HRT drug.[56]

20,000 Unnecessary Deaths Averted in a Five-Year Period When Most Women in US Stopped Using Progestin HRT

"After the Women's Health Initiative's (WHI) (Prempro) study was released, HRT (hormone replacement therapy) use plummeted... and led to a drop in (national) breast cancer rates (for postmenopausal women) with about 100,000 fewer invasive tumors detected than expected, from 2002 to 2007. Using a 10-year mortality rate of about 20 percent, the report calculated that the reduction in postmenopausal women's progestin use may have prevented about 20,000 deaths in the U.S."[57]

Prempro and Birth Control Drug Sales Today

With memories of the National Institutes of Health's (NIH) stunning 2002 National Health Initiative's (NHI) Prempro study fading, and with the landmark 2010 discovery by the Penninger-Glimcher team of *exactly how* progestin or hormonal contraceptive drugs and progestin-laced IUDs cause breast cancer *still* being ignored by the federal government and by mainstream media, the sales of various progestin-based menopausal or "combination HRT" drugs are again on the upswing throughout the United States. In fact, worldwide revenues from all types of HRT drugs are expected to reach $3.3 billion by 2023, based on a compound annual growth rate (CAGR) of 4.2%.[58] Meanwhile, the increasing sales of progestin HRT drugs, combined with our increasing national obesity epidemic among postmenopausal women in the US, are all factors helping maintain today's unnecessary and disastrous breast cancer epidemic among older women.[59]

We've already seen that younger American women continue to experience the highest rates of premenopausal breast cancer in world history.

And as these women (along with the rest of the American public) remain in the dark about this now-proven link between progestin and breast cancer, it is business as usual. Today, the global market for birth control drugs is expected to increase annually by 5.1 percent (CAGR), reaching $26 billion by 2028. This same market was valued at just $13.3 billion in 2018. Younger American women's contribution to this expanding market is expected to continue to represent 40% of worldwide birth control drug sales.[60] This means breast cancer incidence rates and deaths from recurrent metastatic breast cancer, among premenopausal women will continue to increase, as will the cancer industry's income taken from this younger age group each year. Birth control drugs will continue to be a highly profitable "business as usual," so long as women and health care providers remain uninformed about the birth control drug-breast cancer connection.

What could happen to birth control drug sales once the Penninger-Glimcher team's discovery *finally* goes viral? How many fewer women under 50 will stop using these drugs and switch to safer, hormone-free contraceptive alternatives? How many thousands of young women—under 50 years old, under 40 years old, and those still in their teens, twenties and thirties—will find themselves better protected from a breast cancer diagnosis, simply by avoiding these progestin-based contraceptives? How far and how fast will breast cancer rates in our younger women each year begin to drop? How many fewer deaths from de novo and recurrent metastatic breast cancer will pre-menopausal women experience each year?

Only women have a self-interest in this financially powerful issue. Women's groups can now organize to release this information. Our national cancer agencies have a responsibility to keep the public, including our health care providers, the media, and especially women, informed of the dangers inherent in contraceptive drug use.[61] Every woman has the right to have the information she needs to make a fully informed choice about her contraceptive options and breast cancer risk level.

Birth Control Drugs: As American as Apple Pie

Doe-eyed Maura was weary and tense at the same time. The 53-year-old mother of two teens, part-time bookkeeper, an incredible professional house cleaner, and dear friend told me her nasty news. It was 2015. She had just been diagnosed with a stage I breast tumor, based on her mammogram screening.

"Did you ever take birth control pills?" I asked, as we tried to trace possible causes.

"My God, yes," she said. "Since I got out of high school—until three years ago, when I started to go through the pre or peri period...you know, when I stopped my regular periods."

"Did your doctor ever suggest having your tubes tied? Or that Dave have a vasectomy once you had the kids...or once you turned 40?" I asked.

"No!" she said. "We never talked about that stuff."

The US childbearing population comprises about 4.27 percent of the world's childbearing population.[62] But guess what? As we've already seen, the money spent on these drugs by US women accounts for about 40 percent of all birth control drug income worldwide. That's crazy! Why are US women shelling out almost half of the money generated by the worldwide contraceptive drug industry? Two answers: (1) *government-sanctioned, direct-to-consumer advertising*[63] and (2) *government-sanctioned, industry-controlled drug prices.*[64]

Birth Control Drug Sales Skyrocket (1997–current day)

Depending on your age, you may remember when, all of a sudden, Budweiser, Barbies, and Mr. Clean advertisements disappeared from your TV screen, replaced by ads for Yaz, Beyaz, other birth control drugs, diabetes, metastatic cancer drugs and Viagra.[65] This big switch began to happen in 1997, when the pharmaceutical companies convinced then-President Clinton to relax existing direct-to-consumer (DTC) advertising regulations. Now, the big pharma companies had government permission to spend as much money as they wanted on TV, magazine, and internet advertising, encouraging consumers to buy their drugs and medical devices. At the same time, the expanded DTC advertising regulations allow pharmaceutical companies to take their advertising costs as a tax deduction. This has the net effect of increasing industry profits, while lowering our national tax revenues.[66] "In 1997, drug companies spent roughly $17.1 billion to market their prescription drugs. By 2016, that figure was $26.9 billion. Simultaneously, total U.S. consumer and government spending on all prescription drugs skyrocketed from $116.4 billion to $320 billion."[67]

Figure 4.1: World's Childbearing Females

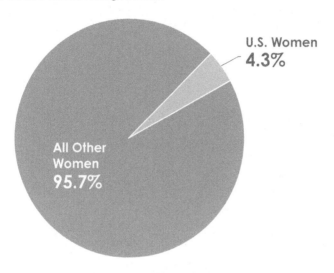

Premenopausal women in the US comprise only 4.3 percent of women globally of childbearing-age.

Jacquie Ostrom, Busting Breast Cancer Study 2012, updated 2020.

Given this new advertising bonanza, birth control drug sales in the US went crazy. Now more than merely an easy, popular, and effective contraceptive method, some of these birth control drugs were advertised as *lifestyle drugs*. Advertisements pushed these progestin drugs as a quick and easy way for millions of teens and women to chemically rebalance their hormones and limit their monthly periods.[68] Suddenly, acne, PMS, and other hormonal imbalance issues in teens and younger women might be solved with a pop of that daily progestin pill.[69]

Today, the United States and New Zealand continue to be the only major countries in the world that allow direct-to-consumer advertising of prescription drugs. In contrast, the European Union, with their variety of government-paid, consumer-oriented, Medicare-for-all healthcare systems, have always opposed such practices. These governments believe such ads dilute physicians' opinions and raise government drug costs.[70]

Figure 4.2: Worldwide Contraceptive Drug Market

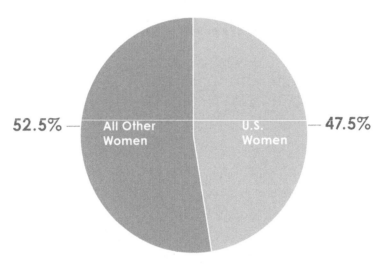

52.5% — All Other Women   U.S. Women — 47.5%

Given the high price of contraceptive drugs in the US, and high percentage of users compared to other countries, women in the US account for about half of international pharma's revenue from hormonal birth control sales.

Jacquie Ostrom, Busting Breast Cancer, 2012 (updated 2020).

As birth control drug sales in the US increased in the 1990s, continuing through 2010, so did breast cancer diagnoses in women under 50 years old. A *Busting Breast Cancer* study, conducted in 2012, illustrated that premenopausal women's risks of developing breast cancer began increasing by an estimated one percent each year in the mid-1980s, or possibly even earlier. By 2008, our study, based on data from three diverse states, shows this rate reached 70 breast tumors diagnosed for every 100,000 women under 50 years old.[71] During the past ten years, US women have begun to increase their use of progestin-based IUDs, instead of progestin-based pills.[72] And so it is not surprising, I suppose, that premenopausal women continue to develop invasive breast cancer at world record-breaking rates. By 2016, the North American Association of Central Cancer Registries (NAACCR) indicated this number was again on the upswing. Today in the United States, breast cancer incidence for women under 50 years old has reached an all-time high of 72 per 100,000 per year.[73]

Meanwhile, the North American contraceptive drug market continues to lead the world. US leadership reflects both the total number of women still utilizing these progestin products and the higher costs that US women and their private and government insurers must pay for these drugs. Are continuing high birth control drug sales just one more ingredient behind that unpublished 2015 National Cancer Institute Study predicting a 50 percent increase in women's breast cancer rates by 2030?[74]

Breast Cancer and Birth Control Drugs: The Statistical Studies

Andrea, a registered nurse from Dallas, emailed me in 2012. Her 39-year-old friend, Sharon, had just died from triple-negative breast cancer. Andrea had read a recent *Busting Breast Cancer* blog post in her search for answers.

"Your website says that birth control drugs are high risk and should be avoided, and that alternative forms of birth control should be implemented," she wrote. "Can you please discuss this with me? I really am trying to do all I can to spread your information. Thanks for listening."

Andrea's friend Sharon had been married to a fundamentalist Christian who did not believe in birth control. Sharon had quietly used Depo Provera injections and Norplant subdermal implants, two types of long-term progestin-based contraceptive drugs, for fifteen years before having a child. Sharon found her aggressive breast tumor a few months after her son was born. She endured the highly toxic and invasive cancer center treatments during two recurrences of her original triple-negative breast cancer diagnosis, before dying four years later.

Even before I began my twelve years of focused research into the possible cultural, environmental and biological causes of this ongoing national breast cancer epidemic, I already believed that progestin-only birth control drugs put women at higher risk for breast cancer than the combination estrogen-progestin drug. Why was it that every few years, I would read another short article that briefly described a new study showing that progestin-only birth control injections or long-term progestin-only patches carried a higher breast cancer risk than other types of contraceptive drugs?[75] In 2010, as I systematically started to review dozens of statistical studies describing health risks for various groups of women, currently using birth control drugs, I began working under the guidance of Dr. Margo Woods, a recently retired professor of nutrition at Tufts Medical School. Dr. Woods had published dozens of epidemiological studies over the years, looking at nutritionally related HIV–AIDS treatments while also studying breast cancer incidence.[76] A decade earlier, she had been part of the National Health Initiative—that $700 million definitive NIH study on health benefits and liabilities facing postmenopausal women when using HRT drugs, including the aborted Prempro or progestin study.[77]

Before I met Dr. Woods in 2010, she and I had separately wondered why the National Institutes of Health had never followed up its startling 2002 progestin drug study with a similar nationwide study of the relationship between birth control drugs and breast cancer. After all, every birth control drug sold in the United States today contains, on average, ten times more progestin than the Prempro HRT drug.[78]

When Margo and I began working together, she mentioned the 2002 Marchbanks study. This was considered by mainstream medicine to be the single most important national birth control drug safety study. The Marchbanks study (known formally as the Women's Contraceptive and Reproductive Experiences or CARE study), was still being cited by every breast cancer agency and corporate-funded breast cancer foundation eight years later. This particular study was always trotted out as the "definitive proof" that there was no connection between progestin birth control drugs and women of all ages developing cancer. Here is how one researcher described this 2002 national study: "The largest modern study, published in 2002, enrolled more than 4500 patients with breast cancer and 4500 controls aged 35 to 64 years from the United States from 1994 to 1998. Key findings included no breast cancer risk among current or former OC users and no risk associated with duration of use or dose of estrogen."[79]

Continuing to work together for many months during 2010 and 2011, Margo and I now questioned how the CARE study could show "no breast cancer risk among current or former OC (oral contraceptive) users." How, exactly, was this feasible, in light of the results from the 2002 Prempro study? Dr. Woods and I decided to begin our work together by unpacking the data from this much-touted Marchbanks study that supposedly showed "no significant breast cancer risk while using birth control drugs."

It did not take the two of us very long to realize that the Marchbanks (or CARE) study was useless for our purposes. The study, amazingly enough, had not included younger women who were *currently* using birth control drugs. The study, headed up by veteran CDC epidemiologist Dr. Polly Marchbanks, had also not included any women under 35 years old. This seemed more than odd, since birth control drug use is highest among women under 35 years old. Specifically, "Almost 1 woman out of 4, aged 15–24 (22.4%), was currently using the pill in 2014, compared with about 1 woman in 12 aged 35–44 (8.7%)."[80] Around 2000, birth control drug use among younger women was even higher,[81] since the only available IUD in the US at the time was the hormone-free Paragard. (Recently, however, all types of IUDs are becoming much more popular.)[82] Correspondingly (and confusingly), only four percent of the 9,200 women in Dr. Marchbanks' study were currently using contraceptive drugs. This was, again, quite strange, because the Marchbanks study's results had long been used by pharmaceutical companies, federal cancer agencies, and corporate-funded breast cancer foundations as *proof* that oral contraceptives are safe for women of all ages, *while using them.*

Why create a national study meant to show the actual risks of "current use of birth control drugs," and then exclude those women (those under age 35) who are the drugs' main customers? And why include only 372 women currently using these drugs, out of the 9,000 women in the study, if you are studying "current use"?[83]

The Marchbanks Study's Headlines: A Perfect Example of Telephone

Remember playing a childhood game called "Telephone"? Or maybe you knew it as "Gossip"? Everyone sits in a circle and the first person whispers a statement into the next person's ear, which is then whispered into the next person's ear. By the time the statement has traveled around the circle, the original statement, "The large dog is on the bed," has turned into something like, "The lousy dough is so big."

As soon as *The New England Journal of Medicine* published Dr. Marchbanks' study in June 2002, the CDC headlined the new report as the largest government analysis to date of any study examining a connection between current use of birth control drugs and breast cancer.

Here is how the CDC's press release described Marchbanks' newly released CARE study:

> *"Women who took oral contraceptives at some point in their lives are no more likely to develop breast cancer between the ages of 35 and 64 than are other women the same age, according to findings from the National Institute of Child Health and Human Development (NICHD) Women's Contraceptive and Reproductive Experiences Study (Women's CARE)."*[84]

In this same press release, Dr. Marchbanks was quoted as saying, "These results are good news. For women 35 to 64 years old, this study provides reassurance that oral contraceptives do not increase the risk of breast cancer."[85]

Once the national media began reporting on the study, each new headline kept inferring or saying outright that a woman's current use of birth control drugs has virtually no impact on breast cancer risk:

- "Study Finds No Association Between Oral Contraceptive Use and Breast Cancer for Women 35 and Over"[86]
- "Study: The Pill Is Not Linked to Cancer"[87]

Fortunately, Marchbanks' fellow epidemiologists were not fooled by the headlines, nor by the design of the actual study. In an unknown number of letters to *The New England Journal of Medicine's* editors, epidemiologists formed a unison chorus complaining that Dr. Marchbanks' database had not focused on women *currently* using birth control drugs, nor did the study focus on *younger* women! These researchers insisted that Dr. Marchbanks' study was not able to prove "no increased risk of breast cancer while using hormonal contraceptives."[88] Why had the CDC seemingly misrepresented their own research?

Thanks to this immediate outcry from her peers, Dr. Marchbanks was forced to release a second statement, published a few months later, again in *The New England Journal of Medicine*. This time, in response to three of these letters to the editor that disputed the CARE study's design and results, which were also published that month by the journal, Dr. Marchbanks came clean. Without admitting guilt for her previous misleading statements or for the study's design, she wrote the following "clarification": "We restricted our study to relatively older women (35 to 64 years old) because we were primarily interested in resolving the longstanding question of whether former use of oral contraceptives would increase the risk of breast cancer later in life."[89]

But never mind. For the next decade, many individual researchers, along with the National Cancer Institute, the CDC, the Susan G. Komen for the Cure Foundation, the American Cancer Society, and other pharmaceutical industry-funded breast cancer groups continued to trot out Marchbanks' CARE Study as their "proof," assuring American women and their physicians that using progestin-based contraceptive drugs does not significantly increase a young women's risk of developing invasive breast cancer.[90]

As we learned at the beginning of this chapter, the Penninger-Glimcher team lowered the boom on progestin. In 2010, their blue-ribbon team proved the unthinkable. The group showed the scientific world exactly how the progestin in birth control drugs—and in progestin-based HRT drugs—is biologically linked to the origin and acceleration of a lot of breast cancer in many current drug users. Just don't tell the American public what these researchers discovered! The news might demolish the current and expected US birth control drug market.

"Just the Facts, Ma'am": The Birth Control Drugs and Breast Cancer Statistical Studies

For decades, epidemiological research has shown that women who use progestin-only birth control drugs, such as Depo Provera injections and Norplant subdermal implants, are at even higher risk of breast cancer than women who use combination birth control drugs containing both estrogen and progestin.[91] During our time working together in 2010 and

2011, Dr. Woods and I were also able to uncover dozens of epidemiological studies that consistently described how certain groups of women face even higher rates of breast cancer than the general population of progestin drug users. Most of this research has been conducted by recognized breast cancer epidemiologists. Here are short descriptions of a sampling of these studies; each of these is either a meta study (i.e., a study of many studies) or it has been chosen to illustrate a trend we found after reviewing dozens of similar reports.

Women under 35 years old who are using contraceptive drugs have a 91 percent higher risk for developing breast cancer than women who use hormone-free contraception, according to a 2003 study by Dr. Marilyn Althuis of the University of Maryland.[92]

Women under 45 years old who have continually used contraceptive drugs since their teens are twice as likely to develop the aggressive estrogen-negative HER-2/neu breast cancer, compared with women of the same age group who have not been using contraceptive drugs from an early age, according to a 1999 study done by Dr. Marilie Gammon and her research team at the University of North Carolina at Chapel Hill.[93]

Women under 45 years old who used contraceptive drugs for more than a year are two-and-a-half times more likely to develop triple-negative breast cancer, compared with women who are not using contraceptive drugs, according to research published by Dr. Jessica Dolle's team in 2009 at the Fred Hutchinson Cancer Research Center in Seattle, Washington. That same year, Dr. Dolle's group also found that the longer a *woman of any age group* continues to use contraceptive drugs, the more likely she is to develop the often fast-growing triple-negative cancer over any other type of breast cancer.[94] Finally, as we've already seen, those under 45 years old who use the progestin-only Depo-Medroxyprogesterone Acetate (DMPA) have a 2.2-fold increase in breast cancer incidence, compared to their peers who do not use this injectable progestin contraceptive, according to a study by Dr. Christopher Li, another leading breast cancer epidemiologist at Seattle's Hutchinson Cancer Center.[95]

African American women of any age who use birth control drugs have a 15 percent higher risk of developing invasive breast cancer than Euro-American women who are also using birth-control drugs, according to a study by Boston University epidemiologist Lynn Rosenberg.[96] Other studies by Dr. Rosenberg show that African American women of any age who use contraceptive drugs have a greater risk of developing triple-negative breast cancer than African American women who are not using hormonal contraceptives.[97]

Women born with a mutated BRCA gene. About five percent of North American women are born with either a damaged BRCA1 or damaged BRCA2 tumor suppressor genes. According to the University of Toronto breast cancer epidemiologist Dr. Steven Narod, these individuals (or *BRCA women*) who live in North America take on an additional 50 to 80 percent increased risk of developing invasive breast cancer in their lives if they use contraceptive drugs before age 30, or if they use contraceptive drugs for more than five years, compared with other North American BRCA women who do not use contraceptive drugs during these same time periods.[98]

Women who have never given birth (non-parous women). In 2006, Dr. Christopher Khalenborn, a dedicated family practitioner and antiabortion activist, published his highly transparent landmark meta-study (a study of studies) in the academic journal *Mayo Clinic Proceedings*. Dr Khalenborn illustrated, for the first time, that women who used birth control drugs prior to a full-term pregnancy increase their risk of developing breast cancer by at least 44 percent, compared to their peers who did not use hormonal contraceptives before their first full-term pregnancy. Like many such studies that criticize birth control drugs, Dr. Khalenborn's study was never mentioned in any US media outlet.[99]

Progestin Causes Breast Cancer: A Long and Muffled History

At a yard sale in 2012, I picked up *What the Dog Saw and Other Adventures*, a book of essays by popular *New Yorker* writer Malcolm Gladwell.[100] Happily flipping through my new 50-cent purchase, I found the piece "John Rock's Error: What the Co-inventor of the Pill Didn't Know About Menstruation Can Endanger Women's Health." I sucked in my breath and began to read.

It turns out that John Rock, an inventor of the first contraceptive drug approved by the US Food and Drug Administration in 1960, could only make an effective and profitable birth control drug if he combined an animal estrogen with a synthetic, patented form of the progesterone hormone *progestin*.[101] This chemical would stop unwanted pregnancies. But Rock always wondered how this new chemical might affect young women's health. By 1983, Dr. Malcolm Pike, a South African medical statistician, and his associate, Dr. Brian Henderson, published the first study to show an increased rate of breast cancer in young women who used these new progestin drugs. Their study showed that a group of very young Euro-American women in Los Angeles who began using these progestin-based drugs before they turned 25 years old experienced a fourfold increase in invasive breast cancer diagnoses before their thirty-seventh birthdays.[102]

Big pharma was reportedly outraged by the epidemiologists' findings. In 1984, *New York Times* health reporter Lara Marks published a dramatic story describing Dr. Pike being publicly hounded by disgruntled pharma representatives for his critical study of their birth control drugs.[103]

"We were all trying to work out, how the hell we could fix the Pill. We thought about it day and night," researcher Malcolm Pike told Gladwell as the two Malcolms discussed Rock's original progestin pill and Pike's first decades of research on contraceptive drugs. Gladwell wrote: "Pike saw nothing natural about subjecting the breast to that heavy a dose of progestin. In his view, the amount of progestin...needed to make an effective contraceptive was much greater than the amount needed to keep the reproductive system healthy."[104]

Those Birth Control Pill Packet Inserts: What Do They Say Today?

I had only been using birth control drugs for a few years, back in the early 1970s, before I switched to a hormone-free IUD for the next ten years. What made me stop and say, "No!" to those birth control drugs so quickly?

- Was it my doctor who turned me against them? Nope. My doctor had prescribed them.

- Was it the fact I had developed a grapefruit-sized benign ovarian cyst, seemingly overnight, after only a few years on the pill? Well, that certainly gave me pause and an impetus to begin my research.

- Was it the information in that thin, folded, single-page insert that came with my monthly pill packet? Certainly not. Back then, the FDA didn't yet require pharmaceutical companies to include current research on the drug's adverse health effects in that monthly packet.[105]

I eventually remembered what finally got me to swear off the pill. It was a little booklet, *For Physicians' Use*, that my Harvard Square doctor had illegally given me. I had ignored the booklet until developing that ovarian cyst.[106]

I also remembered, with a chuckle, that while the booklet itself wasn't illegal, his giving me the information and the prescription were! Back then, the Catholic-dominated Commonwealth of Massachusetts, where I was living, did not allow physicians to prescribe birth control drugs, or even give birth control information, to unmarried women like me! In fact, it wasn't until a US Supreme Court ruling in 1972 struck down the Massachusetts law that it became legal for physicians and pharmacies to distribute contraceptives to wanton single women, such as myself.[107] Hard to imagine, isn't it?

In any event, that physician's booklet, in matter-of-fact terms, said the drug increased my risk of developing high blood pressure, strokes, and invasive breast cancer. It also listed research studies done in the late 1960s that backed up all these statements. That was my last day of taking what we blithely called "the Pill."[108]

I quickly had a hormone-free IUD inserted in my uterus. My employer's insurance plan covered the $15 or $30 cost of this simply-designed, tiny copper coil (or "T"), along with my gynecology visit to insert the device. That copper coil provided me effective and virtually no-cost contraception for the next *ten years*! Back then, at least ten percent of American women were successfully using this same inexpensive, long-lasting copper coil (or another inexpensive, hormone-free IUD make or model).[109] By the late 1970s, the State Department's Population Control Program was purchasing hundreds of thousands of these simple, but incredibly effective, copper coils—known in the US today as the very expensive, $800–$1000 (at monopoly-based prices), hormone-free *Paragard*. Back then, however, this simple copper-coil medical device, created and patented by the nonprofit Population Council, cost less than $1.00 to manufacture. Each year, the US Agency for International Development purchased hundreds of thousands of these copper coils for about 50 cents each, for distribution to family planning clinics throughout Africa, Asia, and South America.[110]

The inexpensive IUD's popularity was shattered during the 1970s when a simple design flaw in a single IUD model, the Dalkon Shield, manufactured by A.H. Robins Company, caused infections in users. This situation enabled the pharmaceutical industry to mount an effective anti-IUD campaign among the US public. By the late 1970s and throughout the 1980s, the one-size copper coil, known today as the *Paragard*, was vertically integrated into a monopoly product overnight by Big Pharma, its price now set at $600.[111] The Paragard had become, and would remain for decades, the only IUD available on the US market.[112] Now American women were virtually limited to a single method of affordable effective reversible contraception, hormonal-based birth control drugs.

Beginning in the mid-1960s with the introduction of "the Pill," at least one small group of women was publicly worried about the various health effects women were experiencing while using this new type of chemical hormonal contraceptive.[113] In 1969, writer and women's health activist Barbara Seaman published her best-selling book, *The Doctors' Case Against the Pill*. Within a year, Senator Gaylord Nelson (D—Wisconsin), having read Seaman's hard-hitting narrative, immediately called for Senate hearings to examine the safety of these contraceptive drugs.[114] The Nelson Hearings resulted in helpful federal regulations, although these were not enacted until nine years later! The regulations require pharmaceutical companies to provide women with up-to-date medical information on these drugs. This information must be inserted into every birth control drug packet. The information packet must describe both the most up-to-date benefits and potential adverse medical issues connected to using these hormonal contraceptives. The FDA also requires these packet inserts to be "intelligible to the average reader."[115]

What do these packet inserts actually say today, I wondered. Is the FDA actually doing its job of clearly informing women about the known breast cancer risks when using these progestin birth control drugs? I decided to find out.

House-sitting in Key West back in the summer of 2010, I was looking for an afternoon break from all of this computer research. I called the nearby CVS on Truman and asked if I could pick up packet inserts for their four most popular brands of contraceptive drugs. The pharmacist was happy to give me company-published inserts for Yaz, Yasmin, BeYaz, and Ortho Tri Lo.

After biking home, I unfolded a huge, thin sheet of paper for Bayer Labs' *Beyaz* birth control pill. There, on the sun-drenched deck, I began scanning the very narrow columns, filled with very fine print. This was certainly not a user-friendly item; this took bright light and concentration. As I knelt on both knees, slowly working my way down the very long columns of tiny text, my outrage slowly started to compete with Key West's intense September sun. It was difficult to make sense out of Big Pharma's doublespeak.

Bayer Labs' insert, dated 2010, said (and this is the full, direct quote), "Women who currently have or have had breast cancer should not use Beyaz because breast cancer is a hormonally sensitive tumor. There is substantial evidence that COCs [combination oral contraceptives] do not increase the incidence of breast cancer.[116] Although some past studies have suggested that COCs might increase the incidence of breast cancer, more recent studies have not confirmed such findings." Huh? Adding to my simmering rage, Bayer's insert did not cite a single research study they were describing to back up their convoluted phrases. I was stunned.

Bayer's insert for their Yazmin brand was equally outrageous. First came more obfuscating language: "Various studies give conflicting reports on the relationship between breast cancer and oral contraceptive use. Oral contraceptive use may slightly increase your chance of having breast cancer diagnosed, particularly after using hormonal contraceptives at a younger age; women who currently have or have had breast cancer should not use oral contraceptives because breast cancer is a hormone sensitive tumor." Unbelievably, Bayer also did not mention the names of any of these studies it was referencing. How could a woman check out these research studies' definitions of "slight increase" or "conflicting"?

Ortho's narrative for its Ortho Tri-Cyclen Lo tablets also tried to downplay the documented links between *current use* of contraceptive drugs and an increased risk of developing breast cancer: "Various studies give conflicting reports on the relationship between breast cancer and oral contraceptive use; tell your health care provider if you have a history of breast cancer, etc." But unlike Bayer, Ortho cited 65 research studies. Upon a second look, however, all of these 65 studies on contraceptive drugs and breast cancer risks were dated between 1971 and 1983! None of the research done on current-day formulas (post 1980), such as the studies discussed earlier in this chapter, was included in Ortho's insert. Why was the FDA being so horribly negligent? Were any legislators or women's groups asking the FDA to finally follow the law and revise these information sheets to reflect the *known* health risks inherent in using these progestin-based birth control drugs?

Finishing up this chapter years later, I checked a few more inserts to see if they offered women any up-to-date research on the breast cancer risks of using these progestin drugs. In effect these "information sheets" currently include general platitudes about the drug's safety and no mention of a single research study. What about Planned Parenthood? Are they willing to counsel women on the risks and benefits of today's birth control drugs? What does this national network of nonprofit women's health clinics tell women about these progestin drugs and breast cancer? How do they inform or counsel women today when it comes to making safe contraceptive choices? Do they include the 2010 Penninger-Glimcher team's study? Do they describe the now-proven biological and increased statistical risks of developing breast cancer while a woman is using any type of hormonal drug or medical device?[117]

You, too, may be shocked and disappointed to find that Planned Parenthood's website doesn't contain a single study, or even a single sentence, about the increased risks of developing breast cancer while using birth control drugs or progestin-laced IUDs. Instead, Planned Parenthood appears to encourage women to use these hormonal contraceptives, both for birth control and for optimal health! Their website actually lists ten non-contraceptive benefits—from using these drugs. Go figure.

Planned Parenthood's Advice to Women Regarding Birth Control Drugs

Possible Side Effects and Risks: Possible side effects that usually last only the first three months include breast tenderness, headaches, irregular bleeding, and nausea. Some women also experience changes in their sex drive. Rare but serious health risks include blood clots, heart attack, stroke, increased blood pressure, liver tumors, gallstones, and jaundice—women who are over 35 and smoke are at a greater risk for some of these problems.

Non-Contraceptive Benefits of the Pill: Use of combined hormone oral contraceptives has many non-contraceptive benefits. These advantages include:

- reduced symptoms of endometriosis
- decreased chances of ectopic pregnancy
- less menstrual flow and cramping
- quick return of ability to become pregnant when use is stopped
- reduced acne
- reduced bone thinning
- reduced iron deficiency anemia related to menstruation
- reduced premenstrual symptoms
- reduced risk of ovarian and endometrial cancers
- shorter and more regular periods.

Planned Parenthood[118]

In the midst of so many studies that clearly outline the risk of using progestin contraceptives and other progestin drugs, I want to be clear: I am not recommending that birth control drugs or any other progestin drugs be banned; that is not my goal. I am, however, calling on the FDA and federal cancer agencies to immediately inform women and their doctors about exactly what biologists finally understand about how all progestin-based birth control drugs and menopausal drugs (including

Prempro, Activella, Femhrt and Ortho-Prefix) can significantly increase the risk of invasive breast cancer in women while they use these drugs.

The Terrific Truth about Hormone-free IUDs

"If your goal is to prevent a pregnancy...using an IUD would be the best way to do this."

—Dr. Tina Raine-Bennett Chair, Committee on Adolescent Health Care,Long-Acting Reversible Contraception Working Group, American College of Obstetricians and Gynecologists, October 2012[119]

In the fall of 2012, Dr. Penninger was quietly being given that $7.4 million Innovator Award to help develop a new breast cancer treatment drug to prevent or treat progestin-created breast cancer. At this same time, Dr. Raine-Bennett, of the American College of Obstetricians and Gynecologists, was encouraging American women to use an IUD instead of progestin-based contraceptive drugs. But Dr. Raine-Bennett, like 99% of others in the US, remained unaware of the Penninger-Glimcher team's shocking 2010 progestin discovery. Instead, a recent university study had shown that if women forget to refill their birth control drug prescription, an IUD becomes a more effective birth control option. These medical devices, inserted and removed by a health practitioner, remain surefire contraception for years at a time.[120]

Dr. Raine-Bennet's statement also drew attention to this recent Washington University study on birth control choices. College women,18 to 20 years old, had been offered their choice of free contraception for the next three years. Of the students surveyed, 71 percent chose an IUD.[121]

That's right, take away all of the expensive advertising for birth control drugs, and women are quite happy to use IUDs instead, especially if IUDs are affordable and fit well. But few women—and few physicians—understand that only hormone-free IUDs do not raise a woman's risk of developing breast cancer.[122]

Meanwhile, any woman in the US who wants to use a hormone-free IUD must pay that whopping $800 plus $200 clinic fee, to have this "one-size-fits-all" hormone-free Paraguard contraceptive device inserted. American women can thank the FDA for the outrageous price tag on this

50-cent copper coil. The twenty-year monopoly of the one and only hormone-free IUD sold in the US was created and continues to be enforced by the FDA.[123] No wonder so many uninsured and underinsured women in the US continue to purchase monthly packs of the progestin-based contraception drugs, when they can't come up with the $1,000 needed for a Paragard.

Why Does a 50-cent Medical Device Cost American Women $1,000?

Ten years ago, I discovered that Paragard was the only IUD on the US market—and its maker was charging women a price that reflected its monopoly status. I emailed the marketing director of Mona Lisa, a long-time European manufacturer of inexpensive and reliable IUDs that offered numerous models and sizes. "It would be good to offer American women something other than the overpriced, one-size-fits-all, hormone-free, $800 copper-coil Paragard," I wrote. "This will enable any number of uninsured, low-income women to stop using birth control drugs."

Their European marketing director emailed me back. "The problem is that copper IUDs are listed as pharmaceuticals in the US, whereas all over the world they are classified as medical products. New drugs (including IUDs classified as a drug) must undergo a 10-year double blind placebo-controlled study before it can gain FDA approval. To see our T-product in the US market with the features it has (e.g., in-situ time of 10 years), we at first would have to go for a 10-year study. That's the reason why we and other companies failed in registration of other IUDs in [the] US," Elizabeth Adomaitis wrote.[124]

Nothing has changed over the past two decades since the FDA reclassified the coil. Is this because the pharmaceutical lobby remains able to influence the FDA when it comes to birth control drugs and copper-coil IUDs? Would complaints and demands from enough grassroots women's groups make a difference? Can we find a majority of senators and representatives who are finally willing to put a woman's need for a variety of models, sizes and brands of affordable, hormone-free IUDs ahead of the pharmaceutical industry's need to keep birth control drug sales strong, by blocking a woman's ability to have an affordable, personally fitted hormone-free IUD in her uterus? Simply reclassifying hormone-free IUDs as medical devices will immediately allow dozens of various makes, models, and sizes of *affordable*, European-made hormone-free IUDs to be available to American women.[125]

Once this FDA regulatory change takes place, how much—and how soon—will we see breast cancer rates in premenopausal women begin to fall? Such grassroots political action will be exciting to watch as individual women, joining together, demanding change, are simultaneously able to help lower breast cancer rates, many women at a time!

Is an IUD in Your Vacation Plans?

Until women can pressure the FDA to reclassify hormone-free IUDS, other FDA regulations on pharmaceutical drugs continue to make access to this type of safe and effective contraception even more difficult for *uninsured* American women. For example, if you are able to purchase an affordable ($10) copper coil IUD in Canada, Mexico, or France, make sure you have it inserted there. Don't bring it back with you! The FDA prohibits Planned Parenthood or any licensed health practitioners from "administering foreign-purchased drugs."[126] In plain English, this means that current FDA regulations *prohibit a US health practitioner from inserting your newly imported, affordable, copper-coil IUD into your uterus!* Sadly, I can't make this stuff up.

Note: *Most of the increased use of IUDs among US women since 2007 represents those using the Mirena or another progestin-laced IUD brand. The one and only hormone-free IUD available, Paragard, as mentioned, represents a very small percentage of all IUDS inserted into women in the United States in recent years.*

Table 4.1: A Dozen Reasons Why Using A Hormone-Free IUD Makes Sense

Birth control Drugs	Hormone-Free IUDs
May increase risk of blood pressure	DOES NOT increase risk of blood pressure
May increase risk of blood clots	DOES NOT increase risk of blood clots

Smoking increases adverse effects	NO increased adverse effects from smoking
Lower sex drive	DOES NOT affect sex drive
Increased mood changes	DOES NOT affect moods
Higher breast cancer risk for non-parous women (those who have never had a full term pregnancy)	DOES NOT increase breast cancer risk in non-parous women (those who have never had a full-term pregnancy)
Cannot use while breastfeeding	Can use while breastfeeding
Must take daily	DO NOT take daily, weekly, monthly or annually
Can cause unbalanced hormone levels	DOES NOT affect hormone levels
Increases weight	DOES NOT increase weight
Must fill prescriptions regularly	NO prescriptions to fill

S. Wadia-Ells

A New Hormone-Free Contraceptive: "Smart Women's Choice"

Dr. Sherrill Sellman is a longtime functional medicine educator. Her pioneering and ongoing work helps women balance their hormones naturally and safely, with her podcasts, books, articles and lectures. She recently recommended I research a new kid on the block: a unique hormone-free and chemical-free birth control option for women.[127] "Smart Women's Choice" is an *inexpensive* vaginal cream, described as a new and more comfortable choice for couples who currently prefer to use condoms. The cream was discovered by accident many years ago by biochemist Dr. Francoise Farron, who used this "home-grown" method successfully for many years. Now 96 years old, Dr. Farron has become the unsung hero of many couples, who won't leave home without her afford-able "Smart Women's Choice" cream. How exactly does this cream work?

According to the video by Dr Farron, available on the Smart Women's Choice website, SWC is different from other contraceptives. It immobi-lizes the sperm in the vagina. An immobilized sperm cannot make the journey to the fallopian tubes, the only place where an egg can be fer-tilized. Without fertilization, it is impossible to become pregnant. SWC does not impact a woman's hormonal system. Instead, by immobilizing the sperm, the egg cannot be fertilized."[128]

Some Final Words

In this chapter, we've seen the development of today's birth control drugs, along with those "combination" menopausal relief drugs, all con-taining the chemical hormone *progestin*. We've also seen a landmark biological discovery, somehow kept from the public's eye since its publi-cation in 2010, illustrating how current-day progestin birth control and menopausal drugs are able to help cause and accelerate breast cancer in current users. We also reviewed a representative sampling of epide-miological studies on all of these subjects. Meanwhile, we learned that breast cancer rates in premenopausal women throughout the United States have continue to increase most years, since the 1990s, just as birth control drug sales have increased, given their heavy advertising. Also, the FDA's 1999 reclassification of all copper-coil IUDs as pharmaceuti-cal drugs, continues to block inexpensive European-made, hormone-free IUDs from the US market, creating today's ridiculous $800 monopoly price of the 50-cent hormone-free Paragard IUD. Thus, the FDA contin-ues to force US women to choose birth control drugs as their cheapest long-acting reversible contraceptive (LARC) option.

If you thought this discussion of the breast cancer risks of using birth control drugs and progestin IUDs was shocking, wait till you see what comes next! In Chapter 5, we'll consider another area of medical "sci-ence" that needs some debunking for the sake of breast cancer preven-tion. Shocking as it may seem at first, I'm going to encourage you to forgo mammograms and opt for thermograms, breast self-exams, clini-cal breast exams, and for some women, regular whole-breast ultrasound tests, or MRIs. Sound crazy? What if I told you that a Swiss medical board has now called for closing all mammogram clinics in that country and banning the creation of new mammogram centers? Confused? Intrigued? Read on.

CHAPTER ENDNOTES

1   Lina S. Morch et al., "Contemporary Hormonal Contraception and the Risk of Breast Cancer," *New England Journal of Medicine* 377 (December 7, 2017): 2228–39, https://doi.org/10.1056/NEJMoa1700732. Author's note: Study funded by birth control manufacturer, Novo Nordisk Foundation.

2   Daniel Schramek et al., "Osteoclast Differentiation Factor RANKL Controls Development of Progestin-driven Mammary Cancer," *Nature* 468, no. 7320 (November 4, 2010): 98–102, https://doi.org/10.1038/nature09387.

3   Thomas N. Seyfried, *Cancer as a Metabolic Disease: On the Origin, Management and Prevention of Cancer,* (New York, John Wiley and Sons) 2012; Also see Chapter 1.

4   Daniel Schramek et al., "Osteoclasts Differentiation Factor RANKL Controls Development of Progestin-driven Mammary Cancer," *Nature* 468, 98–102 (2010). https://doi.org/10.1038/nature09387.

5   RANKL: Receptor Activator of Nuclear Factor Kappa B Ligand (*molecular biology*)

    RANK: Receptor Activator of NF-B Ligand (from Acronymfinder.com).

6   Institute of Molecular Biotechnology, "How HRT and the Pill Can Lead to Breast Cancer: New Research Suggests Possible Treatment," *Science Daily* (October 1, 2010), https://www.sciencedaily.com/releases/2010/09/100929132051.htm.

7   Erika Gebel Berg, "The Chemistry of the Pill," *ACS Central Science* 1, no.1 (2015): 5–7, https://doi.org/10.1021/acscentsci.5b00066.

8   There are at least three progestin-based intrauterine devices available on the US market. Brand names are Mirena, Skyla, and Kyleena. Paragard is the only IUD available in the US that does not contain progestin.

9   The most helpful book on this topic remains John Lee, Virginia Hopkins & Jesse Hanley, *What Your Doctor May Not Tell You About Premenopause: Balance Your Hormones and Your Life from Thirty to Fifty* (New York: Warner Books, 1999).

10   J.P. Bonde, "Work at Night and Breast Cancer: Report on Evidence-based Options for Preventive Actions," *Scandinavian Journal of Work and Environmental Health* 38, no.4 (February 20, 2012): 380–90, https://doi.org/10.5271/sjweh.3282; Claudia M. Hunter and Mariana G. Figueiro "Measuring Light at Night and Melatonin Levels in Shift Workers: A Review of the Literature." *Biological Research for Nursing* 19, no. 4 (2017): 365–374, https://doi.org/10.1177/1099800417714069; S.M. Hill et al., "Melatonin and Associated Signaling Pathways that Control Normal Breast Epithelium and Breast Cancer," *Journal of Mammary Gland Biology and Neoplasia* 3 (September 16, 2011): 235–45A, https://doi.org/10.1007/s10911-011-9222-4. Sasha Tait, et al., "The Role of Glucocorticoids and Progesterone in Inflammation, Autoimmune Diseases and Infectious Diseases," *Journal of Leukocyte Biology* 84, No. 4 (October 2008): 924–31. https://doi.org/10.1189/jlb.0208104.

11   A.S. Tait, C.L. Butts and E.M. Sternberg, "The Role of Glucocorticoids and (Progesterone) Progestins in Inflammatory, Autoimmune, and Infectious Disease," *Journal of Leukocyte Biology* 84, no. 4 (July 2008): 924–931, https://doi.org/10.1189/jlb.0208104. Author's note: This article is also an example of how researchers often use the terms progestin(s) and progesterone interchangeably, making it very difficult to understand studies that point out the distinct differences between the chemical named *progestin* and the *natural progesterone hormone*. As reprinted on Applied Health.com, "Hormones do Effect [sic] the Immune System- Balanced Hormones= Active Immune System," *Journal of Applied Health* no. 118, https://appliedhealth.com/hormones-do-effect-the-immune-system/.

12   Philip J. Cowen and Michael Browning. "What Has Serotonin to Do with Depression?" *World Psychiatry* 14, no. 2 (2015): 158-60. doi:10.1002/wps.20229;

I.D. Glick and S.E. Bennett, "Psychiatric Complications of Progesterone and Oral Contraceptives," *Journal of Clinical Psychopharmacology* 1(6), November 1981: 350-67, https://journals.lww.com/psychopharmacology/Citation/1981/11000/Psychiatric_Complications_of_Progesterone_and_Oral.3.aspx.

13 Lauren Streicher, "When Taking the Pill Takes Away Your Sex Life," https://drstreicher.com/dr-streicher-blog/2015/8/when-taking-the-pill-takes-away-your-sex-life; Nerea M. Casado-Espada et al., "Hormonal Contraceptives, Female Sexual Dysfunction, and Managing Strategies: A Review," *Journal of Clinical Medicine* 8, no. 6 (June 25, 2019): https://doi.org/10.3390/jcm8060908.

14 Schramek et al., "Osteoclast Differentiation Factor RANKL," p. 98, https://doi.org/10.1038/nature09387; Lina S. Morch et al., "Contemporary Hormonal Contraception," p. 2228.

15 In vivo: experiments, often using mice, done within controlled laboratory setting.

16 RANK/RANKL are proteins.

17 Schramek et al., "Osteoclast Differentiation Factor RANKL," 98-99, https://doi.org/10.1038/nature09387.

18 Thomas N. Seyfried and Laura M. Shelton, "Cancer as a Metabolic Disease," *Nutrition & Metabolism* 7, no.7. (Jan. 2010), https://doi.org/10.1186/1743-7075-7-7.

19 See Chapter 3.

20 See Chapter 1.

21 Breast Cancer FY2012 Integration Panel, https://cdmrp.army.mil/bcrp/panels/panels12; V. Sigl, L. Jones and J.M. Penninger, "RANKL/RANK: From Bone Loss to the Prevention of Breast Cancer." *Open Biology* 6, no 11 (2016): 160230. https://doi.org/10.1098/rsob.160230; Breast Cancer Research Program, "RANKL/RANK Control BRCA1 Mutation-Driven Mammary Tumors," October 29, 2018, https://cdmrp.army.mil/bcrp/research_highlights/18josef_penninger_highlight.

22 Email from R. Sherman to author, May 31, 2019. Custom-generated data sheet. (See Chapter 9).

23 Rowan T Chlebowski & Garnet L Anderson, "Menopausal Hormone Therapy and Breast Cancer Mortality: Clinical Implications," *Therapeutic Advances in Drug Safety* 6, no.2 (2015): 45-56, https://doi.org/10.1177/2042098614568300.

24 See Newswise.com's media list: https://www.newswise.com/media/list.

25 Institute of Molecular Biotechnology, "Breast Cancer Advance Wins $7.4m US for Austrian Research Institute," newswire.com, Oct 22, 2012, https://www.newswise.com/articles/breast-cancer-advance-wins-7-4m-us-for-austrian-research-institute.

26 Susan Wadia-Ells, "Birth Control Drugs: Learn the Terrible Truth," in *Busting Breast Cancer: Volume 1* (BookBaby: Kindle Edition, 2012), https://www.amazon.com/Busting-Breast-Cancer-Control-Terrible-ebook/dp/B00AB6AM2Y.

27 M.C. Pike and B. Henderson, "Breast Cancer in Young Women and Use of Oral Contraceptives: Possible Modifying Effect of Formulation and Age at Use," *Lancet* 2, no. 8356 (October 22, 1983): 926-30, https://doi.org/10.1016/s0140-6736(83)90450-6; Nancy Krieger et al., "Decline in U.S. Breast Cancer Rates After the Women's Health Initiative: Socioeconomic and Racial/Ethnic Differentials," *American Journal of Public Health* 100, no. Suppl 1, S1 (April 2010): S132–39, https://doi.org/10.2105/AJPH.2009.181628.

28 American Cancer Society, "Breast Cancer Facts & Figures:2007-2008; ACS, "Breast Cancer Facts and Figures: 2009-2010; ACS, Also; phone conversation between author and ACS Data Development Office on breast cancer statistics related to women under 45 years old for 2011-2012, November 8, 2012.

29 Susan D. Wagner, "Why is Breast Cancer Increasing in Younger Women? You Probably Won't Like This Answer," March 7, 2013, *Modern Ghana*, https://www.modernghana.com/lifestyle/4429/4/why-is-breast-cancer-increasing-in-younger-women-y.html.

30 NIH, "Decrease in Breast Cancer Rates Related to Reduction in Use of Hormone Replacement Therapy," NIH.gov, April 18, 2007, https://www.nih.gov/news-events/news-releases/decrease-breast-cancer-rates-related-reduction-use-hormone-replacement-therapy.

31 Mary Rogan, "The Greatest Scientist of Our Time," *Esquire*, January 29, 2007. https://www.esquire.com/news-politics/a948/esq0701-july-penninger/.

32 Teiji Wada et al., "RANKL-RANK Signaling in Osteoclastogenesis and Bone Disease," *Trends in Molecular Medicine* 12, no. 1 (January 2006): 17–25, https://doi.org/10.1016/j.molmed.2005.11.007; Gina Colata, "Most Osteoporosis Drugs Don't Build Bone. This One Does," *The New York Times*, April 9, 2019, https://www.nytimes.com/2019/04/09/health/osteoporosis-evenity-bone-amgen.html.

33 Amgen, "Amgen Preclinical Study Demonstrated Anti-Tumor Activity in Mammary Tumor Model," press release, http://investors.amgen.com/news-releases/news-release-details/amgen-preclinical-study-demonstrated-anti-tumor-activity-mammary.

34 E. Gonzalez-Suarez et al, "RANK ligand mediates progestin-induced mammary epithelial proliferation and carcinogenesis," *Nature* 468 (2010):103–07, https://doi.org/10.1038/nature09495.

35 Kate Kelend, "Signs that Amgen Bone Drug May Block Breast Tumours," *Regulatory News* (September 29, 2010), https://www.reuters.com/article/cancer-breast-amgen/signs-that-amgen-bone-drug-may-block-breast-tumours-idUKLDE68R29E20100929.

36 US Securities & Exchange Commission, *Form 8-K/A. Bristol Myers Squibb Company*, January 20, 2015.

37 American Chemical Society, "A Step Toward a Birth Control Pill for Men," March 13, 2016, https://www.acs.org/content/acs/en/pressroom/newsreleases/2016/march/male-pill.html; Christina Wang and Ronald S. Swerdloff, "Hormonal Approaches to Male Contraception," *Current Opinion in Urology* 20, no. 6 (2010): 520-24, https://doi.org/10.1097/MOU.0b013e32833f1b4a; Ari Altstedter, "Male Contraceptive Blocked by Drug Companies who Make Billions from the Female Pill," April 4, 2017, *Independent*, https://www.independent.co.uk/news/business/news/male-contraceptive-block-drug-companies-examples-female-pill-injection-india-startup-big-pharma-a7665511.html.

38 Financial Times Markets, "GlaxoSmithKline PLC Directorate Change," July 21, 2017, 7553L, https://markets.ft.com/data/announce/full?dockey=1323-13303472-7GJ53KHTGQ6MEJQH57D0F66HGD.

39 Sacha Pfeiffer and Todd Wallack, "Few Hours, Soaring Pay for Corporate Board Members," *The Boston Globe*, Dec 2, 2015, See: Steven Clifford, *The CEO Pay Machine: How it Trashes America and How to Stop It* (New York: Blue Rider Press, 2017), 253; Rosanna Landis Weaver, "The 100 Most Over-paid CEOs," 40, https://corpgov.law.harvard.edu/2017/03/02/the-100-most-overpaid-ceos/.

40 Margaret Maziarz et al., "Streamlining the Analysis of Oral Contraceptives Using the ACQUITY UPLAC H-Class System," Waters Corporation, May 2013, https://www.gimitec.com//file/720004698en.pdf, accessed March 16, 2019.

41 "Harvard Allies with Merck & Co. on Osteoporosis Research," *Genetic Engineering and Biotechnology News*, April 9, 2008, https://www.genengnews.com/news/harvard-allies-with-merck-co-on-osteoporosis-research/; Melissa Bailey, "Recruited to Lead Harvard Med, 'Fearless' Scientist Chose Dana-Farber," March 1, 2016, statnews.com. https://www.statnews.com/2016/03/01/laurie-glimcher-dana-farber/.

42 Carey K. Anders et al., "Breast Cancer Before Age 40 Years," *Seminars in Oncology* 36, no.3 (2009): 23749, https://doi.org/10.1053/j.seminoncol.2009.03.001; Elizabeth M Ward et al., "Annual Report to the Nation on the Status of Cancer, Featuring Cancer in Men and Women Age 20-49 Years", *Journal of the National Cancer Institute* 111, no. 12, (December 2019): 1279-97, https://doi.org/10.1093/jnci/djz106.

43 Dana Farber, "Young and Strong Program for Young Women with Breast Cancer", https://www.dana-farber.org/young-and-strong-program-for-young-women-with-breast-cancer/.

44   Rosanna Landis Weaver, "The 100 Most Over-paid CEOs," p 40, https://corpgov.law.harvard. edu/2017/03/02/the-100-most-overpaid-ceos/; Lisa Rapaport, "Breast Cancer Treatment Costs Higher for Younger Women," *Health News* (May 11, 2017) https://www.yahoo.com/news/breast-cancer-treatment-costs-higher-younger-women-205234692.html; Helen Blumen, Kathryn Fitch and Vincent Polkus, "Comparison of Treatment Costs for Breast Cancer, by Tumor Stage and Type of Service," *American Health & Drug Benefits* 9, no. 1 (February 2016), PMCID: PMC4822976.

45   This is, of course, a wide range, based on the results of dozens of studies conducted over past decades. It's important to bear in mind that each woman's risk level also depends on age, amount of excess body fat, and several other significant factors described throughout this book, including a woman's Vitamin D3 blood level, her chronic stress level, and her BRCA gene mutation status and the type of mutation she inherits within her BRCA 1 or BRCA2 mutation status. Also see: Chapter 8.

46   This is an example of one of thousands of academic papers published each year that use the terms "progesterone" and "progestin" interchangeably: W.K. Petrie and R.C. Hovey, "A Local Basis for Progesterone Action During Mammary Tumroigensis - no longer RANK and file," Breast Cancer Research 13, no.1 (Jan 2011): 301, https://doi.org/10.1186/bcr2802.

47   John Lee and Virginia Hopkins, *Dr. John Lee's Hormone Balance Made Simple*, (New York: Grand Central Publishing, 2006); John Lee, David Zava and Virginia Hopkins, *What Your Doctor May Not Tell You About Breast Cancer*, (New York: Grand Central Publishing, 2003).

48   Sherill Sellman, *Hormone Heresy: What Women Must Know About Their Hormones* (Tulsa, OK: Get Well International), revised and updated edition (October 30, 2000)m https://www.amazon.com/ Hormone-Heresy-Women-About-Hormones/dp/0958725209.

49   Lara Briden, "The Crucial Difference Between Progesterone and Progestins," October 6, 2015, larabriden.com; Jerilynn C. Prior, "Progesterone is NOT a Progestogen/Progestin: It's Estrogen's Unique Biological Partner," Centre for Menstrual Cycle and Ovulation Research, https://www. cemcor.ubc.ca/resources/progesterone-not-progestogenprogestin—it's-estrogen's-unique-biological-partner; Women Living Better, "Progesterone and Progestins," womenlivingbetter.org.

50   James H Clark, "A Critique of Women's Health Initiative Studies (2002-2006)." *Nuclear Receptor Signaling* 4, no. e023 (October 30, 2006), PMCID: PMC1630688.

51   Melody Petersen, "Wyeth Stock Falls 24% After Report," *The New York Times*, July 10, 2002, https://www.nytimes.com/2002/07/10/us/wyeth-stock-falls-24-after-report.html, accessed April 5, 2019, http://media.corporate-ir.net/media_files/NYS/WYE/reports/AR02.pdf; P. Levinsimes, "Prempro Hormone Replacement Therapy Linked to Breast Cancer and Other Serious Health Problems," https://www.levinsimes.com/prempro-hormone-replacement-therapy-linked-to-breast-cancer-and-other-serious-health-problems/, https://www.levinsimes.com/prempro-hormone-replacement-therapy-linked-to-breast-cancer-and-other-serious-health-problems/, last updated April 2019.

52   Nancy Krieger et al., "Decline in U.S. Breast Cancer Rates After the Women's Health Initiative: Socioeconomic and Racial/Ethnic Differentials," *American Journal of Public Health* 100, no. Suppl 1, S1 (2010): S132–39, www.doi.org/10.2105/AJPH.2009.181628. These decreases were only seen in the most prevalent types of breast cancer: hormone positive.

53   National Institutes of Health, "Decrease in Breast Cancer Rates Related to Reduction in Use of Hormone Replacement Therapy," April 18, 2007, https://www.nih.gov/news-events/news-releases/ decrease-breast-cancer-rates-related-reduction-use-hormone-replacement-therapy.

54   Peter M. Ravdin et al., "The Decrease in Breast Cancer Incidence in 2003 in the United States: Special Report," *The New England Journal of Medicine* 356 (April 18, 2007): 1670-74, https://doi. org/10.1056/NEJMsr070105.

55 Reuters, "Pfizer to Pay $6.3 Mn to Patient in Prempro Lawsuit," November 20, 2009, https://www.reuters.com/article/pfizer-prempro-idCNN2024658320091121; Ronald V. Miller, "$1.5 Million Prempro Verdict," January 27, 2007, https://www.aboutlawsuits.com/prempro-settlement-payments-breast-cancer-29138/.

56 Jef Feeley, "Pfizer Paid $896 Million in Prempro Settlements," June 19, 2012, https://www.bloomberg.com/news/articles/2012-06-19/pfizer-paid-896-million-in-prempro-accords-filing-shows-1-; "Prempro Settlements to Result in $1.2B Payments for Breast Cancer: Report," June 20, 2012, https://www.aboutlawsuits.com/prempro-settlement-payments-breast-cancer-29138/; Jef Feeley, "Pfizer to Pay $1.8 Million in Prempro Punitive Damages," *Insurance Journal*, August 8, 2013, https://www.insurancejournal.com/news/national/2013/08/08/301181.htm [as reprinted in *Insurance Journal*].

57 Rowan T. Chlebowski, "Breast Cancer after Use of Estrogen Plus Progestin in Postmenopausal Women," *New England Journal of Medicine* 360 (February 5, 2009): 573-87, https://doi.org/10.1056/NEJMoa0807684; Rowan T. Chlebowski and Garnet L. Anderson, "Menopausal Hormone Therapy and Breast Cancer Mortality: Clinical Implications," *Therapeutic Advances in Drug Safety* 6, no.2, (2015):45-56, https://doi.org/10.1177/2042098614568300; NIH, "Decrease in Breast Cancer Rates Related to Reduction in Use of Hormone Replacement Therapy," NIH.gov, April 18, 2007, https://www.nih.gov/news-events/news-releases/decrease-breast-cancer-rates-related-reduction-use-hormone-replacement-therapy.

58 Market Research Future, "Menopause Treatment Research Report: Global Forecast till 2023," January 2019, https://www.marketresearchfuture.com/reports/menopause-treatment-market-4579; Transparency Market Research, "Hormonal Contraceptives Market to Surpass US$ 30 billion by 2026: Rise in PCOS to Boost the Market," October 01, 2018, https://www.globenewswire.com/news-release/2018/10/01/1587944/0/en/Hormonal-Contraceptives-Market-to-Surpass-US-30-000-Mn-by-2026-Rise-in-PCOS-to-Boost-the-Market-Transparency-Market-Research.html.

59 Marian L. Neuhouser et al., "Overweight, Obesity, and Postmenopausal Invasive Breast Cancer Risk: A Secondary Analysis of the Women's Health Initiative Randomized Clinical Trials,", *JAMA Oncology* 1, no. 5 (2015): 611-21. https://doi.org/10.1001/jamaoncol.2015.1546.

60 "Global Oral Contraceptive Pills Market Value to Surpass USD 26 Billion by 2028, Finds Bekryl Market Analysts," January 2019, weny.com, https://www.weny.com/story/39825022/global-oral-contraceptive-pills-market-value-to-surpass-usd-26-billion-by-2028-finds-bekryl-market-analysts; ResearchAndMarkets, "Global Hormonal Contraceptives Market Report 2020: Market was Valued at $13.36 Billion in 2018 and is Expected to Grow to $15.39 Billion," December 09, 2019, https://www.businesswire.com/news/home/20191209005689/en/Global-Hormonal-Contraceptives-Market-Report-2020-Market.

61 CDC.gov, "Current Contraceptive Status Among Women Aged 15-49: United States, 2015-2017," National Center for Health Statistics, https://www.cdc.gov/nchs/products/databriefs/db327.htm.

62 Worldometers.info, "U.S. Population" and "World Population," http://www.worldometers.info/world-population/us-population/.

63 Elizabeth Siegel Watkins, "How the Pill Became a Lifestyle Drug: The Pharmaceutical Industry and Birth Control in the United States Since 1960," *American Journal of Public Health* 102, no. 8 (2012): 1462-72, https://doi.org/10.2105/AJPH.2012.300706.

64 Yasmeen Abutaleb & Erica Werner, "Trump's support for bipartisan Senate drug pricing bill may not be enough to push it into law: Senate leaders have yet to embrace the legislation despite widespread public angst about health-care costs." *The Washington Post*, Feb. 18, 2020, https://www.washingtonpost.com/health/2020/02/18/trumps-support-bipartisan-senate-drug-pricing-bill-might-not-be-enough-push-it-into-law/; C. Lee Ventola, "Direct-to-Consumer Pharmaceutical Advertising: Therapeutic or Toxic?" *Pharmacy and Therapeutics: A Peer-reviewed Journal for Formulary Management* 36, no. 10 (2011): 669-84, PMCID: PMC3278148.

65 Dustin Rowles, "The 15 Most Memorable Television Commercial Campaigns from the 1990s," PAJIBA.com (blog), October 26, 2010, https://www.pajiba.com/seriously_random_lists/the-most-memorable-television-advertising-campaigns-of-the-1990s-.php.

66 C. Lee Ventola, "Direct-to-Consumer Pharmaceutical Advertising: Therapeutic or Toxic?" *P&T: A Peer-Reviewed Journal for Formulary Management* 36, no. 10 (September 30, 2001), 672, PMCID: PMC3278148.

67 Katherine Ellen Foley, "Big Pharma Spent an Additional $9.8 Billion on Marketing in the Past 20 Years. It Worked," *Quartz*, January 9, 2019, https://qz.com/1517909/big-pharma-spent-an-additional-9-8-billion-on-marketing-in-the-past-20-years-it-worked/.

68 Elizabeth Watkins, "How the Pill became a Lifestyle Drug," 1462–72.

69 Ibid.

70 T. van Lierop, "Direct-to-consumer Drug Advertisement in Europe," *Lancet* 369 (2007): 1790, https://doi.org/10.1016/S0140-6736(07)60815-0; G. Velo and U. Moretti, "Direct-to-consumer Information in Europe: The Blurred Margin Between Promotion and Information," *British Journal of Clinical Pharmacology* 66, no.5 (2008): 626–28, https://doi.org/10.1111/j.1365-2125.2008.03283.x.

71 See Chapter 9.

72 Jennie Yoost, et al., "Understanding Benefits and Addressing Misperceptions and Barriers to Intrauterine Device Access Among Populations in the United States," *Patient Preference and Adherence*. 8 (July 3, 2014,) 947-57, https://doi.org/10.2147/PPA.S45710.

73 Elizabeth Ward et al., "Annual Report to the Nation on the Status of Cancer, 1999–2015, Featuring Cancer in Men and Women Ages 20–49," *Journal of the National Cancer Institute* (May 30, 2019): 11, djz106, https://doi.org/10.1093/jnci/djz106; Personal correspondence with Recinda Sherman, Program Manager, Data Use and Research, North American Association of Central Cancer Registries, May 2019.

74 P.S. Rosenberg et al., "U.S. Breast Cancer Cases Expected to Increase by 50% by 2030: Abstract 1850," presentation at the American Association for Cancer Research Annual Meeting, April 20, 2015, Philadelphia PA. https://www.healio.com/hematology-oncology/breast-cancer/news/online/%7B48afbf98-6cae-41f2-b1b4-56beb2bfa581%7D/breast-cancer-incidence-will-increase-by-50-by-2030.

75 Christopher I. Li et al., "Effect of Depo-medroxyprogesterone Acetate on Breast Cancer Risk Among Women 20-44 Years of Age," *Cancer Research* (February 27, 2012), https://doi.org/10.1158/0008-5472.CAN-11-4064;Aboutlawsuits.com, "Depo-Provera Shot Side Effects May Increase Breast Cancer Risk: Study," (April 5, 2012), https://www.aboutlawsuits.com/depo-shot-side-effects-breast-cancer-25699.

76 Margo Woods et al., "Effect of a Dietary Intervention and N-3 Fatty Acid Supplementation on Measures of Serum Lipid and Insulin Sensitivity in Persons with HIV," *American Journal of Clinical Nutrition*, September 2009, https://doi.org/10.3945/ajcn.2009.28137; "Margo N. Woods's Research While Affiliated with Tufts University and Other Places," researchgate.net, https://www.researchgate.net/scientific-contributions/39881839_Margo_N_Woods.

77 J.B. Barnett, et al., "Waist-to-hip Ratio, Body Mass Index (BMI), and Sex Hormone Levels Associated with Breast Cancer Risk in Premenopausal Caucasian Women," *Journal of Medical Sciences* 2, no.4 (2002): 170–76, https://doi.org/10.3923/jms.2002.170.176.

78 The progestin in birth control drugs takes over or replaces the natural progesterone your body makes. The progestin used in some hormone replacement drugs protects against the development of uterine cancer. Most birth control drugs have about ten times the amount of progestin in them than Prempro and other progestin/estrogen HRT drugs. See: "HRT vs. Birth Control Pills: The Ultimate Guide," https://www.earlymenopause.com/information/topics/hrt-vs-birth-control/.

79   Polly Marchbanks et al., "Oral Contraceptives and the Risk of Breast Cancer," *The New England Journal of Medicine* 346, no. 26 (June 27, 2002): 2025-32, https://doi.org/10.1056/NEJMoa013202.

80   K. Daniels, J. Daugherty and J. Jones, "Current Contraceptive Status Among Women Aged 15-44: United States, 2011-2013," *NCHS Data Briefs* 173 (December 2014): 1-8. PMID: 25500343.

81   Kaiser Family Foundation, "Contraceptive Use and Methods in the U.S. (Fact Sheet)," June 2002, www.kff.org, https://www.kff.org/wp-content/uploads/2013/01/contraception-fact-sheet-pdf-3244.pdf.

82   D. Hubacher and M. Kavanaugh, "Historical Record-setting Trends in IUD Use in the United States," *Contraception*, 8, no. 6, (May 26, 2018): 467-470, https://doi.org/10.1016/j.contraception.2018.05.016. The land of choice has more limited options when it comes to contraception," *The Atlantic*, April 18, 2017, https://www.theatlantic.com/health/archive/2017/04/why-america-has-fewer-iuds-than-other-countries/523077/.

83   Marchbanks et al., "Oral Contraceptives and the Risk of Breast Cancer," p. 2028, https://doi.org/10.1056/NEJMoa013202.

84   Centers for Disease Control, "Study Finds No Association Between Oral Contraceptive Use and Breast Cancer for Women 35 and Over," press release, June 26, 2002, https://www.cdc.gov/media/pressrel/r020626.htm.

85   Ibid.

86   Centers for Disease Control, "Study Finds No Association Between Oral Contraceptive Use and Breast Cancer for Women 35 and Over," press release," June 26, 2002, CDC Office of Enterprise Communication, www.ede.gov/media/pressrel/r020626.html.

87   "Study: The Pill Is Not Linked to Cancer," ABC News, June 26, 2002, www.abcnews.go.com.

88   C.G. Ellen and M.B. Grant, "Oral Contraceptives and the Risk of Breast Cancer: Correspondence," *The New England Journal of Medicine* 347, no. 18 (October 31, 2002): 1448-49, https://doi.org/10.1056/NEJM200210313471813.

89   Polly Marchbanks, "Correspondence: Oral Contraceptives and the Risk of Breast Cancer, the author's reply," *The New England Journal of Medicine* 347, no. 18 (October 31, 2002): 1449, https://doi.org/10.1056/NEJM200210313471813.

90   P.M. Casey, J.R. Cerhan, and S. Pruthi, "Oral Contraceptive Use and Breast Cancer Risk," Mayo Clinic Proceedings 83, no.1 (January 2008): 89, http://www.mayoclinicproceedings.org/article/S0025-6196(11)61122-1/pdf.

91   Christopher I. Li, et al., "Effect of Depo-medroxyprogesterone Acetate on Breast Cancer Risk Among Women 20 to 44 Years of Age," *Cancer Research* 72, no.8 (2012): 2028-35, https://doi.org/10.1158/0008-5472.CAN-11-4064; Carol Sweeny, et al., "Oral, Injected and Implanted Contraceptives and Breast Cancer Risk Among U.S. Hispanic and Non-Hispanic White Women," *International Journal of Cancer* 121, no.11 (July 26, 2007): 2517-23, https://doi.org/10.1002/ijc.22970.

92   M.D. Althius et al., "Hormonal Content and Potency of Oral Contraceptives and Breast Cancer Risk Among Young Women," *British Journal of Cancer* 88, no.1 (January 13, 2003): 50-7, https://doi.org/10.1038/sj.bjc.6600691.

93   M.D. Gammon et al., "Oral Contraceptive Use and Other Risk Factors in Relation to HER-2/neu Overexpression in Breast Cancer Among Young Women," *Cancer Epidemiology Biomarkers & Prevention* 8, no. 51 (May 1999): 413-39, https://cebp.aacrjournals.org/content/8/5/413?ijk.

94   Jessica M. Dolle et al., "Risk Factors for Triple-Negative Breast Cancer in Women Under the Age of 45 Years," *Cancer Epidemiology Biomarkers & Prevention* 18 no.4 (2009): 1157-66, https://doi.org/10.1158/1055-9965.EPI-08-1005. Also see Chapter 7.

95   Li et al., "Effects of Depo..." 228.

96 Lynn Rosenberg, et al., "A Case-control Study of Oral Contraceptive Use and Incident Breast Cancer." *American Journal of Epidemiology* 169, no. 4 (2009): 473-9, https://doi.org/10.1093/aje/kwn360.

97 Lynn Rosenberg et al., "Oral Contraceptive Use and Estrogen/Progesterone Receptor-Negative Breast Cancer Among African American Women," *Cancer Epidemiology, Biomarkers and Prevention* (July 20, 2010): 2073–79, https://doi.org/10.1158/1055-9965.EPI-10-0428. Also see Chapter 7.

98 Steven A. Narod et al., "Oral Contraceptives and the Risk of Breast Cancer in BRCA1 and BRCA2 Mutation Carriers," *Journal of the National Cancer Institute* 94, no. 23 (December 4, 2002): 1773–79, https://doi.org/10.1093/jnci/94.23.1773.

99 Christopher Khalenborn et al., "Oral Contraceptive Use as a Risk Factor for Premenopausal Breast Cancer: A Meta-analysis," *Mayo Clinic Proceedings* 81 (2006): 1290–1302, https://doi.org/10.4065/81.10.1290; James R. Cerhan, "Oral Contraceptive Use and Breast Cancer Risk: Current Status," *Mayo Clinic Proceedings* 81, no. 10 (2006): 1287–89, https://doi.org/10.4065/81.10.1287.

100 Malcolm Gladwell, *What the Dog Saw and Other Adventures* (Boston, MA: Little, Brown and Company, 2009).

101 Edgar B. Herwick III, "How 'The Pill' Was Born in Massachusetts," WGBH.org, June 24, 2016, https://www.wgbh.org/news/2016/06/24/local-news/how-pill-was-born-massachusetts.

102 M.C. Pike and B. Henderson, "Breast Cancer in Young Women and Use of Oral Contraceptives: Possible Modifying Effect of Formulation and Age at Use," *Lancet* 2, no. 8356 (October 22, 1983): 926-30, https://doi.org/10.1016/s0140-6736(83)90450-6.

103 Lara V. Marks, "Study Linking Birth Control Pill to Breast Cancer is Attacked," *The New York Times*, May 8, 1984; Lara V. Marks, *Sexual Chemistry: A History of the Contraceptive Pill* (New Haven, CT: Yale University Press, 2001), https://yalebooks.yale.edu/book/9780300167917/sexual-chemistry.

104 Malcolm Gladwell, "John Rock's Error: What the Co-inventor of the Pill Didn't Know About Menstruation Can Endanger Women's Health," *The New Yorker*, March 10, 2000. See also "John Rock's Error: What the Co-inventor of the Pill Didn't Know About Menstruation Can Endanger Women's Health," in *What the Dog Saw* (Boston, MA: Little, Brown and Company) 2009.

105 Barbara Seaman, "Birth Control," in *Voices: of the Women's Health Movement; Volume One*, Barbara Seaman with Laura Eldridge editors, (New York, Seven Stories Press) 2012, 129-130; Barbara Seaman, The Doctors' Case Against the Pill:25th anniversary edition updated, (New York, Hunter House) 1995; Women's Health Specialists, "Barbara Seaman: A Powerful Writer and Advocate for Women's Health Issues, Co-Founder of the National Women's Health Network, 1935-2008," https://www.womenshealthspecialists.org/about/the-womens-movement/barbara-seaman/; US Food and Drug Administration, "Regulations, Guidance, and Reports Related to Women's Health," FDA.gov; Requirements on Content and Format of Labeling for Combined Hormonal Contraceptives: Guidance for Industry (draft), FDA.gov, December 2017.

106 Elizabeth Siegel Watkins, *A Social History of Oral Contraceptives*, 1950-1970 (Baltimore: The Johns Hopkins University Press, 1998).

107 US Supreme Court, Eisenstadt v. Baird, 405 U.S. 438 (1972), March 22, 1972, https://supreme.justia.com/cases/federal/us/405/438.

108 Barbara Seaman, *The Doctors' Case Against the Pill* (New York: Peter H. Wyden, Inc., 1969).

109 David Hubacher, "The Checkered History and Bright Future of Intrauterine Contraception in the United States," *Perspectives on Sexual and Reproductive Health* (March/April 2002): 98–103, https://www.guttmacher.org/sites/default/files/article_files/3409802.pdf; W.D. Mosher and C.F. Westoff, "Trends in Contraceptive Practice: United States, 1965–1976," *Advance Data from Vital and Health Statistics* 1982 34, no. 2 (March-April, 2002): 98–103; https://www.cdc.gov/nchs/data/

series/sr_23/sr23_010.pdf; W.D. Mosher and C.F. Westoff, "Trends in Contraceptive Practice: United States, 1965–1976," *Vital and Health Statistics* 23, no.10 (1982).

110 Planned Parenthood, "History of the Pill, 2015," plannedparenthood.org; Population Council, "The Copper T 380 Intrauterine Device: A Summary of Scientific Data," https://www.popcouncil.org/uploads/pdfs/1992_CopperT380.pdf.

111 Susan Wadia-Ells, *Birth Control Drugs and Breast Cancer: Learn the Terrible Truth*, 2012.

112 Caroline Beaton, "Why Does America Have Fewer Types of IUDs than Other Countries?" *The Atlantic*, April 18, 2017, https://www.theatlantic.com/health/archive/2017/04/why-america-has-fewer-iuds-than-other-countries/523077/.

113 National Women's Health Network, "The National Women's Health Network's Founders," https://nwhn.org/nwhn-founders/.

114 Public Broadcasting System, "The Pill: Senate Hearings on the Pill," *The American Experience*, https://www.pbs.org/wgbh/americanexperience/features/pill-senate-holds-hearings-pill-1970/, accessed April 5, 2019.

115 Lara V. Marks, *Sexual Chemistry: A History of the Contraceptive Pill* (New Haven, CT: Yale University Press, 2001), https://yalebooks.yale.edu/book/9780300167917/sexual-chemistry;); Andrea Tone, *Devices and Desires: A History of Contraceptives in America* (New York: Hill and Wang, 2001); Planned Parenthood, "Birth Control Pill: A History," June, 2015, 5–6, https://www.plannedparenthood.org/files/1514/3518/7100/Pill_History_FactSheet.pdf, accessed April 5, 2019.

116 COC: combination oral contraceptive. These drugs contain both a chemical estrogen made from the urine of pregnant horses and the chemical progestin.

117 Lina S. Mørch et al., "Contemporary Hormonal Contraception and the Risk of Breast Cancer, *The New England Journal of Medicine* 377 (December 7,2017): 2228-39, https://doi.org/10.1056/NEJMoa1700732.

118 Planned Parenthood, "The Birth Control Pill: A History" (June 2015): 5–6, https://www.plannedparenthood.org/files/1514/3518/7100/Pill_History_FactSheet.pdf, accessed April 5, 2019.

119 CBS, "Medical Group Says Teens Should Use IUDs, Implants as First Contraceptive Method," September 21, 2012, CBS.com, https://www.cbsnews.com/news/medical-group-says-teens-should-use-iuds-implants-as-first-contraceptive-method/.

120 "Adolescents & Long-Acting Reversible Contraception: Implants and Intrauterine Devices," *The American Congress of Obstetricians and Gynecologists*, Committee Opinion, #539 (October 2012), https://doi.org/10.1097/AOG.0b013e3182723b7d. Author's note: The report contains incorrect information: It states that the Lilleth IUD, manufactured by Allergan, is hormone-free. It is not; it contains progestin.

121 Gina M. Secura et al., "The Contraceptive CHOICE Project: Reducing Barriers to Long-acting Reversible Contraception," *American Journal of Obstetrics and Gynecology* 203, no. 2 (2010): 115. e1-7, https://doi.org/10.1016/j.ajog.2010.04.017.

122 Lina S. Mørch et al., "Contemporary Hormonal Contraception," 2228, https://doi.org/10.1056/NEJMoa1700732.

123 Caroline Beaton, "Why Does America Have Fewer Types of IUDs..." 3.

124 Email to author from Elizabeth Adomaitis, Mona Lisa N.V. Graaf de Theuxlaan 25Bus 2B-3550 Heusden-Zolder, September 29, 2010.

125 See Chapter 10.

126 US Food and Drug Administration, "Imported Drugs Raise Safety Concerns," March 1, 2018, https://www.fda.gov/drugs/drug-information-consumers/imported-drugs-raise-safety-concerns.

127 Sherill Sellman, ND, "Empowering Women to Achieve Hormonal Balance and Optimal Health at Any Age," https://drsherrillsellman.com.

128 Smart Women's Choice, https://www.smartwomenschoice.com.

5 STEP 4:
No More Mammograms!
Choose Self-Exams, Clinical Exams, Ultrasound, MRI and Thermography

"No pitifully small picket line, no poorly attended meeting, no tossing out of an idea to an audience and even to an individual, should be scorned as insignificant.

The power of a bold idea uttered publicly in defiance of dominant opinion cannot be easily measured. Those special people who speak out in such a way as to shake up not only the self-assurance of their enemies, but the complacency of their friends, are precious catalysts for change."

—Howard Zinn,
You Can't Be Neutral on a Moving Train: A Personal History of Our Time

Ice-cold plates come together. Metal slabs flatten your breast tissue with 15 to 20 pounds of pressure.[1] Ionizing radiation shoots through the pressed-thin flesh. And research tells us that inflammation from cumulative radiation, absorbed from regular mammograms, is just one of many reasons why mammograms can hurt more women than they help.[2] Yes, *inflammation*—remember, we saw that's a metabolic cause and universal hallmark of all cancer.[3]

But unnecessary inflammation is just the tip of this iceberg that's made up of too many women's mammogram stories. It's just the tip of this hard, nasty, cold-cash-driven iceberg of too many women's unnecessary pain.

When will women's growing fury about mammograms become hot enough to melt this profitable iceberg? "Welcome to Cancerland," the brilliant writer Barbara Ehrenreich says to each of us in her classic *Harper's* essay. "Welcome to Cancerland: A Mammogram Leads to a Cult of Pink Kitsch."[4]

What If Everything Your Doctors Told You About Breast Cancer Was Wrong?

"Don't look down." Therese Taylor repeats this mantra when she's rising out of bed in the morning. "Don't look down," she says when she's standing in the shower. "Don't think about what you've lost."

She's lost so much. Her breast. Her identity as a healthy person. Her uncomplicated sex life. Her faith in the medical profession.

Taylor has gained something, too: a fury that's uncomfortable to express when other women are dying from breast cancer and her doctors tell her she's *lucky*. She feels rage. Her doctors implied she had cancer and said if she cut off her breast, she would live. Now she knows it was never that simple.

No one—not her physician, or her surgeon, or the pathologist, or her nurse, or anyone else—ever took the time to explain what her mammogram and biopsy had actually found.

Her doctor had said, "It's indicative of cancer." But the fact is that the abnormality on Taylor's mammogram—ductal carcinoma in situ, or DCIS—*is not* considered a cancer by many experts, and it had only a small chance of ever progressing into an invasive cancer. The probability that it would kill her was even slimmer—about 3 percent. The thing in her breast was *not* a ticking time bomb. And were it not for the mammogram, she probably never would have known it was there.

Excerpt from Christie Aschwanden, "What If Everything Your Doctors Told You About Breast Cancer Was Wrong?" Mother Jones, October 6, 2015.

I did not want to include the subject of mammography in this book about effective breast cancer prevention. I stopped having mammograms decades ago; the test has nothing to do with breast cancer prevention. After all, no number of mammograms can stop breast cancer from developing in your body. "Early detection is not prevention...We've got to stop presenting mammography screening as the answer." That's what Dr. Susan Love, the famous breast surgeon and best-selling author, told her audiences all the way back in 1994.[5]

Earlier chapters have described effective prevention steps to help keep breast cancer from developing in your body. This chapter points out how to help women prevent the development of breast cancer by staying aware of any inflammation in their breast tissue or throughout their entire body; something that mammography is not capable of doing. The chapter also describes a number of new or improved radiation-free, non-invasive technologies that can be used for screening and/or identifying palpable tumors throughout the breast. Finally, it chronicles the political and financial control that the breast cancer industry continues to wield over women in the US, trying to limit women's choices over safe, noninvasive and more effective breast screening and breast diagnostic options. Sadly, almost three decades after renegade breast surgeon Susan Love began trying to raise awareness of the problems inherent in mammography technology, the industry's successful hard sell for mammograms goes on; especially in the United States.

Mammograms: Today's Mechanism for Creating and Fueling Our Breast Cancer Epidemic

Today's cancer industry, as described in Chapter 1, does not understand why or how a woman develops breast cancer. Therefore, most woman remain frightened of developing this disease. Most remain willing to have radiologists x-ray the tissue throughout their breasts. Women want to know, "Has this terrifying beast, named breast cancer, invaded my flesh yet?" Yes, the ongoing ignorance of today's oncologists enables and encourages the breast cancer industry to breed fear and submission among so many women.

Financially, mammograms have become the most important part of today's national breast cancer treatment market. This is because mammograms are the most powerful feeder mechanism for the cancer industry's financial achievements and goals. We are told that regular mammography exams generate $7.8 billion a year in the US, while the additional diagnostic tests, surgeries, radiation treatments and drugs generated by mammogram reports generate many excess billions in revenues each year. How so? More than half of all women treated for growing invasive breast tumors each year do not have growing invasive breast cancer, or their pea-size tumor has not progressed and might never progress to becoming a danger to that woman's life.

Mammograms are the only diagnostic test that can tell a woman if she has dots of calcification in her breast tissue, or if she has a few different-looking or atypical cells in a breast's milk duct, or if she has a lot of these atypical cells throughout one or more ducts. These diagnoses are defined respectively as microcalcifications, atypia, and ductal carcinoma in situ (DCIS). None of these different diagnoses are invasive breast cancers.

If the name *ductal carcinoma in situ* sounds scary, with that cancer term "carcinoma"[6] tucked into it, the cancer industry has now decided to rachet up women's fear levels even further. Today, oncologists have upgraded the name DCIS to "stage 0 breast cancer." But zero means "no quantity or number, naught," i.e., no cancer. Yet in 2017, oncologists in the US told over 80,000 women that their mammogram report had come back positive; they had developed stage 0 breast cancer.[7] The women were usually urged to begin some type of invasive breast cancer treatment; "just to be sure." With few exceptions, we are told, oncologists usually recommend that these individuals have an invasive procedure called a breast biopsy to examine these cells further. Then oncologists prescribe toxic therapies that are similar to, or exactly the same as, those prescribed for women diagnosed with dangerous, rapidly growing invasive breast tumors. Go figure.

Since mainstream oncologists still don't understand the exact biological steps that take place before a woman develops her first breast cancer cell, their hopeful solutions to a woman's noncancerous and noninvasive stage 0 breast cancer diagnosis is also based on ignorance and fear. Their treatments reflect doctors' desires to try to cover all their bases, shooting blindly into the dark. But they are not shooting at themselves; they are shooting at their patients. What happened to the idea of doctors adhering to the Hippocratic principle of "first do no harm"?

To make sure the mammogram industry remains strong, the breast cancer treatment industry encourages us to "celebrate" *Breast Cancer Awareness* month each October. Their three-decades old *Think Pink* campaign has become the most successful cause marketing campaign and industry-wide public relations project in US history; almost equal to Coca-Cola and McDonald's in its saturation throughout the population.[8] This national "little-girls-love-pink" campaign, since it began in the mid-1980s, has continued to cajole more than 70% of all women forty years old and older into having regular mammograms. Even women in their 90s continue to "think pink," feeling somehow obligated for life, I suppose, to appear for an annual or biannual mammogram. In 2017, an estimated 300 women *90 years and older* were diagnosed with stage 0 breast cancer, while another 1500 women 90 years and older were diagnosed for stage I breast cancer.[9] With few exceptions, both of these diagnoses can only be made by having a regular mammogram, as no tumor exists in a stage 0 diagnosis, or the tumor is so small in most stage I diagnoses that it is not palpable.

Today, once October arrives, who can miss the silly pink ribbons plastered on police cruisers,[10] the pink lights bathing the White House at night,[11] and pink ribbons decorating food packages on supermarket shelves? Many women believe this annual "get-a-mammogram" campaign tries to infantilize women's own sane judgements about our breasts. Are the pretty pink ribbons there to also distract women from focusing on the crushing pressure and the inflammation-producing radiation needed to produce each and every mammogram image?[12] "The effect of this relentless brightsiding is to transform breast cancer into a rite of passage–not an injustice or a tragedy to rail against, but a normal marker in this life cycle, like menopause or graying hair," Barbara Ehrenreich rails in that iconic 2001 *Harper's Magazine* article, "Welcome to Cancerland."[13]

Financially, this entire pink campaign makes excellent sense. This pro-mammogram programming was created in the mid-1980s by the Swiss chemical and pharmaceutical conglomerate AstraZeneca. This is when the company was manufacturing carcinogenic pesticides, as well as the blockbuster breast cancer drug, tamoxifen.[14] Today, the annual pink ribbon campaign is heavily funded by the entire mushrooming US breast cancer industry and its well-funded surrogates, led by the American Cancer Society and the Susan G. Komen Foundation.[15]

According to the longtime breast cancer industry critic Sharon Batt, "When Zeneca created Breast Cancer Awareness Month in 1985, it was owned by Imperial Chemical Industries (ICI), a multibillion-dollar producer of pesticides, paper and plastics. State and federal agencies sued ICI in 1990, alleging that it dumped DDT and PCBs—both banned in the US since the 1970s—in Los Angeles and Long Beach harbors."[16] Thus Batt also reminds us that, "Any mention of what role such chemicals may be playing in our rising breast cancer rates among younger and older women is missing from Breast Cancer Awareness Month promos."[17]

AstraZeneca: One-Stop Shopping

Creating and Treating Breast Cancer Under One Roof

"Syngenta was the result of a merger of the agri-side, Novartis, with AstraZeneca. So, the company that's giving you atrazine, which turns on your aromatase,[18] turns around and sells you an aromatase blocker and says it's a thousand times better than any other breast cancer treatment."[19]

Urged on every October by Breast Cancer Awareness Month, in 2015 some 65.3 percent of US women 40 years and older still continued to have a regular or screening mammogram every two years.[20]

The Metabolic Approach to Cancer = "Goodbye" to All Mammograms

Since 2012, when Dr. Seyfried's landmark text, *Cancer as A Metabolic Disease*, was published, we now have a detailed map tracing the evolutionary biology-based steps that take place each time a healthy cell turns itself into a cancer cell. This means that women no longer need to be terrified about developing breast cancer. That's because we now understand there are many effective lifestyle changes each of us can make to protect our breast cells from going rogue; turning into destructive cancer cells. These prevention steps all protect our breast cells' power batteries from suffocating. These prevention steps are all nourishing. Each step helps keep our breast cells' power batteries vibrant as these cells' mitochondria are able to remain in optimal health.

Meanwhile, as described later in this chapter, new technologies now make mammograms old-fashioned, unnecessary and potentially dangerous. This is wonderful news since mammograms with their steel plates, their RADS[21] being shot into breast tissue, and their ability to overdiagnose, make even the most updated mammogram machines harmful to women's physical and mental health.

Fortunately, not every woman will develop breast cancer during her lifetime. But every woman in the US today is urged, once she turns 40 or 45 years old, to begin regular mammograms. For far too many of us, a single mammogram can lure us across the border into Cancerland.[22] For all of these reasons and more, the information you're about to read about mammograms may make this the most important chapter in this entire book.

Listen Up! The Four National Mammogram Studies That Have Changed Everything

American women are being kept in the dark. Four national studies published between 2013 and 2017 have changed the landscape and the future of mammography forever. All four studies illustrate how mammograms, by themselves, are *irrelevant* and actually *harmful* in the eyes of objective medical researchers and clinicians across Europe and Canada. These governments provide health care to all of their citizens, through a variety of "single-payer" systems. This makes these national governments interested in the need to neither overdiagnose nor overtreat individuals for any type of disease or condition.

In 2014, a study on the safety and usefulness of mammography was conducted by an independent medical panel assembled by the Swiss government. This interdisciplinary board, comprised of a medical ethicist, a clinical epidemiologist, a pharmacologist, an oncologic surgeon, a nurse scientist, a lawyer, and a health economist, was asked to review the international research on mammography. The board's final report recommended the scheduled closing of all mammogram clinics, nationwide. The board also recommended banning the opening of any new mammography clinics across the country.[23]

Here is a summary of this historic Swiss report, along with conclusions from those other national studies out of Canada and Denmark, as well as an all-Scandinavia study. All four reports included the same findings:

- Mammograms do not decrease the incidence of fast-growing, dangerous tumors. Women discover most such tumors with breast self-exams, by accident, or with the help of regular clinical exams.

- Mammograms do not save lives.

- Mammograms cause tens of thousands of women to be overdiagnosed each month, with most of these falsely diagnosed women agreeing to begin what the industry today openly calls "overtreatment."

Today, even women who once felt they had no choice but to follow the recommendations of the so-called medical "experts" (like the American Cancer Society, federal cancer agencies, their Planned Parenthood practitioner, their primary care practitioner, or their OB/GYN), may now decide to stop having mammograms. Even the most cautious among us may finally realize we have sufficient objective information to develop our own personal, well-informed, and independent answer to this all-important question: Should I, or shouldn't I, have regular mammograms?

The 2014 Swiss Medical Board Study

Close All Mammogram Clinics; Do Not Allow New Clinics to Open.[24]
An independent, ad hoc national medical board's report was made public on February 2, 2014. "The published study acknowledged that systematic mammography screening might prevent about one death attributed to breast cancer for every 1000 women screened, even though there was no evidence to suggest that overall mortality was affected. At the same time, it emphasized that harm—in particular, false positive and false negative test results and the risk of overdiagnosis takes place in too many women. The board therefore recommended that no new systematic mammography screening programs be introduced and that a time limit be placed on existing programs."[25]

The 2013 Scandinavian Study[26]

Breast Cancer Screening Was Not Associated with a Reduction in the Incidence of Advanced Cancer

"600,000 women in the analysis in the age range 39 to 74 years... For every 2000 women invited for screening throughout 10 years, one will avoid dying of breast cancer and 10 healthy women, who would not have been diagnosed, if there had not been screening, will be treated unnecessarily. Furthermore, more than 200 women will experience important psychological distress, including anxiety and uncertainty for years, because of false positive findings...Breast cancer screening was not associated with a reduction in the incidence of advanced cancer. It is also likely that 1 in every 3 invasive tumors and cases of DCIS diagnosed in women from their screening, were actually an over diagnosis...Also, a systematic review of over diagnosis in five other countries allowed us to show that about half of the screen-detected breast cancers are over diagnosed."

The 2014 Canadian 25-Year Mammography Study[27]

Once again, a blue-ribbon study showed how this diagnostic test creates many more problems than it solves. When the American Cancer Society and US radiologists, (all advocates for the radiology industry), offered major criticism of the study, Dartmouth College Medical School professor, researcher and best-selling author on the overuse of medical testing, Dr. H. Gilbert Welch, described and defended the study.[28] "In the Canadian trial, one group received a regular physical exam of the breast—a very careful exam performed by specially trained nurses. The other group received the same regular physical exam, plus regular mammography. In other words, the trial tested the usefulness of adding mammography to a physical exam in an effort to detect abnormalities that are too small to feel."[29] According to Dr. Welch, the trial showed that finding these "too-small-to-feel" abnormalities doesn't help women live longer. "If we are going to do mammography, we should be using it to find big, important things—not small unimportant things."[30]

The 2017 Danish Study: Mammograms Offer No Benefits[31]

Researchers looked at all Danish women aged 35 to 84 years old who had a mammogram between 1980 and 2010. One key finding: Breast cancer screening using mammography was not associated with a reduction in the incidence of advanced cancer. Also, 1 in every 3 invasive tumors and cases of DCIS diagnosed in women who underwent mammograms were overdiagnosed. For every 2000 women who are screened in a ten-year period, one will avoid dying of breast cancer and 10 healthy women who would not have been diagnosed if they had not agreed to a mammogram will be overdiagnosed and then overtreated—or treated unnecessarily.

US Media Remain Silent

These four studies clearly and severely denigrate the current practice of mammography. Why don't American women know about these reports? Why haven't Planned Parenthood clinics, the American Cancer Society, the National Cancer Institute, and the Susan G. Komen Foundation shared these landmark studies with the American public? Why hasn't the US press made sure all women know that a national Swiss medical board has recommended closing all mammography clinics nationwide, and—more importantly—why hasn't the US public been told the reasons behind this board's decision? Why has our mainstream media chosen to virtually ignore this important report? After all, women over the age of 40 are told to have regular mammograms and a majority of women continue to follow this directive. Even our public broadcasting network, National Public Radio, has never reported on the Swiss Medical Board's findings, according to the network's listing of past broadcasts on the topic of mammograms.[32] In fact, the only US news sources I have found that published an in-depth look at the Swiss Board's historic decision were Dr. Joseph Mercola's well-researched and wide-ranging health website, mercola.com, an online *Forbes* magazine piece, and Dr. H. Gilbert Welch's opinion piece for CNN.com.[33]

As mentioned, multiple reports calculate that 90 percent of US print, TV, radio, and internet media today are owned and controlled by a small group of billionaires and multibillion-dollar corporations.[34] As a result of this US censorship of any adverse critique of the mammography industry, almost 70 percent of American women over 40 years of age continue to have regular mammograms. Our national media's virtual blackout of these national and transnational mammogram reports from Switzerland, Canada, and Scandinavia offers American women additional proof: The power that today's cancer industry appears to hold over our public health agencies and our mainstream media is endangering the health of US women.

> ## US Mainstream Media is No Friend of American Women[35]
>
> "In 1983, 90 percent of US media were controlled by 50 companies; today, 90 percent is controlled by the Big Six. (AT&T, Comcast, The Walt Disney Company, 21st Century Fox, CBS and Viacom control the spoken and printed word from sea to shining sea.) Although many people are aware of the monopolistic tendencies of the US mainstream media, it's important to understand the level of concentration. It means the vast majority of everything you see and hear on any electronic device or printed publication is 'democratically' controlled by six average white guys and their shareholders."

Overdiagnosing or Overtreating An Estimated 275,000 US Women Annually

Mimi, the stylish and incredibly successful founder and former CEO of a multimillion-dollar design business, was 53 years old when we met in 2009. She had opted to have both of her noncancerous breasts amputated two years earlier. "A mammogram showed I had 'stage 0' breast cancer in my right breast. They said if I had a mastectomy, I wouldn't have to have chemo and lose my hair. When they suggested a double mastectomy, I said 'yes.' I had wanted to have a breast reduction for a long time, anyway. Now I don't have to wear a bra all the time."

When a physician does not understand how a disease begins in a woman's breast, it becomes difficult for such doctors or mainstream cancer centers, even the ones with famous names such as Memorial Sloan Kettering or Dana-Farber, to know how to effectively and nontoxically screen, diagnose and/or treat this disease, let alone prevent it. No wonder most oncologists and breast surgeons continue to take a worst-case approach when a mammogram screening finds atypical cells or a tiny "indolent" (not-growing or slow-growing) pea-sized tumor that has broken through the breast duct wall. As earlier described, they label those atypical cells, "stage 0 breast cancer," and they label any pea-sized tumors "stage I breast cancer."[36]

Types of Overdiagnoses

Macrocalcification and atypical hyperplasia

Today's mainstream cancer industry worries that a diagnosis of *microcalcification* or *atypical hyperplasia*, found only by a mammography report, could be a pre-DCIS, a pre-stage 0 breast cancer condition.[37] Women who receive such diagnoses are often instructed to have additional mammograms or undergo a breast biopsy to understand these abnormalities better; increasing existing inflammation in the breast; such inflammation could stimulate the damaged mitochondria in these abnormal cells to move closer to total suffocation, the creation of atypical cells (DCIS) or possibly the initiation of invasive cancer cells.[38]

Stage 0 Breast Cancer

In 2017 the College of Surgeons' National Cancer Database indicates that 84,300 women in the US were diagnosed with stage 0 breast cancer, or DCIS.[39] This means about 20 percent of all women diagnosed and subsequently treated for breast cancer in the US that year, had atypical cells (DCIS/stage 0 breast cancer). They did not have breast cancer!

Stage I Breast Cancer

Mammograms can create even more problems for another 190,000 women in the US each year. These are women who are diagnosed with a pea-sized or stage I breast tumor.[40] The four national mammogram studies we just reviewed, and other smaller studies, tell us that only about 18 percent of these tiny pea-sized tumors will ever grow into large, dangerous tumors.[41] Instead, almost a quarter of these stage I tumors will disappear on their own,[42] while the majority of such tumors will never grow very quickly, nor will they ever become large or go on to create metastatic tumors.[43] Some *Nervous Nellies* might be hesitant to call the diagnosis of a stage I breast tumor an "overdiagnosis"; however, the most comprehensive studies of such tumors indicate that such tiny pea-sized growths should not be immediately biopsied, nor treated with surgery, radiation, or toxic drugs. Instead, many women with stage I tumors can apparently be put on a "watch and wait" notice.[44] Thankfully, using breast self-exams and clinical breast exams, supported by recent elastography technology[45] and tumor diagnostic testing, using today's expanding array of highly accurate and noninvasive ultrasound equipment,[46] women can continue to monitor tiny tumors on an ongoing basis, under the guidance of their ob/gyn, their primary care practitioner, an open-minded breast surgeon or oncologist or a functional medicine practitioner. Women can also initiate any or all of the five anti-inflammatory and immune-building prevention steps described in this book, if they want to play an active role in maintaining, shrinking or enabling these tiny pea-sized tumors and any atypical cells to disappear.[47]

Studies described in this chapter illustrate how the widespread use of mammograms in the US today results in the cancer industry overdiagnosing and possibly overtreating as many as 54 percent of women who receive a breast cancer diagnosis each year.[48] Eliminating mammograms, as Switzerland, Canada and the Scandinavian countries are now poised to do, would dramatically reduce the cancer industry's current and projected income, sending breast cancer drug stocks plummeting.

The 84,000 women in the US who are overdiagnosed with stage 0 breast cancer each year and most of the estimated 190,000 women who are overtreated for their stage I indolent or soon-to-disappear pea-sized tumors are why some breast cancer researchers, clinicians, and patients now use these unsettling terms: *overdiagnosis* and *overtreatment*.[49] The National Cancer Institute also accepts these concepts as existing within the cancer industry and offers us their official definitions for these two problematic medical industry phenomena.

Table 5.1: How Many Women Are Overdiagnosed and Overtreated in the US (2017)?

STAGE OF BREAST CANCER DIAGNOSED IN 2017 (ALL AGE GROUPS: 20 THROUGH 90 AND OVER)									
	Stage							Totals	
All Age Groups	0	I	II	III	IV	NA	UNK	N	%
Total	84,339	191,149	105,557	29,060	18,659	324	4,999	434,086	100%
%	19.4%	44.0%	24.3%	6.7%	4.3%	0.1%	1.2%	100%	

These numbers reflect an estimate of all primary breast tumors (stages I-III) diagnosed in US women + an estimate all US women diagnosed with DCIS and with de novo metastatic breast cancer during 2017.

Basis of estimates : American College of Surgeon's National Cancer Database "Female Breast Cancer: Diagnosis Year: 2017 (ACS data representing 70% of total numbers in table)

Overdiagnosis: According to the National Cancer Institute

"Finding cases of cancer with a screening test (such as a mammogram or PSA test) that will never cause any symptoms. These cancers may just stop growing or go away on their own. Some of the harms caused by overdiagnosis are anxiety and having treatments that are not needed."[50]

Overtreatment: According to the National Cancer Institute

"Overtreatment is treatment of a cancer that would have gone away on its own or never caused any symptoms. These cancers are usually found on a screening test. Overtreatment may lead to problems and harmful side effects from cancer therapies that are not needed."[51]

The Costs of and the Profits from Overtreatments

Once a mammogram has identified either atypical cells (stage 0) or a stage I pea-sized tumor breaking through a woman's breast duct, individuals are usually encouraged to have a breast biopsy and then a procedure called *breast conserving* surgery, also called a *lumpectomy*. This type of breast surgery is a huge industry unto itself, predicted to grow to $10 billion annually by 2024 in the US alone. An uninsured woman in the

US is charged between $10,000 and $20,000 per lumpectomy.[52] Women treated with a lumpectomy, even for stage zero and stage I breast cancer, are often given dozens of subsequent radiation treatments.

Overdiagnosis in Breast Cancer Screening: Time to Tackle an Underappreciated Harm[53]

"Pathologically diagnosed breast cancer is heterogeneous; whereas some tumors grow rapidly, others grow slowly, and still others may never grow. Tumors that grow slowly or not at all can lead to overdiagnosis. Unfortunately, mammography screening programs cannot distinguish between fatal and harmless breast cancer. Breast cancer overdiagnosis can only harm the affected woman."

Privately insured women, diagnosed with DCIS (stage zero breast cancer) like Mimi, are often encouraged to have one or both of their *noncancerous* breasts amputated. In medical terms, this procedure is called *prophylactic mastectomy*. Most women are then urged to have their amputated breast(s) immediately replaced (or, in medical terms, *reconstructed*).

Today, reconstruction after a single or double amputation is the most expensive treatment option, and often includes the most complications. However, it has become more popular, especially with younger women who are diagnosed with stage 0 breast cancer, since the actress Angelina Jolie publicly shared her decision, in 2015, to have such a prophylactic procedure.[54] With this choice, women are promised symmetrical (i.e., matched) breasts of their preferred cup size, with or without nipples, fixed in place and permanently numb. According to Dr. Susan Love, "We've promoted it, saying it looks good, but we don't talk about what it's going to feel like. To the feeler, it doesn't feel the same. To the feelee, it doesn't feel at all."[55]

Going Flat: Some women are saying "no" to reconstruction. They are saying "no" to the culture's fetish for breasts. They are firmly standing with the Womanist icon Audre Lorde, who in 1980 described her lack of interest in using the falsie that the American Cancer Society's visiting volunteer provided. She describes her refusal as not wanting to allow the breast cancer industry "to elevate one's mammary glands to the most significant aspect by which a woman is defined."[56]

In her 1980 landmark book *The Cancer Journals*, Lorde writes, "This emphasis upon the cosmetic after surgery reinforces this society's stereotype of women, that we are only what we look or appear, so this is the only aspect of our existence we need to address. Any woman who has had a breast removed because of cancer knows she does not feel the same. But we are allowed no psychic time or space to examine what our true feelings are, to make them our own. With quick cosmetic reassurance, we are told that our feelings are not important, our appearance is all, the sum total of self."[57]

From The Cancer Journals

"For me my scars are an honorable reminder that I may be a casualty in the cosmic war again radiation, animal fat, air pollution, McDonald's hamburgers and red dye no. 2, but the fight is still going on, and I am still a part of it. I refuse to have my scars hidden or trivialized behind lambswool or silicone gel...I refuse to hide my body simply because it might make a woman-phobic world more comfortable.

...Prothesis offers the empty comfort of "Nobody will know the difference." But it is that very difference which I wish to affirm, because I have lived it, and survived it, and wish to share that strength with other women. If we are to translate the silence surrounding breast cancer into language and action against this scourge, then the first step is that women with mastectomies must become visible to each other. For silence and invisibility go hand in hand with powerlessness. By accepting the mask of prosthesis, one-breasted women proclaim ourselves as insufficient, dependent upon pretense. We reinforce our own isolation and invisibility from each other, as well as the false complacency of a society which would rather not face the results of its own insanities. In addition, we withhold that visibility and support from one another which is such an aid to perspective and self-acceptance.

Audre Lorde, The Cancer Journals

As the worldwide market for breast implantation and breast augmentation is expected to reach $4.6 billion by 2025,[58] more and more women are also heeding Lorde's words, turning their backs, maintaining their short- and long-term health and "going flat." Their goal is to refuse the artificiality, the treatments, the distress, discomfort and, for some, the chronic pain that many reconstructive surgeries can create, sometimes plaguing women for the rest of their lives, even once they undergo explant surgery.[59] Instead, women want to calm their bodies, minds and stress levels as they create their own new normal, their new personal definition of optimal health.

Today a number of organizations offer personal, psychological, legal, medical and fashion support to women who choose to go flat after a mastectomy, or after an explant. These group's websites, Facebook pages and podcasts are filled with information specific to the needs of this emerging and growing number of women. The creative and strident names of these newly emerging activist groups, such as *Not Putting on a Shirt, Flat Closure Now, Flat is Where It's At, and I Don't Need Two,* all reflect Audre Lorde's insistence that women must take charge.[60] Women must insist that society change to fit our needs, not remain subservient to today's government and cancer industry's authorities. Lorde would also be proud of the journalist, Catherine Guthrie's 2019 memoir: *Flat: Reclaiming My Body from Breast Cancer.*[61]

Before Lorde's death from recurrent metastatic breast cancer in 1992, fourteen years after having a mastectomy to treat a localized or early-stage breast tumor,[62] Lorde urges women to not be fearful of "going flat," to help society become more aware of today's new "normal." And so Lorde asks, "...what would happen if an army of one-breasted women descended on Congress and demanded that the use of carcinogenic, fat-stored hormones in beef-feed be outlawed?"[63]

The fashion model and artist Matuschka began having periodic mammograms beginning in her late twenties.[64] Her mother had died from breast cancer when Matuschka was just thirteen years old.[65] Two decades later, when Matuschka was thirty-seven years old, a regular mammogram diagnosed a stage I breast tumor in her left breast. She was told a mastectomy was her only effective treatment option.[66] She proceeded. Also refusing to shield her personal truth from the public eye, the artist created a self-portrait which later appeared on the cover of *The New York Times Magazine* on August 15, 1993.[67] The powerful image of the stately model's mutilated body caused a collective gasp across the country. Americans were forced to acknowledge, if only for a moment, the obvious physical mutilation being done to tens of thousands of women each year, in the name of effective treatment. There are no pink ribbons, nor happy smiling faces attached to this self-portrait, merely endurance.[68]

Figure 5.1: Beauty Out of Damage

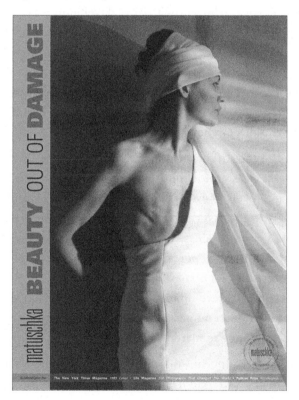

This self-portrait of the artist Matuschka appeared on the cover of The New York Times Magazine, August 15, 1993.

Image used with permission of the artist.

Are Tamoxifen or Arimidex Helpful or Hurtful Prevention Drugs?

Tamoxifen is a breast cancer drug, sometimes prescribed as a recurrence prevention measure, usually for women who have been treated for DCIS or an invasive hormone-positive breast tumor. The drug helps block unbalanced or toxic estrogen from entering a woman's breast cells. Studies show the drug can lower the incidence of recurrent metastatic breast cancer. Three other drugs, Arimidex (anastrozole), Aromasin (exemestane) and Femara (letrozole) are also considered to be similar prevention drugs, for women who have been treated for an early stage breast cancer diagnosis (stage I-III), to try and lower their risk of developing an early-stage or a metastatic recurrence. These drugs block a woman's normal production of aromatase, a building block or precursor of estrogen. Tamoxifen is usually prescribed for premenopausal women, while aromatase inhibitors are more often prescribed for postmenopausal women. Some women are prescribed both types of drugs, taking tamoxifen for a number of years, before switching to Arimidex or another aromatase inhibitor.

The goal of both types of these endocrine therapy drugs is to protect a woman's breast cells' mitochondria from being assaulted by unbalanced (i.e., toxic) levels of estrogen entering her breasts, and by helping prevent any existing breast cancer cells from being stimulated by toxic estrogen levels.[69] Nevertheless, as described in Chapter 1 and Chapter 9, US clinicians continue to report that 20–40 percent (two to four women in ten) who are treated for an early-stage breast cancer in the US today continue to eventually develop terminal or metastatic (stage IV) breast cancer, while lower percentages of breast cancer patients continue to develop an earlier-stage recurrence.[70]

Both types of these endocrine-disrupting prevention drugs also carry adverse side effects. Tamoxifen can apparently assault the mitochondria in a woman's uterine muscle cells and in the endometrial lining of her uterus. Thus, the drug increases a woman's risk of developing both endometrial cancer[71] and uterine sarcomas.[72] Research has also discovered that using tamoxifen increases the risk for older postmenopausal women to develop a hormone-negative, triple-negative breast tumor, if they go on to develop a second primary breast cancer diagnosis after being treated for an early stage hormone-positive breast cancer.[73] The aromatase blocking drugs also have numerous adverse side effects. These range from joint issues to increased heart attacks and strokes.[74]

Meanwhile, as we learned from those four national and transnational mammogram studies described earlier in this chapter, along with a separate statistical study from Canada, women diagnosed with stage 0 breast cancer (DCIS) have the same life span as women who have never been diagnosed with any stage of breast cancer.[75] In other words, a woman diagnosed with stage 0 breast cancer does not risk dying any sooner than women who never received a stage 0 breast cancer diagnosis. No wonder this diagnosis of stage 0 breast cancer is now considered an "overdiagnosis"...a much ado about nothing.

Three Heroes: Questioning Authority

Here are three brave physicians, willing to speak their truth to the power of today's $20 billion or larger US breast cancer industry; an industry currently expecting to almost double its income by 2025. Thankfully, these three medical insiders are willing to openly question, analyze and publish critical studies, trying to enact policies that can help tamp down today's epidemic of overdiagnoses and overtreatment, including the number of overtreated women who develop rMBC.

Our first hero is Dr. Laura Esserman, director of the Carol Franc Buck Breast Care Center at the University of California, San Francisco. Dr. Esserman is not against the use of mammography. But, this outspoken breast surgeon recommends that women who are diagnosed with these atypical cells *not* begin immediate treatment for their DCIS (stage 0) breast diagnosis.[76] "Ductal carcinoma in situ (DCIS) lesions, in and of themselves, are not life-threatening. Although in situ lesions are not tumors, they are usually treated in a manner similar to that of an invasive cancerous tumor. But there is little evidence to support that this practice has improved mortality."[77] In an article with fellow surgeon, Dr. Christina Yau, Dr. Esserman goes on to say, "For many DCIS lesions, there is only a 5 percent chance of invasive cancer developing over 10 years. That's like the average risk of a 62-year-old. We don't do heart surgery when someone comes in with high cholesterol. What are we doing to these people?"[78]

At the grassroots level, more and more women who have been overdiagnosed and overtreated for DCIS (stage 0 breast cancer) are now informing themselves and also speaking out, thanks to the blog *DCIS 411*.[79] Created by a San Diego woman who was overdiagnosed and overtreated for DCIS because of a routine mammogram when she was 44 years old, Donna Pinto's popular blog serves as an important source of information by and for women on this subject.

Figure 5.2: Types of treatments chosen by women diagnosed with DCIS (non-invasive breast cancer) in a single year at the Carol Franc Buck Breast Care Center, UCSF

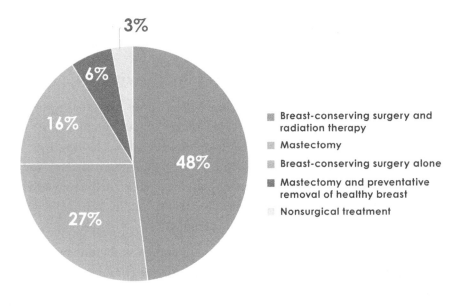

- Breast-conserving surgery and radiation therapy
- Mastectomy
- Breast-conserving surgery alone
- Mastectomy and preventative removal of healthy breast
- Nonsurgical treatment

"Nonsurgical treatment" probably refers to taking tamoxifen for a number of years or not accepting any clinical treatment.

Adapted from C.J. Wells et al., "Evolving Paradigm for Imaging, Diagnosis, and Management of DCIS," Journal of the American College of Radiology 2013, 10(12), 918-923, doi:10.1016/j.jacr.2013.09.011.

Our second hero is Dr. H. Gilbert Welch, a longtime Professor of Medicine and Community & Family Medicine at Dartmouth Medical School, a long-time researcher at Dartmouth's Institute for Health Policy and Clinical Practice and a best-selling New York Times author on the over-testing now done by the US medical community. Dr Welch is currently a senior researcher at the Brigham and Women's Hospital, part of Harvard Medical School.[80] During the past few decades, Dr. Welch has published groundbreaking research analyzing the extensiveness of the overdiagnoses happening to women each year as a result of having regular mammograms.[81] His conclusions are based on data that continue to show us some unsettling facts behind today's breast cancer epidemic throughout the US.

Despite the massive number of mammograms performed on women, and the increasing number of women currently treated for subsequent stage 0 and stage I breast cancer diagnoses each year, mammography screenings have not decreased women's death rate from breast cancer. Also, the increased detection of these noncancerous stage 0 "atypical cells" and stage I tumors has not lowered the rate of fast-growing, stage III tumors, nor the number of women diagnosed with de novo metastatic breast cancer.[82] So what are the benefits of having a mammogram?

Effect of Three Decades of Screening Mammography on Breast Cancer Incidence

"Screening can result in both the benefit of a reduction in mortality and the harm of overdiagnosis. Our analysis suggests that whatever the mortality benefit, breast-cancer screening involved a substantial harm of excess detection of additional early-stage cancers that was not matched by a reduction in late-stage cancers. This imbalance indicates a considerable amount of overdiagnosis involving more than 1 million women in the past three decades— and, according to our best-guess estimate, more than 70,000 women in 2008 (accounting for 31% of all breast cancers diagnosed in women 40 years of age or older)..."

Archie Bleyer, MD and H. Gilbert Welch, MD, MPH, "Effect of Three Decades of Screening Mammography, 1998-2005"[84]

Figure 5.3: Overdiagnosis occurs when screen-detected cancers are either non-growing or so slow-growing that they would never cause medical problems

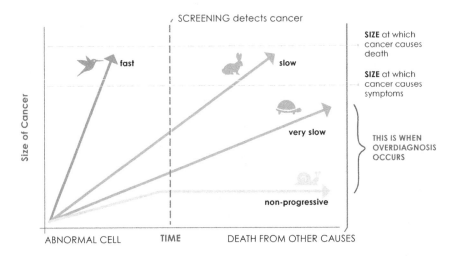

National Cancer Institute
OVERDIAGNOSIS
Occurs when screen-detected cancers are either
non-growing or **slow-growing**
that they would never cause medical problems

Dr. H. Gilbert Welch describes breast tumors as being either *birds, rabbits, turtles* or *snails*. Birds are the very fast-growing tumors that harm women once they travel to vital organs. *Rabbits* are slower-growing tumors. *Turtles* and *snails* are growing at such a slow pace, they are not harmful. These same tumors may disappear on their own accord.

From prevention.cancer.gov, NCI Division of Cancer Prevention. Permission courtesy of H. Gilbert Welch, Dartmouth Medical School.

Our third hero is an open-minded gynecologist, and a longtime *New York Times* best-selling author of numerous books on forward-thinking and commonsense health practices for women. Dr. Christiane Northup, a practicing ob/gyn, understands that women who are diagnosed with stage 0 breast cancer (DCIS) do not have invasive breast cancer! She, like Dr. Welch, does not encourage the use of mammograms. In a 2017 article she wrote, "Autopsies on healthy women in their 40s who died in car accidents found that fully 40% of these women had evidence of DCIS in their breasts. This is NOT cancer. And in the vast majority of women, it will never become cancer. But DCIS is now picked up on at least 15% of the newer digital high-resolution mammograms. And it's being called stage zero breast cancer, and often being overtreated with modalities that have significant side effects such as radiation, surgery, and tamoxifen. This leads everyone to believe that they 'beat breast cancer because they caught it early enough.' I've said for years that there's got to be a better way."[84]

Instead, Dr Northup strongly advocates that women become aware of any ongoing inflammation in their breast tissue; a precursor to breast cancer, by having regular thermograms, described later in this chapter. When it comes to finding fast-growing, significant tumors, she encourages women to lovingly practice breast self-exams and to have regular clinical breast exams.[85]

Premenopausal Women and Mammograms: A Destructive Practice

Environmental research has shown, for decades, that all types of toxic assaults, including mammograms and other types of radiation on a younger woman's breast cells, can often initiate breast cancer.[86] As described in Chapter 1, once a person is able to understand the metabolic approach to cancer, it becomes clear that radiation of any amount can easily help suffocate the fragile mitochondria within younger women's developing or still immature breasts.[87]

And timing is everything. Just ask the highly respected, environmentally focused prevention organizations Silent Spring Institute,[88] Breast Cancer Prevention Partners,[89] and the Collaborative on Health and the Environment.[90] These leading national breast cancer research and education groups have long studied and reported on how it is the *timing* of a radiation attack, the *timing* of toxic chemical attacks, and the *timing* of other inflammatory assaults on a premenopausal woman's breast cells that determine the level of damage that is inflicted. The timing of any radiation attack on a premenopausal woman's breast tissue is more important than how much radiation, or the dose, or the length of these attacks.

Nevertheless, the United States appears to be the only major nation in the world whose medical industry continues to instruct all premenopausal women to have regular mammograms once they reach the age of forty.[91]

By 2015, almost 60 percent of all women in the US between the ages of 40 and 50 had subjected their premenopausal breast tissue to inflammatory rays from mammograms within the previous two years.[92] Are mammograms just one more reason why premenopausal women in the US continue to lead the world in breast cancer incidence?[93]

Here are a few facts, taken from numerous studies that illustrate the heightened sensitivity of teens' and younger women's breast cells' to assaults from all types of radiation:

- Premenopausal women who undergo high levels of medical radiation to the chest during treatment for Hodgkin's lymphoma face an 82% *increased relative risk* of developing breast cancer in the coming twenty years.[94]

- When the atomic bomb was dropped on Hiroshima in 1945, the teenage girls and women under 40 years old who lived just a half-mile from the bomb site experienced much higher rates of breast cancer throughout their lives than the older women living in that same community on that horrific day in history.[95]

- A small percentage of women in the US, just one in 600, is born with damage to one of the two tumor protection BRCA genes located in each of our breast cells.[96] When these genes are fully functioning, they can activate proteins that help control a number of metabolic functions, including cell growth and cell death (helping prevent breast cancer from ever developing). These BRCA1 and BRCA2, genes, located in each of our breast cells, take their names from the words BReast CAncer, since they were first discovered within breast cells.[97] We also have a third cancer protection gene in our breast cells, called P53.[98] If any one of these three genes is malfunctioning, a woman can lose one or more of the cancer-protective abilities of that specific gene. This can make it more difficult, but not impossible, for such a woman's body to destroy a cancer cell, should it begin to form in her breast.[99]

As described in Chapter 8, two to four percent of women in the US are born with either a malfunctioning/mutated BRCA1 gene or a malfunctioning/mutated BRCA2 gene. A higher percentage, about 5 to 10 percent of all breast cancer cases in the US today are diagnosed in women who have one of these mutated tumor-suppressor genes. The cancer is usually diagnosed while these women are premenopausal.[100] It is therefore not surprising that statistically, premenopausal women born with a mutated BRCA gene who have been exposed to the small but significant amount of radiation delivered by a single mammogram end up having a higher rate of breast cancer than other premenopausal BRCA women who have not been exposed to even a single mammogram.[101]

Dense Breasts: Another Scare Tactic

As of 2016, the average height for American women, age 20 and older, was just under 5 feet 4 inches (about 63.7 inches) tall.[102] This is a demographic fact. As of 2016, the percentage of American women with dense breasts was between 40 and 50 percent.[103] This is another demographic fact. Having *dense breasts* means you have more fibrous tissue than fatty tissue in your breasts. Women with more fatty tissue than fibrous breast tissue are defined as having *non-dense breasts*. These are all just basic demographic, physiological facts about American women. Nothing more.

Radiologists are clear: The technology used in current-day mammograms cannot accurately identify tumors in women who have dense breasts. Apparently, dense or fibrous breast tissue is indistinguishable from tumors of any size, and also indistinguishable from atypical cells in a mammography image. This leads to errors called *false positive* or *false negative* readings. In other words, a mammogram says you have a tumor, but you don't: *false positive*. Or your mammogram says you don't have a tumor, but then you find a tumor: *false negative*.[104]

Instead of informing women, straight out, they should not have a regular mammogram if they have dense breasts, the industry likes to switch the conversation to a different subject. The industry continues, instead, to tell women that "dense breasts are a risk factor for breast cancer." But is this statement true?

To answer this question, I went looking for the best statistical and biological research explaining what it is exactly that leads to the conclusion that "dense breasts are a risk factor for breast cancer"—and how much of a risk we're talking about. Try as I might, I couldn't find a clear answer to these questions, amidst all of this well-funded research that began decades ago.

In the past, statistical dense breast studies were all based on dozens of radiologists using different types of highly subjective dense breast image charts. Radiologists each had different methods of determining what constituted "dense breast tissue."[105] Needless to say, results of these studies were never the same.[106]

In 2018, using a new mechanism that can objectively measure breast density, Norwegian researchers were finally able to standardize this concept of "dense breasts."[107] Using this measurement tool for the first time, researchers found only a *slight* difference between the two groups' breast cancer rates.[108] Specifically, in a group of over 100,000 women with dense breasts, only about one additional woman was diagnosed with breast cancer in every 1,000 women examined, compared to every group of 1,000 women who did not have dense breasts. Specifically, the rate of cancer was 6.7 per 1,000 exams for women with dense breasts, compared to 5.5 per 1,000 exams for those with non-dense breasts. Here's another way of stating this finding: For every 1,000 women in the study who had dense breasts, 6.7 women were diagnosed with invasive breast cancer, and for every 1,000 women in the study who did not have dense breasts, 5.5 women were diagnosed with breast cancer; that's a difference of 1.2 women per 1,000.

Nevertheless, it still appears difficult for those embedded in the mammogram industry to give up their mantra that "dense breasts are a risk factor for breast cancer." Dr. Liane E. Philpotts, chief of breast imaging at Yale University's Smilow Cancer Hospital, reviewed the Norwegians' data. According to Dr. Philpotts, "This study really shows that women with dense breasts did have more cancers. It wasn't a huge amount. It was a small increase, but it was an increase."[109]

What do the biologists have to say about all this? Have any researchers yet been able to find a biological reason why dense breast tissue might help create the development of that first cancer cell, as compared to fatty breast tissue? What are the proven or known biological reasons behind the industry's nonstop claim that "dense breasts are a risk factor for developing cancer?" After all, remember that a full 40-50 percent of women in the US have dense breasts!

Over a period of decades, epidemiologists and biologists have been given hundreds of thousands of dollars to conduct studies that begin with the premise that "dense breasts are a risk factor for breast cancer." Still, no researcher has yet been able to pull this rabbit out of the hat. To help prove my point, a 2017 review study from the University of North Carolina looked at 74 dense breast laboratory studies published since the 1970s.[110] In their concluding statement, the UNC biologists state the objective of their research: "to determine why women with high-density breast tissue have a higher risk for developing breast cancer." Their findings: "there are many gaps in the understanding...underlying the strong association of dense breast tissue with initiation of breast cancer."[111] In other words, this meta study concludes, "We just don't know."

Today's mainstream cancer industry continues to come up empty when they try to give us any biological justification for their claim that "dense breast tissue is a risk factor for developing cancer." Of course, this isn't terribly surprising, since today's same genetic-based cancer industry has never been able to tell *any* woman why she develops a breast cancer diagnosis in the first place.

Finally, a Dutch study published in 2018 provides further assurance to women that dense breasts do not increase their risk of dying from breast cancer. This study compared the death rate of women with dense breasts who had been diagnosed with invasive breast cancer against the death rate of women without dense breasts who had also been diagnosed with invasive breast cancer. The study found "no clear association is apparent between breast density and breast cancer death."[112]

It seems two independent juries have now reached similar verdicts. Based on the findings of both recent studies done by Norwegian and Dutch researchers, women can rest assured that having dense breasts does *not* increase their risk of developing nor dying from breast cancer. Better for women to focus on the five effective prevention steps described in this book, than to obsess over the density of their breasts! At least these five prevention steps are lifestyle habits, women can control—starting with just saying "no" to the dangers of even a single mammogram.

State and Federal Laws and Guidelines Regarding Dense Breasts

In 2004, a health practitioner discovered a breast tumor during Dr. Nancy Cappello's annual physical exam. The tumor was diagnosed as stage III. Although Dr. Cappello, an educator from Connecticut, had undergone a regular mammogram every year for many years, her mammogram results had never identified the existence of this tumor. Once Nancy Carvello was diagnosed, however, a doctor mentioned that her dense breasts were probably the reason her numerous mammograms had been unable to identify the tumor's existence.

This experience motivated Dr. Cappello and her husband Joseph to initiate the passage of the first state dense breast notification law in the US.[113] The Cappellos' goal was to require mammogram clinics to notify a woman if she has dense breasts, and to state that a mammogram is not the best breast diagnostic test for her to use, since mammography is often unable to identify irregularities in dense breast tissue.[114] Today, the Connecticut law reads, in part, "If your mammogram demonstrates that you have dense breast tissue, which could hide small abnormalities, you might benefit from supplementary screening tests, which can include a breast ultrasound screening or a breast MRI examination, or both, depending on your individual risk factors."[115]

Thanks to the Cappellos' determination, at least 38 states and the District of Columbia have also now passed some type of breast density identification law. None of these laws, however, mentions the fact that mammograms are not the best test for women to use if they have dense breasts, since mammograms are often unable to diagnose any size tumor in dense breast tissue. Go figure.[116]

In 2019, a federal law was passed that requires the FDA to also address the topic of dense breasts and the fact that mammograms are not an appropriate test for women with dense breasts. But similar to all current state laws which do not make this fact clear, the FDA seems determined to also protect today's mammogram industry. What does this proposed guideline say? The federal agency's current proposal encourages women to continue to have mammograms, while also giving them this popular, but misleading, information: "Dense breasts are an important risk factor for breast cancer."

Fortunately, there are at least a few independent national breast cancer organizations that work on behalf of women's safety, determined to counter any misinformation about dense breasts that government and cancer industry authorities keep spreading. In 2019, Breast Cancer Action's executive director, Karuna Jaggar, tried to help women understand the truth about dense breasts and breast cancer risk: "It's often suggested that dense breasts are a problem, when the reality is that dense breasts are perfectly normal and healthy. In fact, the very concept of breast density emerged as a result of mammography screening. There is nothing uncommon or abnormal about having dense breasts."[117]

Beyond Mammograms: Use Breast Self-Exams and Clinical Breast Exams to Diagnose Fast-Growing, Cancerous Breast Tumors

Year after year, in country after country, study after study has always shown that women find most fast-growing or dangerous tumors themselves, "by accident," by using regular breast self-exams (BSEs), through breast massage, and during lovemaking.[118] Clinical breast exams (CBEs), included in a woman's regular physical or ob/gyn exam, are also how a large number of aggressive or fast-growing breast tumors are found.[119] The recently developed SureTouch technology, using noninvasive elastography technology, can now be employed as part of a clinical exam to improve health practitioners' accuracy in screening for significant palpable lumps.[120]

Once a hard lump is found, it is important to determine or diagnose, noninvasively, whether the lump is cancerous or not. New ultrasound whole-breast technologies and MRIs can make such a diagnosis. Yes, given the availability of these various low- and high-tech screening and *noninvasive* diagnostic tests, mammograms have now become unnecessary. Mammograms are simply the outdated center of a harmful $7.8 billion-dollar-a-year US industry, that offers too many women the headaches of being overdiagnosed and often overtreateded for noninvasive cancer (no cancer) or for tumors that would never go on to harm a woman in any way.

In addition, mammograms are not a trustworthy test when used for that 40 to 50 percent of US women who have dense breasts. No wonder the Swiss Medical Board has called for the closing of all current mammogram clinics throughout their country and the banning of new clinics opening in the future.[121]

In the US, however, the mammogram industry, aligned with private and government health insurance plans, appears determined to force as many mammograms on as many US women as possible. Without being able to force women to have regular mammograms, the breast cancer treatment industry in the US would not be able to overdiagnose an estimated 84,000 women each year with atypical cells or DCIS. Without mandatory mammograms, this same industry would not be able to overdiagnose as many as 190,000 other women with pea-sized, usually non-palpable, usually slow-growing breast tumors. Self-exams and clinical exams will usually miss such unimportant tumors, until they begin to grow. These are the tumors that cautious physicians and surgeons such as Dr. Welch and Dr. Esserman consider to be "important" and should be treated.

Today, women can use noninvasive metabolic therapies to shrink or stop any size tumor's growth, without fear of exacerbating their breast's current condition by overtreatment. Such overtreatment includes undergoing breast biopsies or other types of invasive surgery, radiating the affected breast, or beginning toxic hormone-blocking drugs, such as tamoxifen. In contrast, metabolic therapies include using a ketogenic diet to starve an active tumor of one of its major fuels (glucose), burning off all excess body fat, using whole-body detoxification methods, initiating or expanding meditation or yoga and moving away from highly stressful living and work relationships along with other cortisol-lowering lifestyles. Women overdiagnosed in the US each year, (those identified by a mammogram as being Stage 0 or stage I), currently represent an estimated 275,000 women, or 63 percent of all women who are being annually diagnosed with "breast cancer." Yes, the mammogram industry is an effective feeder system for today's breast cancer overtreatment industry.

Susan G. Komen for the Cure and The American Cancer Society: Loyal Partners with the US Mammogram Industry

In the fall of 2014, while living in Key West, I was invited by the Susan G. Komen Foundation's South Florida office to apply for one of the organization's community grants. At the time, I had created a small nonprofit group that was helping fund the ongoing research for this book project. I agreed to join a conference call that would describe the Komen application process for interested grant recipient organizations throughout South Florida and the Keys. During the conference call with the Komen representative in Miami, we were all quietly told that no group was eligible to receive any Komen grants (ranging from $1,000 to $100,000 annually) for any purpose if the organization taught, endorsed, or even mentioned the practice of breast self-exams.

This was quite a surprise to learn! The following paragraph is taken directly from the Komen Foundation's FY2015 guidelines. It describes the group's strange policy, literally telling women not to touch our own breasts!

Guidelines for Grant Recipients, Appendix D

Breast self-exam must not be taught or endorsed. According to studies, teaching breast self-exam (BSE) has not been shown to be effective at reducing mortality from breast cancer. Therefore, Komen will not fund education projects that teach or endorse monthly breast self-exams or use breast models. As an evidence-based organization, we do not promote activities that are not supported by scientific evidence or that pose a threat to Komen's credibility as a reliable source of information on the topic of breast cancer.[123]

Several years later, little seems to have changed. Here is Komen's ongoing, jaw-dropping policy, taken directly from the organization's FY 2019 Community Grants Guidelines for Grant Recipients:

Funds May Not Be Used for the Following Purposes: **Education regarding breast self-exams/use of breast models.** According to studies, teaching breast self-exam (BSE) has not been shown to be effective at reducing mortality from breast cancer.[123]

If you think that Komen's misstatements about the effectiveness of mammograms and their anti-breast self-exam policy is bad, we now move from the absurd to the ridiculous. Since 2015, the American Cancer Society has recommended that women no longer do breast self-exams, *nor have annual clinical breast exams!* Truly, I can't make this stuff up.

American Cancer Society Releases New Breast Cancer Guidelines[125]

Breast exams, either from a medical provider or self-exams, are no longer recommended. Research has not shown a clear benefit of regular physical breast exams done by either a health professional (clinical breast exams) or by yourself (breast self-exams). There is very little evidence that these tests help find breast cancer early when women also get screening mammograms.

Meanwhile, leading researchers, such as Dr. Welch, who study the overdiagnosis taking place through the use of mammograms today, consider annual clinical breast exams (CBE) as an excellent breast cancer screening practice. "A significant number of cancers would have been missed if CBE (clinical breast exam) had not been performed. Compared with cancers detected by mammography alone, those detected by CBE had more aggressive features. Clinical breast examinations are a very low-cost test that could improve the detection of breast cancer and could prompt breast ultrasonography in the case of a negative mammogram."[125]

In spite of this knowledge, very little funding appears to be available from the US government or from other cancer industry-friendly sources to conduct studies documenting the benefits or liabilities of regular clinical breast exams. As confirmation of this fact, in their "2013 Recommendations on Breast Cancer Screening," the US Preventive Services Task

Force (USPSTF) tells us, "Few data are available to evaluate harms associated with CBE."[126]

Standing Up to Komen and the American Cancer Society

Many national breast cancer organizations continue to ignore Komen's and the Cancer Society's self-serving, truly embarrassing, and rabidly pro-mammography industry policies. Jeopardizing tens of thousands of dollars in annual Komen grant monies, a number of breast cancer groups continue to educate women about the importance and practice of breast self-exam techniques, while also recommending annual clinical breast exams. The Maurer Foundation, located in Hauppauge, New York, on Long Island (where, for the past three decades, environmental studies have documented very high rates of breast cancer), continues to encourage women to do self-exams and have clinical breast exams.[127] The National Breast Cancer Foundation and Breastcancer.org also continue to recommend regular breast self-exams and annual clinical breast exams.

Meanwhile, the California-based Helen Knoll Foundation[128] informs college women that breast cancer incidence in those under forty years old is now at world-record highs throughout the US. This unique group also teaches young women breast self-exam techniques and recommends annual clinical breast exams. Young Survival, the leading national education and support organization for women under forty who have been diagnosed with breast cancer, also continues to ignore these strange anti-BSE and anti-CBE policies created by Komen and the American Cancer Society.[129]

Thank heavens so many national, regional and local breast cancer prevention and support groups are willing to question these so-called breast cancer authorities. These women-focused groups continue to help women understand the importance of using regular breast self-exams and annual clinical breast exams as the two most important tools most women have, when they want to screen their breasts for rapidly growing, dangerous breast tumors. But isn't it strange to have our leading "breast cancer awareness" organizations virtually forbid us women, and our health practitioners, from touching our own breasts?

Early Breast Cancer Prevention Requires Thermography

Functional and metabolic health practitioners, including Dr. Nasha Winters, co-author of *The Metabolic Approach to Cancer*, and Dr. Christiane Northup, author of *Women's Bodies; Women's Wisdom*, recommend women have regular breast thermograms to help them effectively monitor their current level of breast inflammation. Breast and whole-body inflammation are both preconditions for the development of invasive breast cancer. Once a thermogram-reading indicates inflammation exists, a woman now has time to begin cleansing her breast cells, along with the cells throughout the rest of her body. Such internal cleansing can be done by following this book's many prevention steps, especially those described in Chapter 2 and Chapter 6.

Ten years ago, Dr. Northup was already promoting the importance of thermography to women of all ages. "Thermography is safer and more useful for younger and older women than annual or periodic mammograms. Thermography is the most comprehensive breast diagnostic test available. Studies show that a thermogram identifies precancerous cells earlier, and produces unambiguous results, which cuts down on additional testing—and it doesn't hurt the body. Isn't this what women really want?"[130]

When combined with breast self-exams and regular clinical breast exams, thermography, a heat-based diagnostic test, can be used to diagnose inflammation and rapidly growing cancerous tumors throughout the breasts. It is also radiation-free and noninvasive. It can be used to safely diagnose the breast health of both premenopausal and postmenopausal women. Today, two very different types of thermography are available: infrared imaging of the breasts and regulation or whole-body thermography.

Numerous companies manufacture and train health practitioners in the use of infrared cameras for *infrared breast imaging*.[131] It is therefore widely available. Using the second, more recent technology, known as *regulation thermography*, a health practitioner scans the entire body with a heat-sensitive device in order to measure levels of heat throughout the breasts and other organs. Dr. Daniel Beilin, one of the developers of this computer-based body-imaging process, tells us, "the infrared sensor system incorporates historical knowledge of infrared thermography and noninvasive assessment with modern mathematical algorithms to create a whole-body graphic image and report...Regulation thermography is not unlike the cardiologist's treadmill test. More information about health can be obtained from watching how the body behaves dynamically, than with static blood tests or X-rays, that often miss disorders in their developing stages...By assessing the functional capacity of the body's regulation system, it can provide physicians with increased diagnostic and pre-diagnostic capabilities."[132]

Both types of these heat-based technologies, while quite different from one another, are equally popular throughout Europe, and other regions outside of the US. Both technologies are becoming more popular in the US, as women turn away from mammograms. Both thermography technologies are incredibly helpful in diagnosing levels of precancerous inflammation within a woman's breast tissue, while also identifying very fast-growing (hot) tumors. As Dr. Northrup has noted, *"thermography is the best early breast cancer diagnostic test available to women today."*[133] Both types of thermography can also be used to indicate if diagnostic tests, such as noninvasive ultrasound imaging or magnetic resonance imaging (MRI),[134] are required.

Metabolic oncologist Dr. Nasha Winters advocates thermography when women are ready to take an active role in their health and want to be able to understand their current breast health, i.e., the level of inflammation in their breast tissue. For women who want to diagnose palpable growths within their breasts, or have had a prior breast cancer diagnosis, Dr. Winters recommends using a high-definition ultrasound test, such as the SonoCiné, or the next-generation nontoxic MRI called *Prenuvo*.[135] She also calls a breast MRI "the gold standard for a woman who has had breast cancer, and is due for a follow-up screening."[136]

Meanwhile the AMA, the American College of Radiology, the Susan G. Komen Foundation,[137] the FDA, and other radiology industry advocates continue to denounce the capabilities of any and all types of thermal imaging. The FDA's most recent statement, published in 2019, tells us, "the scientific literature is inadequate to validate the clinical role of thermography."[138] Their statement also lauds mammography as the only reliable breast cancer diagnostic procedure available to women.

Yes, here it is again. The Komen Foundation is continuing to use the power of its purse to try to block women's health clinics from uttering the term *thermography*, let alone offer women this noninvasive early breast cancer diagnostic service. Grants applicants continue to be told they are disqualified from receiving a Komen grant if they teach women about thermography, let alone offer either type of thermography test.[139]

Summing Up: Questioning Authority Again!

Today's epidemic of overdiagnosis and overtreatment, almost always triggered by regular mammogram screenings, is quite profitable to mammogram clinics and cancer treatment centers. As mentioned earlier, the 9,000 mammogram clinics throughout the US today are generating about $7.8 billion a year in revenue.[140] Next, the first year of overtreatments given to the estimated 84,000 or more women overdiagnosed each year with stage 0 breast cancer costs an average of $60,637 per woman, for a total of about $5 billion. The estimated 190,000 women currently being diagnosed with stage I breast cancer each year are being charged even more—an average of $82,000 each, during their first two years of overtreatment, for a total of $15 billion.[141]

US clinicians tell us the 20–40 percent of women initially treated for an early-stage breast cancer go on to develop metastatic breast cancer (recurrent metastatic breast cancer or rMBC).[142] This terminal stage of the disease carries the highest annual treatment cost: $182,655 for the first 24 months of treatment. European studies indicate that about 8 to 10 percent of women initially treated for early stage breast cancer also suffer at least one early-stage recurrence of their original breast tumor.[143] Any of these recurrent diagnoses, of course, brings additional treatment expenses. No wonder US women, once diagnosed, often face financial disaster, including bankruptcy. For stage I breast cancer patients who were overtreated and then developed rMBC, their financial tsunami usually stems from a regular mammogram.[144]

In this chapter, we also learned that Switzerland is now considering a scheduled shutdown of all mammography clinics nationwide, while banning the opening of new centers. Meanwhile, Canada and Scandinavia may soon decide to follow Switzerland's lead. We also found studies illustrating how thermography is highly recommended for women of all ages who want to safely identify precancerous or inflamed breast tissue. Noninvasive breast self-exams and clinical breast exams are both important screening tests to find fast-growing or important tumors. New ultrasound technology is available to diagnose any fast-growing, dangerous breast tumors that are found, while new MRI technology is also recommended for women who want to screen and diagnose any recurrent disease. All of this means that women can safely do away with having any regular mammograms. Alleluia!

We then learned about a physician-researcher, a gynecologist-author and a leading breast surgeon who are publicly questioning the overdiagnoses and overtreatment happening to hundreds of thousands of women in the US each year, based on their regular mammogram reports. Each of these physicians continues to place women's best interests first, as they courageously critique and openly disagree with today's monolithic mammogram industry and its ability to overdiagnose and/or overtreat hundreds of thousands of women in the US each year. Meanwhile, the breast cancer industry appears to continue to control federal regulations, insurance coverage policies and the industry's non-profit surrogates, including the American Cancer Society and Susan G. Komen for the Cure; all enforcing today's fiction that mammography is the premiere and mandatory breast cancer prevention, screening and diagnostic test for all women.[145]

This chapter also looked at studies that dispel the fear and confusion the cancer industry and its government partners continue to create, funding never-ending research studies, and never-ending hollow claims that "dense breasts are a risk factor for breast cancer."

Finally, we reviewed the thirty-year-old annual "get a mammogram" pink ribbon campaign that seems to choke the US culture each October. Since chemical and pharmaceutical industries created and have continued to heavily support this "Breast Cancer Awareness Month," this massively successful campaign has helped build, maintain, and expand today's breast cancer epidemic by overdiagnosing and/or overtreating possibly a quarter of a million women in the US each year.[146]

Yes, welcome to "Mammogramland," located on the border of Cancerland. In my mind, and in the minds of those National Swiss Medical Board members, it's best to stay away from the border.[147]

Figure 5.4: How soon will this house of cards fall?

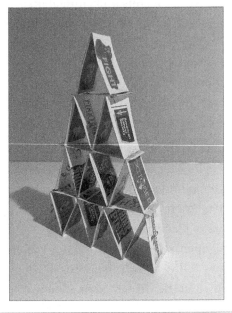

House of Cards, by Steve Linden, paper and glue on cardstock, 2017.

Hopefully, this chapter has helped reduce some stress for you as you learned some basic facts, such as "dense breasts don't condemn you to a cancer diagnosis," and that it is possible to avoid the dangers of overdiagnosis and overtreatment by taking control of your own health using a variety of noninvasive and early breast diagnostic exams. That's good! As the next chapter shows, eliminating our chronic stress can be the single most important part of an effective breast cancer prevention regime. *Busting Breast Cancer*'s simple Prevention Step #5 is all about eliminating what's unhealthy from our minds and our bodies. While we're eliminating stress from our minds, we'll also cleanse our bodies' cells of unwanted toxins. Let's learn how!

CHAPTER ENDNOTES

1   Siva Teja Kakileti et al., "Advances in Breast Thermography," Chapter Five, in *New Perspectives in Breast Imaging* (Karachi, Pakistan BoD–Books on Demand, 2017), 93. https://doi.org/10.5772/intechopen.69198.

2   Diana L Miglioretti et al., "Radiation-Induced Breast Cancer Incidence and Mortality From Digital Mammography Screening: A Modeling Study," *Annals of Internal Medicine* 164, no. 4 (2016): 205–14, https://doi.org/10.7326/M15-1241; G. J. Heyes et al., "Enhanced Biological Effectiveness of Low Energy X-rays and Implications for the U.K. Breast Screening Programme," *British Journal of Radiology* 69, no. 939 (March 2006): 195–200, https://doi.org/10.1259/bjr/21958628.

3   Monica Neagu et al., "Inflammation and Metabolism in Cancer Cell: Mitochondria Key Player, Review Article," *Frontiers in Oncology* (May 14, 2019), https://doi.org/10.3389/fonc.2019.00348; D. Hanahan and R.A. Weinberg, "Hallmarks of Cancer: The Next Generation," *Cell* 144, no.4, (March 4, 2011): 646–74, https://doi.org/10.1016/j.cell.2011.02.013; Yousef Ahmen Fouad and Carmen Aanei, "Revisiting the Hallmarks of Cancer," *American Journal of Cancer Research* 7, no.5 (2017): 1016–36, PMCID - PMC5446472; Buddhini Samarasingle, "The Hallmarks of Cancer 8: Tumor-Promoting Inflammation," Guest Blog, https://blogs.scientificamerican.com/guest-blog/the-hallmarks-of-cancer-8-tumor-promoting-inflammation/.

4   Barbara Ehrenreich, "Welcome to Cancerland: A Mammogram Leads to a Cult of Pink Kitsch," *Harper's*, (November 2001), 43–53, https://harpers.org/archive/2001/11/welcome-to-cancerland/.

5   Sharon Batt, *Patient No More: The Politics of Breast Cancer* (Charlottetown, PEI, Canada: Gynergy Books, 1994), 394.

6   Carcinoma: Cancer that begins in the skin or in tissues that line or cover body organs. Examples are carcinoma of the breast, colon, liver, lung, pancreas, prostate, or stomach, https://www.medicinenet.com/script/main/art.asp?articlekey=20677.

7   The American College of Surgeons' Commission on Cancer's 2017 National Cancer Database was used as the basis for this national estimate of cases. https://www.facs.org/quality-programs/cancer/ncdb.

8   V. L. Vaccaro, "Cause Marketing Partnerships, Diffusion of Breast Cancer Awareness & the Komen Case," Kean University, University of Wollongong, Research Online, Wollongong, Australia, 2008. https://ro.uow.edu.au/insm08/9/.

9   Data based on American College of Surgeons' National Cancer Database, extended to cover 100% of the population, 2017, https://www.facs.org/quality-programs/cancer/ncdb.

10 "Florida Cities' Pink Police Cars Support Breast Cancer Awareness," *Government Fleet*, October 1, 2014, https://www.government-fleet.com/125687/fla-city-designs-pink-police-car-for-breast-cancer-awareness.

11 TMZ.com, "White House Lights Up in Pink for Breast Cancer Awareness Month," October 1,2017, https://www.tmz.com/2017/10/01/white-house-lights-up-pink-breast-cancer-awareness-month/.

12 Sandy M. Fernandez, "History of the Pink Ribbon," Think Before You Pink, https://thinkbeforeyoupink.org/resources/history-of-the-pink-ribbon/.

13 Barbara Ehrenreich, "Welcome to Cancerland," *Harper's Magazine*, November 2001, 43-53.

14 Pesticide Action Network, "Atrazine," https://www.panna.org/resources/atrazine; Newswire, "AstraZeneca Provides $10 Million to American Cancer Society Patient Navigator Program," February 14, 2007, newswire.com, https://www.newswise.com//articles/astrazeneca-provides-10-million-to-american-cancer-society-patient-navigator-program.

15 "AstraZeneca Provides $10 Million to American Cancer Society Patient Navigator Program," February 14, 2007, newswire.com; Charity Navigator, "Susan G. Komen for the Cure," charitynavigator.org.

16 Sharon Batt and Liza Gross, "Cancer, Inc.," *Sierra Magazine*, September/October 1999, https://vault.sierraclub.org/sierra/199909/cancer.asp.

17 Sharon Batt and Lisa Gross, 1999, 1.

18 Aromatase is an enzyme involved in the production of a type of estrogen (estradiol). Aromatase is located in estrogen-producing cells in the adrenal glands, ovaries, placenta, testicles, adipose (fat) tissue, and brain, as per William C. Shiel Jr., "Medical Definition of Aromatase," medicinenet.com.

19 Tyrone Hayes, as quoted in the Land Stewardship Project and Pesticide Action Network North America's Report, "The Syngenta Corporation and Atrazine: The Cost to the Land, People and Democracy," January 2010, https://www.panna.org/sites/default/files/AtrazineReportBig2010.pdf. [Author's note: Tamoxifen blocks estrogen from entering breast cells; it is not an aromatase blocker. But tamoxifen has a similar effect as aromatase blocking drugs.]

20 CDC, "Breast Cancer Screening," *Cancer Trends Progress Report*. https://www.cdc.gov/nchs/fastats/mammography.htm.https://progressreport.cancer.gov/detection/breast_cancer#:~:text=In%202018%2C%2072.8%25%20of%20women,within%20the%20past%202%20years.

21 RADS: A unit of absorbed radiation equal to the amount of radiation that releases an energy of 100 ergs per gram of matter, https://www.britannica.com/science/ionizing-radiation.

22 Barbara Ehrenreich, "Welcome to Cancerland," 43.

23 Collective Evolution, "Swiss Medical Board Condemns Mammogram Screening, Important Facts for Women," Collective-Evolution.com, October 6, 2016, https://www.collective-evolution.com/2016/10/06/switzerland-completely-abolished-mammography-screenings-heres-why-you-should-probably-never-get-one/.

24 Nicola Biller-Adorno and Peter Juni, "Abolishing Mammography Screening Programs? A View from the Swiss Medical Board," *New England Journal of Medicine*, 370 (May 22, 2014): 1965–7, https://doi.org/10.1056/NEJMp1401875.

25 Thermography Center of Sonoma County, "Why Mammography Screening is Being Abolished in Switzerland," *Breast Care*, June 2, 2017, http://thermography-sc.com, https://thermography-sc.com/why-mammography-screening-is-being-abolished-in-switzerland/.

26 K.J. Jorgensen, "Mammography Screening: Benefits, Harms, and Informed Choice," *Danish Medical Journal* 60, no. 4, (April 2013), PMID: 23651722.

27 Steven Narod et al., "Twenty-five-Year Follow-up for Breast Cancer Incidence and Mortality of the Canadian National Breast Screening Study," *British Medical Journal* (2014): 348–366, https://doi.org/10.1136/bmj.g366.

28 H. Gilbert Welch, *Overdiagnosed: Making People Sick in the Pursuit of Health* (Boston, MA: Beacon Press, 2012).

29 H. Gilbert Welch, "Don't Slam Canada for Mammogram Study," February 2, 2014, https://www.cnn.com/2014/02/19/opinion/welch-mammograms-canada/index.html.

30 Ibid.

31 K.J. Jorgensen et al., "Breast Cancer Screening in Denmark: A Cohort Study of Tumor Size and Overdiagnosis," *Annals of Internal Medicine* 166, no. 5 (January 10, 2017): 313–23, https://doi.org/10.7326/M16-0270.

32 "Stories About Mammograms," National Public Radio, https://www.npr.org/tags/125944453/mammogram.

33 Joseph Mercola, "Abolishing Mammography Screening Programs? A View from the Swiss Medical Board," April 30, 2014, https://articles.mercola.com/sites/articles/archive/2014/04/30/mammography-screening-programs.aspx; Geoffrey Kabat, "Should Mammography Be

Abolished?" May 24, 2014, https://www.forbes.com/sites/geoffreykabat/2014/05/24/should-mammography-be-abolished/#4b631dd07e57; H. Gilbert Welch, "Don't Slam Canada for Mammogram Study," https://www.cnn.com/2014/02/19/opinion/welch-mammograms-canada/index.html.

34   Kate Vinton, "These 15 Billionaires Own America's News Media Companies," *Forbes*, June 1, 2016, https://www.forbes.com/sites/katevinton/2016/06/01/these-15-billionaires-own-americas-news-media-companies/#14139887660a.

35   Robert Bridge, "U.S. Mainstream Media is No Friend of the American People," MintPress News., August 20, 2018, https://www.mintpressnews.com/mainstream-media-is-not-your-friend/248025/.

36   J. Koh and M.J. Kim, "Introduction of a New Staging System of Breast Cancer for Radiologists: An Emphasis on the Prognostic Stage," *Korean Journal of Radiology* 20, no. 1 (January 2019): 69-82, https://doi.org/10.3348/kjr.2018.0231.

37   "Understanding Breast Calcifications," https://www.breastcancer.org/symptoms/testing/types/mammograms/mamm_show/calcifications.

38   Gabriele Multhoff, and Jürgen Radons, "Radiation, Inflammation, and Immune Responses in Cancer," *Frontiers in Oncology* 2, no. 58 (June 2012), https://doi.org/10.3389/fonc.2012.00058; Also see Chapter 1.

39   Calculations based on most recent data (2017) from American College of Surgeons National Cancer Database.

40   Ibid.

41   H. Gilbert Welch et al., "Breast Cancer Tumor Size, Overdiagnosis, and Mammography Screening Effectiveness," *New England Journal of Medicine* 375, (October 13, 2016):1438-147, https://doi.org/10.1056/NEJMoa1600249.

42   P.H. Zahl, J. Maehlen, H.G. Welch, "The Natural History of Invasive Breast Cancers Detected by Screening Mammography," *Archives of Internal Medicine* 168, no. 21(2008):2311-16, https://doi.org/10.1001/archinte.168.21.2311.

43   Ibid.

44   Joann G. Elmore and Suzanne W. Fletcher. "Overdiagnosis in Breast Cancer Screening: Time to Tackle an Underappreciated Harm." *Annals of Internal Medicine* 156, no. 7 (2012): 536-7, https://doi.org/10.7326/0003-4819-156-7-201204030-00012.

45   SureTouch, "Introduction to SureTouch for Clinicians," https://suretouch.global, https://static1.squarespace.com/static/58dbb56d6b8f5bc401f33ab9/t/58dd26453e00be49e40abc2d/1490888277585/SureTouch_Physician_Introduction.pdf.

46   Any diagnostic test that does not involve radiating, cutting or poking the tumor is considered to be "nontoxic." Such tests include breast self-exams, clinical breast exams, use of Sure Touch technology, and ultrasound.

47   See: Chapter 7 for Jerilyn's case study.

48   Joann G. Elmore and Suzanne W. Fletcher. "Overdiagnosis in Breast Cancer Screening: Time to Tackle an Underappreciated Harm," 536; also see American College of Surgeons, National Cancer Database, http://oliver.facs.org/BMPub/index.cfm.

49   Estimated incidence numbers based on 2017 American College of Surgeons' National Cancer Database for stage 0 and stage I breast cancer diagnoses.

50   National Cancer Institute, "Overdiagnosis," https://www.cancer.gov/publications/dictionaries/cancer-terms?expand=O.

51   National Cancer Institute, "Overtreatment," https://www.cancer.gov/publications/dictionaries/cancer-terms/def/overtreatment. Author's note: The NCI uses the misleading term "screening test" in their definition of overtreatment, when they are actually referring to the specific use of mammography.

52   ResearchAndMarkets.com, "$10 Billion U.S. Breast Cancer Lumpectomy Market 2018: Treatment Cost & Opportunity Analysis 2024," March 23, 2018, https://www.prnewswire.com/news-releases/breast-cancer-lumpectomy-market-in-the-us-2018-2024—-increasing-breast-cancer-incidence-is-driving-the-market-300618666.html.

53   Joann G. Elmore and Suzanne W. Fletcher, "Overdiagnosis in Breast Cancer Screening: Time to Tackle an Underappreciated Harm," *Annals of Internal Medicine* 156, no. 7 (2012): 536-7, https://doi.org/10.7326/0003-4819-156-7-201204030-00012

54   Alexander Liede et al., "Risk-reducing Mastectomy Rates in the US: A Closer Examination of the Angelina Jolie Effect," *Breast Cancer Research and Treatment* 171, no 2 (2018): 435-442. https://doi.org/10.1007/s10549-018-4824-9.

55   Sharon Batt, *Patient No More*, 394; D. Aygin and H. Cenqiz, "Life Quality of Patients Who Underwent Breast Reconstruction After Prophylactic Mastectomy: Systematic Review," *Breast Cancer* 25, no. 5 (September 2018): 497–505, https://doi.org/10.1007/s12282-018-0862-8; Cleveland Clinic, "What You Should Know About Numbness After Mastectomy: Surgeons Are Researching Ways to Retain and Restore Sensation," May 22, 2017, https://health.clevelandclinic.org/dont-let-numbness-take-you-by-surprise-after-your-mastectomy/.

56   Audre Lorde, *The Cancer Journals* (Argyle, NY: Spinsters Ink, 1980), 57.

57   Audre Lorde, *The Cancer Journals*, 57.

58   Global Market Insights, "The Breast Implants Market to Hit $4.6 Billion by 2025," Press Release, March 11, 2019, https://www.pressrelease.com/news/the-breast-implants-market-to-hit-4-6-billion-by-2025-global-market-20828921.

59   R.S. Roth et al.," Chronic Postsurgical Pain Following Breast Reconstruction: A Commentary and Critique," *Breast Cancer Research and Treatment* 169, no.2 (2018):209-16, https://doi.org/10.1007/s10549-018-4687-0; Explant is a term that describes having a breast implant removed.

60   Flat Closure Now, "Going Flat After Explant," https://www.flatclosurenow.org/explanting#:~:text=Explant%20surgery%20has%20the%20same,the%20pectoralis%20muscle)%20is%20pneumothorax; Not Putting on a Shirt, "Going Flat at Explant," https://notputtingonashirt.org/explant/.

61   Catherine Guthrie, *Flat: Reclaiming My Body from Breast Cancer* (New York: Skyhorse Publishing, 2018). Also see: Catherine Guthrie, "I'm Flat and I'm Proud: Why More Breast Cancer Survivors Are Going Flat," O, The Oprah Magazine, October 2017, https://catherineguthrie.com/wp-content/uploads/2013/05/GoingFlat.OMag_Breast_Cancer_2017-copy.pdf.

62   Audre Lorde, *The Cancer Journals*, 1980, 29-33.

63   Ibid, 16.

64   Matuschka, www.matuschka.net/.

65   Beauty Out of Damage, http://www.beautyoutofdamage.com.

66   Matuschka, personal interviews with author, July 25, 2009 and April 3, 2020.

67   Pia Peterson, "The Times Magazine Cover That Beamed a Light on a Movement," *The New York Times*, August 15, 2018, Section A, Page2; https://www.nytimes.com/2018/08/15/insider/breast-cancer-mastectomy-photo.html.

68   Matuschka, "Beauty Out of Damage," http://www.beautyoutofdamage.com/Aboutphoto.html.

69	R. Gray, "Early Breast Cancer Trialists' Collaborative Group: Effects of Prolonging Adjuvant Aromatase Inhibitor Therapy Beyond 5 Years on Recurrence and Cause-specific Mortality: An EBCTCG Meta-analysis of Individual Patient Data from 12 Randomized Trials Including 24,912 women," Presentation, December 6, 2018, San Antonio Breast Cancer Symposium, https://doi.org/10.1158/1538-7445.SABCS18-GS3-03.

70	A. Lafourcade et al., "Factors Associated with Breast Cancer Recurrences or Mortality and Dynamic Prediction of Death Using History of Cancer Recurrences: The French E3N Cohort," *BMC Cancer* 18, no. 171 (2018), https://doi.org/10.1186/s12885-018-4076-4. Nick Mulcahy, "The Mystery of a Common Breast Cancer Statistic," *Medscape*, August 18, 201, https://www.medscape.com/viewarticle/849644; Joyce O'Shaughnessy, "Treatment Advances in Solid Tumors During the Past Decade: Benchmark Studies Impacting Survival and Quality of Life," *The Oncologist* 10, no. S3, (October 1, 2005):20-9, https://doi.org/10.1634/theoncologist.10-90003-20.

71	F.E. van Leeuwen et al., "Risk of Endometrial Cancer After Tamoxifen Treatment of Breast Cancer," *The Lancet* 343, no. 8895 (February 19, 1994): 448–52, https://doi.org/10.1016/s0140-6736(94)92692-1.

72	Sarcoma: "Committee Opinion No. 601: Tamoxifen and Uterine Cancer," *Obstetric Gynecology* 123, no. 6 (June 2014): 1394–47, https://doi.org/10.1097/01.AOG.0000450757.18294.cf.

73	C.I. Li et al., "Adjuvant Hormonal Therapy for Breast Cancer and Risk of Specific Subtypes of Contralateral Breast Cancer," *Cancer Research* (August 25, 2009), https://doi.org/10.1158/0008-5472.CAN-09-1355. Also, see Chapter 7. *Risk Management* 4, no. 1 (2008):189-204, https://doi.org/10.2147/tcrm.s1566.

74	Jean-Marc A. Nabholtz, "Long-term Safety of Aromatase Inhibitors in the Treatment of Breast Cancer," *Therapeutics and Clinical Risk Management* 4, no. 1 (2008):189-204. https://doi.org/10.2147/tcrm.s1566. Farzin Khosrow-Khavar et al., "Cardiovascular Outcomes in Women with Breast Cancer," Circulation 141, (2020): 549-59, https://doi.org/10.1161/CIRCULATIONAHA.119.044750.

75	Steven A. Narod et al., "Breast Cancer Mortality After a Diagnosis of Ductal Carcinoma in Situ," *JAMA Oncology* 1, no.7 (August 20, 2015): 888–96, w https://doi.org/10.1001/jamaoncol.2015.2510.

76	Nick Mulcahy, "Laura Esserman and Shelley Hwang," *Medscape*, January 21, 2010, https://www.medscape.com/viewarticle/715586; Laura J. Esserman et al., "The WISDOM Study: Breaking the Deadlock in the Breast Cancer Screening Debate," *NPJ Science of Learning* 3, No. 34 (September 13, 2017), https://doi.org/10.1038/s41523-017-0035-5.

77	L. Esserman et al., "Less is More: The Evolving Surgical Approach to Breast Cancer," Educational Session, 2016 American Society of Clinical Oncology, https://meetinglibrary.asco.org/record/50969/edbook.

78	Laura Esserman and Christina Yau, "Rethinking the Standard for Ductal Carcinoma in Situ Treatment," *JAMA Oncology* (August 20, 2015): E1–E3, https://www.scribd.com/document/316970898/2016-EdBook; Marhias Worni et al., "Trends in Treatment Patterns and Outcomes for Ductal Carcinoma In Situ," *Journal of the National Cancer Institute* 107, no. 12 (September 2015): djv263, https://doi.org/10.1093/jnci/djv263; Katie Hafner, "A Breast Cancer Surgeon Who Keeps Challenging the Status Quo," *The New York Times*, September 28, 2015, https://www.nytimes.com/2015/09/29/health/a-breast-cancer-surgeon-who-keeps-challenging-the-status-quo.html; See also Peggy Orenstein, "Our Feel-Good War on Breast Cancer," *The New York Times Magazine*, April 25, 2013, https://www.nytimes.com/2013/04/28/magazine/our-feel-good-war-on-breast-cancer.html.

79	DCIS 411, Helping Women Make Better Health Care Decisions, https://dcis411.com.

80	"Welcoming New Faculty-Gilbert Welch," August 13, 2019, https://bwhsurgerynews.partners.org/welcoming-new-faculty-gilbert-welch-md-mph/.

81 H. Gilbert Welch, "Screening Is Not a Medical Health Imperative - It Is a Choice," https://radiantbodythermography.com/h-gilbert-welch-work.

82 Brigham and Women's Hospital, "Cancer Data Provide Insights Into Occurrence Overdiagnosis, and Treatment Advances, Brigham and Women's Hospital, Oct 2, 2019, https://www.brighamandwomens.org/about-bwh/newsroom/press-releases-detail?id=3448; "Welcoming New Faculty - Gilbert Welch," August 13, 2019, https://bwhsurgerynews.partners.org/welcoming-new-faculty-gilbert-welch-md-mph/.

83 A. Bleyer and H. G. Welch, "Effect of Three Decades of Screening Mammography on Breast-Cancer incidence," *The New England Journal of Medicine* 367, no. 21 (2012): 1998-2005, https://doi.org/10.1056/NEJMoa1206809.

84 Christiane Northrup, "Five Reasons Not to Have a Mammogram," October 9, 2017. https://www.drnorthrup.com/best-breast-cancer-screening-tests/.

85 Christian Northrup, "Transforming the Breast Self-Exam," https://www.drnorthrup.com/transforming-breast-self-exam/; Also see: *Women's Bodies, Women's Wisdom* (New York: Bantam, 2010).

86 Janet Gray et al., "State of the Evidence 2017: An Update on the Connection Between Breast Cancer and the Environment," *Environmental Health* (2017) 16:94, https://doi.org/10.1186/s12940-017-0287-4.

87 See Chapter 1.

88 Mary Beth Terry et al., "Environmental Exposures During Windows of Susceptibility for Breast Cancer: A Framework for Prevention Research," *Breast Cancer Research* 21, no. 96 (August 20, 2019) https://doi.org/10.1016/j.envres.2020.109346; Julia G. Brody, "Everyday Exposures and Breast Cancer," *Reviews on Environmental Health* 25, no. 1 (December 4, 2008), https://doi.org/10.1515/REVEH.2010.25.1.1.

89 Breast Cancer Prevention Partners, https://www.bcpp.org.

90 Collaborative on Health and the Environment, Breast Cancer Working Group, "Consensus Statement on Breast Cancer and the Environment," 2006, https://www.healthandenvironment.org/docs/ConsensusStatementOnBreastCancerAndTheEnvironment.pdf.

91 American Cancer Society, "American Cancer Society Guidelines for the Early Detection of Cancer," https://www.cancer.org/healthy/find-cancer-early/cancer-screening-guidelines/american-cancer-society-guidelines-for-the-early-detection-of-cancer.html.

92 Centers for Disease Control, "Trend Tables: Table 70: Use of Mammography Among Women Aged 40 and Over, By Selected Characteristics: United States, Selected Years 1987-2015," https://www.cdc.gov/nchs/data/hus/2016/070.pdf.

93 *Busting Breast Cancer*, "Breast Cancer Rising in Women Under 50," 2012 (see Chapter 9); E. Ward et al., "Annual Report to the Nation on the Status of Cancer, Special Section on Cancer Among Adults Age 20-49," *Journal of the National Cancer Institute*, djz106 (May 30, 2019), http://doi.org/10.1093/jnci/djz106.

94 Joaira Bakkach et al., "Secondary Breast Cancer After Hodgkin Lymphoma: A Case Report and Literature Review," *ecancermedicalscience* 12, no. 810 (February 14, 2018), https://doi.org/10.3332/ecancer.2018.810; Veronica Manzo et al., "Breast Cancer After Hodgkin Lymphoma: The Price of Success," *Oncology Journal* 30, no. 12 (December 15, 2016), https://www.cancernetwork.com/oncology-journal/breast-cancer-after-hodgkin-lymphoma-price-success; Boston University School of Public Health, "Risk Ratios and Rate Ratios (Relative Risk)," http://sphweb.bumc.bu.edu/otlt/MPH-Modules/EP/EP713_Association/EP713_Association3.html.

95 Dorothe Schaue et al., "Radiation and Inflammation," *Seminars of Radiation Oncology* 1 (January 25, 2015): 4-10. https://doi.org/10.1016/j.semradonc.2014.07.007.

96 Gayle Sulik, "Angelina Jolie and the One Percent," *Scientific American*, May 20, 2013, https://blogs.scientificamerican.com/guest-blog/angelina-jolie-and-the-one-percent/.

97 Kumaravel Somasundaram, "BRCA1 and BRCA1 Genes and Inherited Breast and/or Ovarian Cancer: Benefits of Genetic Testing," *Indian Journal of Surgical Oncology* 1, no. 3 (2010): 245–49, https://pubmed.ncbi.nlm.nih.gov/22693372/.

98 It is unknown what percentage of the population is born with a mutated P53 gene. But younger women who develop triple-negative breast cancer often lose the tumor protection function in their P53 gene. Also, see Raman Preet Kaur et al., "Role of P53 Gene in Breast Cancer: Focus on Mutation Spectrum and Therapeutic Strategies," *Current Pharmaceutical Design* 24, no. 30 (2018): https://doi.org/10.2174/1381612824666180926095709; A. Amadou et al., "Revisiting Tumor Patterns and Penetrance in Germline TP53 Mutation Carriers: Temporal Phases of Li-Fraumeni Syndrome," *Current Opinions in Oncology* 1 (January 30, 2018): 23–29, https://doi.org/10.1097/CCO.0000000000000423.

99 See Chapter 8.

100 Stanford University, "BRCA1 & BRCA2 Genes," https://stanfordhealthcare.org/medical-conditions/cancer/hboc/brca-1-and-2.html.

101 Anouk Pijpe et al., "Exposure to Diagnostic Radiation and Risk of Breast Cancer Among Carriers of BRCA1/2 Mutations: Retrospective Cohort Study (GENE-RAD-RISK)," *British Medical Journal (Clinical Research Edition)* 345 e5660. 6 (September 2012), https://doi.org/10.1136/bmj.e5660.

102 "Average Height for Women: America, World, Weight & More," https://www.healthline.com/health/womens-health/average-height-for-women.

103 Shayan S. Nazari and Pinku Mukherjee, "An Overview of Mammographic Density and its Association with Breast Cancer," *Breast Cancer* 25 (October 12, 2018): 259–67, https://doi.org/10.1007/s12282-018-0857-5.

104 Ibid.

105 Jacques Brisson et al., "Wolfe's Parenchymal Pattern and Percentage of the Breast with Mammographic Densities: Redundant or Complementary Classifications?" *Cancer Epidemiology, Biomarkers & Prevention* 12, no. 8 (August 2008): 728–32, https://doi.org/10.1093/oxfordjournals.epirev.a036105; I.T. Gram et al., "Percentage Density, Wolfe's and Tabár's Mammographic Patterns: Agreement and Association with Risk Factors for Breast Cancer," *Breast Cancer Research* 7, R854 (2005): https://doi.org/10.1186/bcr1308.

106 Karla Kerlikowske et al., "Identifying Women with Dense Breasts at High Risk for Interval Cancer: A Cohort Study," *Annals of Internal Medicine* 162, no. 10 (2015): 673–81, https://doi.org/10.7326/M14-1465; Valerie A. McCormack and Isabel dos Santos Silva, "Breast Density and Parenchymal Patterns as Markers of Breast Cancer Risk: A Metanalysis," *Cancer Epidemiology, Biomarkers & Prevention* (June 2006), https://doi.org/10.1158/1055-9965.EPI-06-0034.

107 Solveig Hofvind et al., "Density in a Screening Setting: Worse Outcomes for Women with Dense Breasts," *Radiology* 288, no. 2 (June 26, 2018): https://doi.org/10.1148/radiol.2018172972.

108 Radiological Society of North America, "Breast Density Alone Not a Risk Factor for Cancer, Study Suggests," *ScienceDaily*, December 2, 2015, www.sciencedaily.com/releases/2015/12/151202084226.htm.

109 Liane E. Philpotts, "Machine Detection of High Breast Density: Worse Outcomes for Our Patients," *Radiology* (June 26, 2018), https://doi.org/10.1148/radiol.2018180827.

110 Shayan S. Nazari and P. Mukherjee, "An Overview of Mammographic Density and Its Association with Breast Cancer," *Breast Cancer*, 25 (2018): 259–67, https://doi.org/10.1007/s12282-018-0857-5.

111 Ibid.

112 Daniëlle van der Waal et al., "Breast Density and Breast Cancer-specific Survival by Detection Mode." *BMC Cancer* 18, no., 1 (April 5, 2018): 386, https://doi.org/10.1186/s12885-018-4316-7.

113 Are You Dense Advocacy, Inc., "Connecticut's Landmark Breast Density Legislation," https://www.areyoudenseadvocacy.org/news/connecticuts-landmark-breast-density-legislation.

114 Joseph Cappello, phone interview with author, February 18, 2019.

115 Are You Dense Advocacy, Inc., https://www.areyoudenseadvocacy.org, Click on state of Connecticut in the map to see the law.

116 US Food and Drug Administration, "Mammography: What You Need to Know," https://www.fda.gov/consumers/consumer-updates/mammography-what-you-need-to-know.

117 Breast Cancer Action, "Breast Cancer Action Challenges the FDA's Proposal Requiring Women Get Breast Density Information After Mammograms," March 28, 2019, https://bcaction.org/2019/03/28/breast-cancer-action-challenges-the-fdas-proposal-requiring-women-get-breast-density-information-after-mammograms/.

118 Mara Y. Roth et al., "Self-Detection Remains a Key Method of Breast Cancer Detection for U.S. Women," *Journal of Women's Health* 20, no. 8 (August 2011): https://doi.org/10.1089/jwh.2010.2493.

119 Huan Jiang et al., "Estimation of the Benefit and Harms of Including Clinical Breast Examination in an Organized Breast Screening Program," *The Breast* 43 (February 2019): 105-112, https://doi.org/10.1016/j.breast.2018.11.012; H. Gilbert Welch, "Don't Slam Canada," 2014, https://www.cnn.com/2014/02/19/opinion/welch-mammograms-canada/index.html; Damian Dovarganes, "Contentious Canadian Study Says Mammography Doesn't Cut Deaths from Breast Cancer," *The Canadian Press/AP*, February 12, 2014, https://nationalpost.com/news/canada/contentious-canadian-study-says-mammography-doesnt-cut-deaths-from-breast-cancer.

120 Cary S. Kaufman et al., "Digital Documentation of the Physical Examination: Moving the Clinical Breast Exam to the Electronic Medical Record," *Journal of Surgery* 192, no.4 (October 1, 2006):444-49, https://doi.org/10.1016/j.amjsurg.2006.06.006; Cancer Connect, "SureTouch Improves Accuracy of Manual Palpation in Detection of Breast Cancer," https://news.cancerconnect.com/breast-cancer/suretouch-improves-accuracy-of-manual-palpation-in-detection-of-breast-cancer-JWDDaQh2bUSmNliZW-b8Og.

121 Laura Esserman et al., "Ductal Carcinoma in Situ: Where We Have Been and Where We Can Be," *The ASCO Post*, October 10, 2015, https://ascopost.com/issues/october-10-2015/ductal-carcinoma-in-situ-where-we-have-been-and-where-we-can-be/; Nick Mulcahy, "Laura Esserman and Shelley Hwang," *Medscape*, January 21, 2010, https://www.medscape.com/viewarticle/715586.

122 Susan G. Komen Foundation, "Community Grants Program Request for Applications" FY 2019, 6, http://chicagoland.info-komen.org/site/DocServer/2019-2020_Komen_Chicago_CG_RFA_FINAL.pdf?docID=17213.

123 Nancy Knoche, "Is the American Cancer Society Putting Money Ahead of Mission?," *Nonprofit Quarterly*, March 28, 2011, https://nonprofitquarterly.org/2011/03/28/is-the-american-cancer-society-putting-money-ahead-of-mission/; also see Devra Davis, *The Secret History of the War on Cancer* (New York: Basic Books, 2006); Daniel B. Kopans, "Arguments Against Mammography Screening Continue to be Based on Faulty Science," *The Oncologist* 19, No. 2 (2014): 107-12, https://doi.org/10.1634/theoncologist.2013-0184.

124 "American Cancer Society Recommendations for the Early Detection of Breast Cancer," cancer.org, February 2019, https://www.cancer.org/cancer/breast-cancer/screening-tests-and-early-detection/american-cancer-society-recommendations-for-the-early-detection-of-breast-cancer.html.

125 L. Provencher et al., "Is Clinical Breast Examination Important for Breast Cancer Detection?" *Current Oncology* 23, no. 4 (2016):e332-39, https://doi.org/10.3747/co.23.2881; Also see Huan Jiang, et al., "Estimation of the Benefit and Harms," *The Breast*, 43 (February 1, 2019): 105-112, https://doi.org/10.1016/j.breast.2018.11.012; Nover et al., "Modern Breast Cancer Detection: A Technological Review," *International Journal of Biomedical Imaging*, December 2009 (4): 902326; https://doi.org/10.1155/2009/902326; Narod, "25 Year Follow-Up," 348–366, https://doi.org/10.1136/bmj.g366.

126 United States Preventive Services Task Force, "Breast Cancer Screening: Published Final Recommendations," December 30, 2013; https://www.uspreventiveservicestaskforce.org/uspstf/document/RecommendationStatementFinal/breast-cancer-screening.

127 Diana Jean Schemo, "Long Island Presses for Answers on Breast Cancer," *The New York Times*, October 5, 1992, https://www.nytimes.com/1992/10/05/nyregion/long-island-presses-for-answers-on-breast-cancer.html.

128 Helen Knoll Foundation, helenknollfoundation.org.

129 Young Survival Coalition, https://www.youngsurvival.org.

130 Christiane Northup, "The Best Breast Test: The Promise of Thermography," *Huffington Post*, October 12, 2010, https://huffpost.com/entry/the-best-breast-test-the-b_752503.

131 International Association of Thermology, https://iamtonline.org/; also, see Meditherm.com.

132 Alfathermo.com, "Download the free PDF," https://alfathermo.com/about/about-alfa.

133 Northup, The Best Breast Test: The Promise of Thermography."

134 National Institutes of Health, "Magnetic Resonance Imaging (MRI)," https://www.nibib.nih.gov/science-education/science-topics/magnetic-resonance-imaging-mri.

135 DCIS 411, "Bye-Bye Mammograms: Hello SonoCiné Ultrasound," January 10, 2017, https://dcis411.com/2017/01/10/bye-bye-mammograms-hello-sonocine-ultrasound/.

136 Correspondence with author, March 15, 2019.

137 The Susan G. Komen Foundation, "A Note About Thermography," https://ww5.komen.org/BreastCancer/EmergingAreasinEarlyDetection.html, June 25, 2-019, [4,86,97-98].

138 Food and Drug Administration, "FDA Warns Thermography Should Not Be Used in Place of Mammography to Detect, Diagnose, or Screen for Breast Cancer: FDA Safety Communication," February 25, 2019, https://www.fda.gov/medical-devices/safety-communications/fda-warns-thermography-should-not-be-used-place-mammography-detect-diagnose-or-screen-breast-cancer.

139 Susan G. Komen, "Community Grants Program," 'Funds may not be used for the following purposes,' 6, http://chicagoland.info-komen.org/site/DocServer/2019-2020_Komen_Chicago_CG_RFA_FINAL.pdf?docID=17213.

140 Cristina O'Donoghue et al., "Aggregate Cost of Mammography Screening in the United States: Comparison of Current Practice and Advocated Guidelines," *Annals of Internal Medicine* 160, no. 3 (2014): 145–53, https://doi.org/10.7326/M13-1217.

141 Helen Blumen et al., "Comparison of Treatment Costs for Breast Cancer, by Tumor Stage and Type of Service," *American Health & Drug Benefits* 9, no.1 (2016): 23–32, PMCID: PMC4822976.

142 Ibid, 123.

143 B. Holleczek et al., "Risk of Loco-regional Recurrence and Distant Metastases of Patients with Invasive Breast Cancer up to Ten Years After Diagnosis–Results from a Registry-based Study from Germany," *British Medical Journal of Cancer* 19, no.520 (2019). https://doi.org/10.1186/s12885-019-5710-5.

144 Julia Malacoff, "Breast Cancer is a Financial Threat No One's Talking About," Shape.com, https://www.shape.com/lifestyle/mind-and-body/breast-cancer-dangerous-financial-threat; Patrick Richard et al., "The Burden of Out of Pocket Costs and Medical Debt Faced by Households with Chronic Health Conditions in the United States," *Public Library of Science One* 13, no. 6 (June 25, 2018), https://doi.org/10.1371/journal.pone.0199598.

145 C. Hardin et al., "Long-term Relationships Between Screening Rates, Breast Cancer Characteristics, and Overdiagnosis in U.S. Counties, 1975–2009," *International Journal of Cancer* 144, no. 3 (February 1, 2019): 476–88, https://doi.org/10.1002/ijc.31904. Epub 2018 November 5; P. Autier and M. Boniol, "Mammography Screening: A Major Issue in Medicine," *European Journal of Cancer* 90, (February 2018): 34-62, https://doi.org/10.1016/j.ejca.2017.11.002; Also see the blog, DCIS411.com.

146 Estimates based on 2017 data from American College of Surgeons' Commission on Cancer, National Cancer Database, http://oliver.facs.org/BMPub/.

147 Ehrenreich, "Welcome to Cancerland," 43; also see Barbara Ehrenreich, *Natural Causes: An Epidemic of Wellness, the Certainty of Dying, and Killing Ourselves to Live Longer* (New York: Twelve, 2018).

STEP 5:
Cleanse the Insides of Your Brain and Body Every Day

"Cancer is a metabolic, environmental and emotional disease."

—Nasha Winters and Jess Higgins Kelley,
The Metabolic Approach to Cancer

"Because they believe in the metabolic theory of cancer, (Thomas) Seyfried and (Domenic) D'Agostino approach cancer therapy from a different angle. Their vision is almost utopian—a therapeutic approach less like combat and more like a gentle rehabilitation and restoration of health. Their vision is not a bombardment based on the "no pain, no gain" mentality. Their description of cancer as an 'ecosystem' is an honest characterization of the complex nature of the disease. As any ecologist would tell you, the best way to alter an ecosystem is to change the entire environment. Focus on changing the entire environment in which the cancer tries to live."

—Travis Christofferson,
Tripping Over the Truth[1]

Imagine you have a home aquarium. One day you notice your fish are looking limp. Do you take their blood pressure and throw them some aspirin, or do you simply clean the tank and its filters, and change the water?

Our body is a lot like that fish tank, and our breast cells are like those fish. If we keep our liquids, pumps, and filters cleaned, lubricated, and free flowing, our fish (our breast cells) will probably thrive. If we ignore these tasks, don't be surprised when our breast cells' oxygen-loving mitochondria start to suffocate.

For more than a decade, the US government has continued to tell us, "one in eight women in the US can expect to develop breast cancer in her lifetime."[2] And, as we saw earlier, in 2015 the National Cancer Institute quietly began predicting that American women will experience a *fifty percent* increase in breast cancer by 2025! Their stated reason? That huge post-World War II baby boomer generation will have reached retirement age by 2030.[3] But what does a woman's aging have to do with such a huge increase in breast cancer risk?

The answer is simple: the aging process causes cellular congestion or inflammation.[4] As we've learned, unmitigated inflammation from many sources eventually causes the mitochondria of our breasts (and other organs) to suffocate. This suffocation ultimately leads to the development of that first cancer cell.[5]

Familiar signs of inflammation are heat, pain, redness, and swelling. These indicate your body is working hard to heal an external abrasion, a sprain, an internal or external surgical incision, or a burn. But when heat, pain, redness, and swelling remain on your skin (as a chronic rash, for example, or as atypical cells in your breast tissue), you are now dealing with *chronic inflammation*.[6] Fortunately, chronic inflammation is a situation that can be reversed. And that's why continuously cleansing or *detoxing* your body makes sense.[7]

Most US medical schools do not teach doctors how to lower inflammation naturally; they use some type of drug. Mainstream physicians often prescribe toxic anti-inflammatory steroids, or nonsteroidal anti-inflammatory (NSAID) medications to do the trick. However, there are other approaches to lowering chronic inflammation. The branch of Western medicine known as *functional* or *holistic medicine* focuses on a patient's entire detoxification needs, seeing the patient as a mind–body whole. In this regard, functional/holistic medicine is similar to many schools of traditional medicine, including Native American medicine, East Indian Ayurveda, European homeopathy, and both ancient Chinese and Japanese healing methods. These traditional schools of medicine understand that curbing inflammation is best done through supporting the body's natural detoxification or cleansing systems.[8] Yes, detox is critical for healing, disease prevention, and maintaining ongoing optimal health.

No wonder aging happens faster in those who don't work every day to limit and help clean out the toxins in their bodies. If you'd like to join the ranks of those who have decided to age as slowly as possible, and also help prevent breast cancer, here are ten tasks you can perform to help cleanse your cells—especially your breast cells—on a regular basis. And the good news is that most of these steps are simple, nourishing, and inexpensive. In this chapter, we'll take a look at what you can do every day to cleanse the insides of your body and your brain.

An Inside Job: Ten Paths to Cleanliness

We already know lots of ways to cleanse the outside of our bodies: brush our teeth, scrub our back, shampoo our hair. That's easy! Now it's time to tackle the insides of our minds and bodies. Some of these ten tasks can help cleanse and oxygenate blood, along with the crucial interstitial fluid (I-fluid) that bathes our breast cells in oxygen and other nutrients.[9] Many of these tasks can also cleanse the cells in our minds and bodies of toxins caused by chronic daily stress.[10]

Detox Task #1: Fill Your Body with Clean Water

You've heard this before: Drink six to eight glasses of clean (filtered) water daily. And you already know why: More than half of your body is comprised of water. So, we begin this chapter by suggesting that you change much of the water in your "fish tank" every day!

But what's in that water you're drinking? The easiest way to keep the inside of your body as clean as possible is to drink water that has been cleansed of chlorine, heavy metals, animal and chemical hormones, fluoride, pesticides, and traces of prescription drugs—which are all too often found in our public water supplies today.[11] Drinking lots of filtered water also keeps our bowels well-hydrated and moving—another basic, but critical, way to keep the fluids and cells throughout our bodies as clean as possible.

Drinking bottled water may protect you from the chlorine, fluoride, and hormones found in too many public water supplies today, but other toxins can leach into the water if you drink from plastic bottles. Better to use glass bottles, bisphenol A (BPA)-free plastic bottles, or no bottles at all, whenever possible.[12] The Silent Spring Institute and Breast Cancer Prevention Partners, both leading independent environmentally focused breast cancer organizations, have long researched and educated women about possible environmental causes of this disease. Their findings and publications are excellent resources for understanding more about BPA and other types of chemical hormonal disrupters, called xenohormones.[13]

Bisphenol A (BPA)

An industrial chemical used to make polycarbonate plastic, epoxy resin linings for food and beverage cans, thermal paper receipts, and other products. It is one of a broad suite of organic chemicals—identified as endocrine disrupting compounds—that are important for breast cancer research. Exposure to BPA has been associated with effects on the developing brain, and on mammary and prostate glands, in laboratory studies.

Silent Spring Institute | *silentspring.org*

First, install a good water filter under your kitchen sink, on the kitchen faucet—or even better, if it's affordable, on the main water line into your home, thus filtering your home's entire water supply. Another alternative is to use a variety of water pitchers that filter your tap water.[14] These are all systems designed to help filter out heavy metals and chlorine from the public water supply coming into your kitchen.

Filter your shower water.
Our skin also absorbs lots of water—and along with it, any pollutants that may be in the water, whenever we shower. Some say the amount absorbed in one ten-minute shower is equal to drinking a gallon of water! Fortunately, a decent shower filter doesn't have to cost more than $30 to $50. Dr. Joseph Mercola's wide-ranging and well-researched natural health website, mercola.com, continues to educate and update consumers on why we need to use water filters in our homes, and what makes one type of filter more effective than another.[15]

Detox Task #2. Keep Your Lymph System and Toxins Moving
Our heart, the biggest muscle in our body, pumps blood 24/7. But our lymph system doesn't come with a comparable built-in pumping station. This is a problem because the lymph system carries nutrients and immune cells around our bodies and helps move toxic or processed (i.e. used) and excess natural hormones and chemical or xenohormones

(along with other types of toxins) into our sweat and urine so they can be eliminated. This means our lymph system depends on us to move our bodies around every day in order to physically push the lymph fluid through the body. So, here are four easy ways to make sure lymph fluids don't stagnate in your breasts. Stagnating fluids, after all, help breast cells' mitochondria suffocate.

1. **Use a dry skin brush before you shower.**
   A dry skin brush gently activates your lymph system before you step into the shower. Lightly brush—almost tickle—your body with this medium-to long-handled, natural-bristle brush. Move the brush in light, downward strokes from your neck down to your heart. Then use light, upward strokes from your toes to your belly. Brush your belly and breasts in a very gentle, circular manner, but avoid brushing your highly sensitive nipples.[16] Dry skin brushing also stimulates your immune cells, exfoliates your skin, and opens up your pores so they'll release even more toxins.

2. **Enjoy regular breast massage.**
   Breast massage is another relaxing way to keep your lymph system moving. Whether done by yourself or your partner, massage is also a wonderful way to gently relieve stress, another cause of whole-body inflammation (discussed later in this chapter).[17] Breast massage can also become a part of your regular breast self-exams (BSEs), (described in Chapter 5).

3. **Engage in no-sweat exercise.**
   Walking the dog, cycling around the block a few times, and joining a gentle exercise or yoga class are all no-sweat exercises that also help pump your interstitial fluid, what I like to call *I-fluid*, through your lymph system and around your cells. I-fluid is extremely important in breast cancer prevention. It is "found in the spaces around cells. It comes from substances that leak out of blood capillaries (the smallest type of blood vessel). It helps bring oxygen and nutrients to cells and to remove waste products from them. As new interstitial fluid is made, it replaces older fluid, which drains towards lymph vessels. When it enters the lymph vessels, it is called lymph. Also called tissue fluid."[18]

Another efficient way to move your lymph system, without sweating, is with a whole-body vibration plate. According to a growing number of studies led by Dave Asprey, creator of *Bulletproof*, a manufacturer of ketogenic-lifestyle products, exercising while using a vibration plate improves blood circulation, lymphatic drainage, flexibility and mobility.[19]

4. Include high-sweat exercise.

Getting your body into a full-blown heavy sweat also helps move your lymph fluid, further cleansing your body of toxins. If you are in good physical shape, choose some type of high exertion exercise that you enjoy doing a few times each week. This workout can be anything from spinning to jogging to hot yoga. All of these practices help eliminate toxins through the sweat glands in your skin.

If you're not able to be physically active, or if you just want to relax and sweat at the same time, think about purchasing a near infrared sauna. This type of sauna raises the internal temperature of your body, produces a solid sweat, and enables you to gain the cleansing benefits of rigorous full-sweat exercise without exercising! Fortunately, some infrared saunas are now portable and can be affordable, costing about $325. Again, Dr Joseph Mercola's website stays up to date on research regarding the best infrared saunas for effective detoxification.[20]

Detox Task #3: Increase Digestive Enzymes and Cell-to-Cell Communication

Here is a two-for-one discovery. Once past menopause, most women have a much harder time manufacturing enough digestive enzymes to enable food to move down and through our digestive tracts where these nutrients are further processed by whatever good bacteria currently reside and are multiplying within our small intestines. Recent science tells us that this personal or unique garden of single-cell flora (microbiota) living inside our gut creates a very important part of our body's ability to fight viruses, bacterial infections and overall healing.[21] The foods we eat every day, and how well we can digest or break these foods into nutrients and then absorb them, determines how well our gut bacteria (also known as our biome) are functioning. In other words, the foods we eat every day are what fuel this major piece of our body's complex immune system.

Digestive enzymes and glycans

Before our digestive system can process food into nutrients, the food must first be chewed and then further broken down by our body's digestive system. Now, I hate to be indiscreet, but if you're over fifty, how frequently do you pass gas? Like many before me, once I reached menopause, my body began having a hard time manufacturing the volume of digestive enzymes enjoyed during my younger days. Orchestral noises seemed to follow me, more often than not, after every meal. So, I carried Beano around with me, terrified to eat anything—raw or cooked. Without that bottle of liquid enzymes to protect me, I knew that an unwanted symphony of low sounds would be passing through my system within the hour. One day, a friend took me aside and told me her postmenopausal secret. "Take this white powder every day, and watch how quickly things quiet down," she whispered.

She told me she had no idea how the white powder worked, or even what it was, but friends in California had recommended it, and her proof was in her silence—no matter what she ate. I thanked her. I tried her magic powder. And it worked! For two decades now, I've been eating a half-teaspoon of that white powder every morning. And day after day, no matter what I eat, raw or cooked, I'm able to digest all types of food in polite silence.

When I finally tracked down the ingredients in that white powder, I found it was a mixture of eight simple carbohydrates, called glycans, all of which are found widely in nature. Glycobiology (the study of the structure, function, and biology of these glycans) is a rapidly growing field, now being relied upon in biomedicine, biotechnology, and basic research. The names of these carbohydrates in my white powder are mannose, glucose, galactose, xylose, N-acetyl glucosamine, N-acetyl galactosamine, fucose (not to be confused with fructose), and N-acetyl-neuraminic acid. My original friend, Beano, apparently contains one of these enzymes—alpha-galactosidase (α-GAL)!

According to New England Biolabs, a leading company involved in this new field of research, one of the many functions of glycans is the facilitation of intercellular interactions, or cell-to-cell communication.[22] In Chapter 3, we learned how our immune system's killer T-cells can eradicate newly formed cancer cells—once our body is powered up with sufficient vitamin D3. Now I understand why this white powder has become my body's best friend and protector over the past few decades.[23] The powder, marketed under the name Ambrotose, apparently also improves cell-to-cell communication.[24] Just as a sufficient level of vitamin D3 in my blood improves my internal Wi-Fi system, these glycans can apparently play a similar role, helping communicate with, and activate my killer T-cells to knock out any cancer cells that begin to develop.[25]

Andrea Lambert, a raw-vegan chef and optimal health coach in Scottsdale, Arizona, often works with individuals who want to follow a ketogenic diet for healing, while also remaining vegan. Lambert recommends eating a variety of mushrooms to improve nutritional absorption and to get the most bang for the buck from the foods eaten each day. She describes this process as improving your *Agni* in order to keep making your own digestive enzymes, no matter what your age or medical situation.[26] Agni, a major concept within the study of East Indian Ayurvedic medicine, is considered to be "the force of intelligence within each cell, each tissue and every system within the body. Ultimately, it is the discernment of Agni that determines which substances enter our cells and tissues, and which substance should be removed as water. In this way, Agni is the gatekeeper of life. In fact, according to Ayurvedic science, when the Agni is extinguished, death soon follows."[27]

I was then delighted to find several published studies showing that chaga mushrooms contain three of the eight glyconutrients or glycans that are also in my magical white powder.[28] So now I take my white powder, and enjoy my chaga tea, along with a very peaceful existence every day.

Detox Task # 4: Build Your Personal Biome—with Pro-Biotics and Pre-Biotics

Probiotics

You are not alone. As mentioned, within your small intestines live a trillion little bacteria that form 70 percent of your immune system.[29] These good bacteria are your personal biome. They have the full-time job of grabbing your chewed-up and partially digested cucumber dill salad, roasted celery root, and grilled salmon, along with the Big Mac you ate yesterday—converting it into:

- Nutrients that are sent off into your I-fluid to feed and energize your cells, and

- Residue that is sent off into your colon to be eliminated.

Since your body is not able to create these little single-cell organisms, you need to eat small amounts of foods each day that actually contain these helpful bacteria. Eating probiotic foods, especially fermented foods that contain these live bacteria, is an easy way to replenish and re-energize your personal colony of these energy-building and immune-boosting workhorses.[30] Just a tablespoon of plain, whole-fat organic yogurt with breakfast, a tablespoon of naturally fermented sauerkraut or fermented beets with lunch, a glass of kombucha in the afternoon, and a tablespoon of spicy kimchi with your chicken stir-fry tonight, can all be helpful. Start inviting more fermented foods—more live, beneficial bacteria—into your tummy, at least once a day, as you consciously work to replenish and strengthen your personalized, gut-based immune militia.

Instead of eating fermented foods to replenish your biome, you can also take probiotic supplements every day—or just use such supplements when you're sick or constipated. But to avoid the high cost of such supplements, it can be enjoyable to explore all different types of probiotic foods, adding small amounts to daily meals.

Here's a list of these "alive" probiotic foods that are easy to find in most supermarkets, co-ops, and health-food stores:

- Plain, organic (grass-fed, if possible) whole-milk (i.e., full-fat) yogurt

- Plain kefir (a fermented milk drink)

- Plain lassi (an Indian yogurt-based drink)

- Fermented pickles (like Bubbies brand—not those made with vinegar)

- Naturally fermented cabbage, beets, cauliflower, etc.

- Kimchi

- Kombucha (beware of less expensive brands that contain excess cane sugar or fruit juices!)
- Tempeh (not tofu, as tofu is not fermented)
- Miso
- Tamari

Prebiotics:

While it's important to replenish your gut bacteria with fermented foods, it's also important to use prebiotics to nourish the good bacteria you already have. These pre-biotic foods include asparagus, garlic, bananas, onions, leeks, and dandelion greens.[31]

Detox Task # 5: Keep Organochlorides (OCs) Out of Your Body

Studies have shown that women diagnosed with breast cancer have 50 to 60 percent higher levels of organochlorides (OCs) in their breast tissue than women who have not developed the disease.[32] Organochlorides are chemical compounds known for their high toxicity, slow degradation, and ability to actually accumulate, generation after generation, in commercially grown livestock, fish, and poultry. This is why organochlorides are known as persistent organic pollutants (POPs).[33] For example, one of the reasons most farmed salmon contains ten times higher levels of POPs than wild salmon is because the fish are usually fed meal that has been made from animal wastes containing these POPs. These toxins are then stored in the salmon's fat. "We recycle waste animal fats back into the food supply. We feed the cow fat to the pigs and the chickens, and we feed the pig and chicken fat to the cows," according to David Carpenter, director of the Institute for Health and the Environment at the University of Albany, New York.[34] Sadly, even farm-raised salmon advertised as "organically grown" may not be that different from other farm-raised salmon.[35]

Meanwhile, organochloride-based pesticides such as atrazine, banned in Europe since 2003, are still widely used by US agribusiness, with field runoff from the pesticides often polluting nearby public water supplies.[36] Banning these types of known carcinogenic pesticides, known to assault our cells' mitochondria,[37] can apparently help make a huge difference in a country's (or a region's) breast cancer rates. One example: when Israel (with the land size of New Jersey) phased out the use of DDT and two other organochloride pesticides in 1976, the country's breast cancer death rate in premenopausal women *dropped thirty percent within a decade.*[38]

Organochlorides also continue to be used in dry-cleaning fluids.[39] Recently, a cluster of breast cancer diagnoses was identified in men who had lived at Camp Lejeune, a Marine base in North Carolina, between the 1950s and 1985. This was the period of time when the base's water supply contained high levels of organochlorides released from a nearby dry-cleaning facility.[40] Other sources of these organochlorides include vinyl products, ranging from rigid pipes to microwavable packaging and plastic wrap. Research and experience show OCs easily slough off into our food and water.[41]

In *Breasts: A Natural and Unnatural History,*[42] science writer Florence Williams offers a compelling read on what has happened to younger American women's breasts, having constantly absorbed organochlorides throughout their lives. She describes how these chemicals operate just like natural estrogen, able to easily enter breast cells. She also describes how both organochlorides and the animal estrogens that we absorb from bovine growth hormones in commercial dairy products, commercial lamb and beef, eggs, nonorganic produce and farm-raised fish can move through the estrogen receptors (or "estrogen-admitting doors") into our breast cells every day.[43] Eating these foods on a daily basis can help create high levels of unbalanced, excess, or toxic types of estrogens throughout our bodies. And so, these food additives also help support today's record-high breast cancer epidemic, currently pummeling women of all ages throughout the US. How much chemical and animal estrogens did your body absorb today?

These animal hormones and xenohormones are also thought to be a cause of the increasing size of many younger women's developing breasts.[44] Did you know it's reported that women in the US currently have the largest average breast size of women in the world? This change has taken place over the past twenty years, increasing the US average bra size from a B cup to a DD cup![45]

Figure 6.1: Dirty Dozen & Clean Fifteen

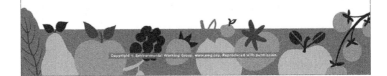

EWG'S 2020
DIRTY 12™

1. Strawberries	5. Apples	9. Pears
2. Spinach	6. Grapes	10. Tomatoes
3. Kale	7. Peaches	11. Celery
4. Nectarines	8. Cherries	12. Potatoes

Copyright © Environmental Working Group, www.ewg.org. Reproduced with permission.

EWG'S 2020
CLEAN 15™

1. Avocados	6. Sweet Peas (Frozen)	11. Broccoli
2. Sweet Corn	7. Eggplant	12. Mushrooms
3. Pineapple	8. Asparagus	13. Cabbage
4. Onions	9. Cauliflower	14. Honeydew Melon
5. Papaya	10. Cantaloupe	15. Kiwi

Copyright © Environmental Working Group, www.ewg.org. Reproduced with permission.

Dirty Dozen = Buy Organic. Clean 15 = Non-organic is okay.

Environmental Working Group: https://static.ewg.org/pdf/EWG_FN-2020_Guide.pdf. Reproduced with permission.

A Review of Breasts: A Natural and Unnatural History

"Because of various factors, which might include obesity and industrial contaminants, breasts are arriving earlier and becoming larger, often to the point of grotesqueness. Brassiere manufacturers who once made cups in sizes A to D have had to extend their range to H and KK. For generations, male thinkers and opinion-shapers from Sigmund Freud to Hugh Hefner have enshrined the female breast as a locus of eroticism and nurturance. In *Breasts*, Williams upends that perspective. She shows us our breasts as museums of deadly detritus[47]—monstrous, menacing, potentially lethal.

M.G. Lorde, "Unnatural Women," The New York Times Book Review, September 14, 2012.[48]

Detox Task #6: Use Only Nontoxic Cosmetics and Personal Care Products

During the past few decades there has been an increasing amount of laboratory research connecting the use of animal hormones and chemical hormones, or "xenohormones," in many personal care products and cosmetics. Hormonal imbalance issues, such as PMS, obesity, and depression, are increasing at epidemic levels throughout the US population. And some of these issues may be caused by the brand of cosmetics, lotions, shampoos, and conditioners you use.

Epidemiological studies and publications by the Silent Spring Institute, the Center for Environmental Ecology at the University of Pittsburgh, and author and activist Stacy Malkin, among others,[48] have looked at the use of ethnic hair relaxers and skin creams containing estradiol, a strong type of estrogen taken from sheep placenta. Their work questions what role these strong hormones may play in the development of breast cancer in African American women and others who use placenta-based products on their hair.[49] To stay up to date on this research, Breast Cancer Prevention Partners compiles these and other environmentally based breast cancer studies in their periodic encyclopedic report, *State of the Evidence*.[50] Meanwhile, the majority of US senators and representatives still refuse to vote in favor of laws banning xenohormones from personal care products.[51] Even California has yet to pass its own safe cosmetics bill.[52] In contrast, the European Union passed their first comprehensive law prohibiting the use of 1,328 such toxins in cosmetics and personal care products a decade ago.[53] Once again, it appears that large campaign contributions from the chemical and personal care industries, allowed to fund US elections, continue to influence the voting choices of most legislators from both major political parties.[54]

According to the Campaign for Safe Cosmetics, "Unlike the United States, EU law requires pre-market safety assessments of cosmetics, mandatory registration of cosmetic products, and government authorization for the use of nanomaterials and prohibits animal testing for cosmetic purposes."[55] Today, chemical preservatives such as parabens, which extend a cosmetic's shelf life, continue to be found in most personal care products and cosmetics that fill major chain store pharmacies across the country.[56] Best to buy your toothpaste, shampoo and lipstick from food co-ops and other health food stores that care more about your health than maximizing profits.

Trying to help protect US consumers, the nonprofit Environmental Working Group has created a free online database, Skin Deep. This invaluable resource offers a 10-point evaluation on the safety of more than 60,000 personal care products.[57] Meanwhile, the Campaign for Safe Cosmetics and co-founder Stacy Malkin, author of the landmark book *Not Just a Pretty Face: The Ugly Side of the Beauty Industry*, and co-director of In The Public Interest,[58] continue to advocate against the use of toxic fragrances, toxic preservatives, and toxic animal and chemical hormones that continue to pollute American women's bodies.[59]

Detox Task # 7: Balance Your Hormones Naturally

How is estrogen involved in the development of breast cancer? Here is how Dr. Angela Poff, a leading metabolic cancer researcher at the University of South Florida, describes how unbalanced estrogen entering breast cells can promote the growth of any existing cancer cells: "... you also need activation of signaling pathways that promote survival, cause new blood vessels to grow, resist apoptosis, induce proliferation, etc. Estrogen and other hormones can promote, and one could say 'fuel' tumor growth by activating those signaling pathways. Those hormones still promote tumor growth through known signaling pathways. This is unrelated to what specific metabolites are being fermented or oxidized for ATP production."[60]

In other words, according to Dr. Poff, high (i.e., unbalanced) estrogen levels help accelerate the growth of existing cancer cells. In this way the excess hormone can "fuel" or feed existing cancer cells. Meanwhile, as described in Chapter 1, glucose and glutamine still remain cancer cells' two primary fuels; both are required to keep cancer cells alive.

Many women today complain of hormonal imbalance issues. Depending on one's age, the effects of this condition can range from premenstrual syndrome (PMS), acne, and infertility,[61] to depression, migraines and hot flashes. If a woman is premenopausal, physicians will often prescribe a progestin birth control drug, instead of encouraging lifestyle changes, such as weight loss, a low-sugar and low-starch diet, exercise, and meditation.[62] If the patient is menopausal or post-menopausal, they may prescribe a progestin-based HRT drug.[63]

Although these drugs may quickly offer relief, by replacing natural unbalanced hormone levels with fixed levels of chemical hormones, for premenopausal women and supplementing the decreasing hormone levels of post-menopausal women, the Penninger-Glimcher research described in Chapter 4, clearly shows how all of these progestin drugs can both initiate and accelerate breast cancer while a woman continues to use them.[64]

We're fortunate to have a number of books that can help women understand the importance of keeping the progesterone and estrogen in our bodies in balance. Chief among these is a series of books written by and/or based on the work of Dr. John Lee, Dr. David Zava, and Virginia Hopkins. These include *What Your Doctor May Not Tell You About Premenopause; What Your Doctor May Not Tell You About Breast Cancer; What Your Doctor May Not Tell You About Menopause;* and *Dr. John Lee's Book on Hormone Balancing*, along with Dr Sherrill Sellman's *Hormone Heresy: What Women Must Know About Their Hormones and What Women Must Know to Protect Their Daughters From Breast Cancer*, in addition to Dr. Nasha Winters' and Jess Higgins Kelley's *The Metabolic Approach to Cancer.*

These practitioners all recommend that women have a urine-based estrogen metabolite test or a saliva-based hormone balancing test to understand the extent and type of hormone imbalance they may be experiencing. Once this information is known, some practitioners, such as Dr. Winters, who specializes in treating cancer with metabolic therapies, recommends lifestyle changes centering on food and removing hormones from your household environment, including filtering the water you drink and shower with, and using hormone-free body care products.[65] Some, but not all functional medicine practitioners may also recommend the use of natural plant-based hormones, either ready-made[66] or specifically formulated to the individual's test results.[67] Some of these authors also explain why using a weaker form of natural plant-based estrogen (called *estriol*), once a woman has passed menopause, is sometimes beneficial, while the stronger type of estrogen (*estradiol*), is only useful in some situations. Other practitioners in this group do not endorse the use of bioidentical or plant-based hormones.

The Estrogen Metabolite Test

Dr. Heather Eliasson, an epidemiologist at Harvard Medical School and a researcher at Brigham and Women's Hospital's Channing Center, found that regardless of excess body fat or BMI, some premenopausal women who have trouble eliminating their body's toxic, processed, or used natural estrogen and progesterone have higher breast cancer rates than other women.[68] As we'll also see in Chapter 8, it is often very difficult for women born with a defective or mutated BRCA1 tumor suppressor gene to naturally eliminate these toxic hormones from their bodies.

Dr. Anna Cabeca, a functional health practitioner who specializes in women's health, recommends this test to all women. "I offer the estrogen metabolite test to all my patients because it enables them to evaluate their personal risk for developing breast, ovarian, and colon cancer, based on how their body is detoxifying (eliminating) estrogen. I tell my patients that no matter how you get the hormones, whether it is from what your body produces naturally, what hormones you take in, such as with hormonal therapy, or what you get from your environment, such as with xenoestrogens, it is important to know what your body is doing with it. With that knowledge patients can be put in charge of their own health and [make lifestyle changes to] reduce their risk. This is very empowering."[69]

Zava Labs, an affordable and user-friendly metabolic testing resource, and Canyon Ranch, an upscale health spa, have both offered or recommended the estrogen metabolite test to clients for decades.[70]

The Estrogen Balancing Test

Another way to find out if your hormones are currently balanced or unbalanced, is to take a saliva-based hormone-balancing test. Also offered by ZRT Laboratory and others, this test can be ordered by you or by your physician. ZRT also offers patient-friendly test reports that clearly explain your current hormonal balance or imbalance. Balancing your hormone levels, especially with the guidance of one or both of these tests while under the care of a functional health practitioner, can help address current premenopausal, menopausal or postmenopausal complaints and protect you from any increased breast cancer risk that may exist.[71]

The Battle to Save Natural Plant-Based Hormones

Plant-based hormones, also called bioidentical hormones, are less toxic than the chemical and animal hormones used in pharmaceutical drugs today. Unfortunately, it appears that the pharmaceutical industry is trying to block the sale of these natural products in the US. Here we again find that Congress continues to give the food and pharmaceutical industries' powerful lobby group, the National Academy of Medicine (NAM), the responsibility of advising the Food and Drug Administration on the safety and sale of these natural plant-based hormones (estradiol, estriol and progesterone)! As described in Chapter 2 and Chapter 3, our national food policy and national standards for vitamins and minerals, including the vitamin D3, also continue to be controlled by this private industry lobby, with the lofty, but deceptive name the *National Academy of Medicine*.[72] In each of these situations, putting NAM in charge of any nutritional or health-related policy is akin to asking the fox to guard the hen house. If NAM does recommend the FDA block the sale of estriol, US women will be forced to use only the stronger estradiol-based products, increasing their risk of developing breast cancer, rather than offering women the choice of using the safer and weaker plant-based estriol.[73]

Detox Task #8: Reduce the Recurrence of Hormone-Positive Breast Cancer

US women are anything but safe when treated for an early-stage breast cancer diagnosis by today's mainstream cancer centers. This is because, while undisclosed to the US public, breast cancer clinicians report that anywhere from 20–40 percent of women initially treated in the US for early-stage breast cancer (I, II, or III), go on to develop terminal recurrent metastatic breast cancer.[74] A smaller percentage of women, possibly 8 to 10 percent, initially treated for an early-stage diagnosis develop an early-stage recurrence of their initial diagnosis within the following ten years. Again, such data is not released to the US public.

The largest and most recent recurrence studies I have found are from the Netherlands and Germany. Researchers in both countries show early-stage recurrence around 8 percent, with metastatic recurrence around 25 percent.[75] Women who are premenopausal and those who are diagnosed with early-stage hormone-negative tumors appear to have higher recurrence rates within the group and quicker recurrence time. But these statistics, unfortunately, do not tell the entire grim story, as some women, especially those initially diagnosed with slow-growing hormone-positive tumors, are not diagnosed with recurrent metastatic breast cancer until more than a decade has passed since their initial mainstream cancer treatment.

As mentioned, since the 1980s the drug tamoxifen and a few other drugs all classified as endocrine therapy continue to be prescribed to patients after they have completed their treatments for stage 0 or for stage I, II or III breast tumors. These drugs are therefore classified as *adjuvant* drugs, meaning "serving to aid or contribute; enhancing the effectiveness of medical treatment, or for use after initial disease treatment has ended."[76]

Studies tell us these drugs, when used for five to ten years after initial treatment ends, can reduce recurrence rates by 40 to 50 percent, with only 20 percent of women developing recurrent metastasis.[77] If these data are correct, it means that rMBC recurs in an estimated 40 percent of women who undergo today's mainstream cancer treatment for stage I, II, or III hormone-positive breast tumors, but who do not take these endocrine therapies.

Today, data describing each patient's date and type of first recurrence is submitted by physicians and cancer centers, as required by state medical licensing boards and by the American College of Surgeons' Commission on Cancer (CoC), to state cancer registries that are certified by the private North American Association of Central Cancer Registries (NAACCR), and to the CoC. The NAACCR certifies state cancer registries, qualifying them to receive their federal funding, while the CoC certifies their approved hospitals and cancer centers throughout the US, Washington DC, and Puerto Rico. CoC-certified hospitals treat about 70 percent of all cancer patients who undergo today's mainstream cancer therapies in the US annually. None of this recurrent breast cancer data, however, is released to the public.

The Adverse Effects of Using Endocrine Drugs

As mentioned in Chapter 5, taking tamoxifen for five years or longer can raise an older postmenopausal woman's risk of developing a triple-negative breast tumor, but only *among that group of women who ever develop a second primary tumor*.[78] The drug can also increase sexual dysfunction, bone loss, musculoskeletal symptoms, cardiovascular disease, brain fog, hot flashes, venous thromboembolism, risk of cataracts, and fatty liver disease.[79] A recent study also tells us that tamoxifen is able to cause permanent cognitive impairment in some premenopausal women after they have used the adjuvant drug for four or more years.[80]

Detox Task #9: Cleanse Your Mind

The Buddhists have the right idea. Instead of saying, "Aunt Wilma died yesterday," Buddhists say, "Aunt Wilma left her body yesterday." Buddhism, Hinduism, Christianity and other religions understand that we are greater than our physical bodies. But you don't have to be Buddhist or Hindu to realize that keeping your mental state calm and clear helps keep your physical body healthy, while you are still alive—still "in the body."

My spiritual teacher, Mata Amritanandamayi, known to the world as "Amma" (or, as *The New York Times* calls her, "the hugging saint"), describes the goal of meditation as becoming mindless. This means detaching from our emotions as much as possible. Instead, we become witnesses to the events of our lives while remaining grounded within our center.[81] To paraphrase many of her teachings, the past is a cancelled check; *the past is dead; and we do not have absolute control over what will happen in the next minute.* This means that all we actually can affect is this immediate moment. So, it's best to plan, relax, and then do our best possible work, and not worry! Instead, simply focus on being within, and on witnessing or acknowledging this present moment.[82]

From a biological or physiological perspective, daily meditation can actually help lower the amount of acidic cortisol hormones that our adrenal glands dump into our bodies when we're upset, worried, or stressed. And we know that these chronically high levels of cortisol hormones can also assault those precious mitochondria in our breast cells.[83] More and more research shows that quieting our minds, even for fifteen minutes or a half-hour once or twice each day, can lower the amount of cortisol hormones surging through our bodies—literally for hours![84]

The relationship between mind and body is the focus of Bruce Lipton's decades-old best-selling book, *The Biology of Belief: Unleashing the Power of Consciousness, Matter & Miracles.* His writing does a wonderful job of outlining how the energy and biology of our bodies, including the energy and biology of our minds, can physically heal or hinder us. The renowned cell biologist goes on to describe how the "miracle of prayer" and "the placebo effect" are not just in our minds. Rather, they reveal the ability of our minds to have an actual biological or physical effect on our bodies.[85] That's exciting!

In her two end-of-life memoirs,[86] Elizabeth Edwards, the highly respected and politically outspoken spouse of former senator and two-time Democratic presidential candidate John Edwards, describes her lifestyle choices and unabated emotional issues during the last half of her life. She recounts various types of high-stress events, which Lipton has shown are able to create and maintain chronic inflammation throughout a person's body. Edwards's frank writing describes her paralyzing grief over the sudden death of her 16-year-old son and her continuing passion for junk food, while also remaining more than fifty pounds overweight for the last decades of her life. She also reports being given daily hormone shots months after her son's death, in order to successfully carry a daughter to full term at age 48; then delivering a son, again using hormone shots, when she was age 51. A few years after these births, Edwards recounts learning the news that her husband had recently fathered a child with another woman.

Written in a dispassionate tone, her books stoically chronicle these episodes of overwhelming chronic stress. But neither book indicates that Edwards understood anything about the critical need to make lifestyle choices or to practice effective ways to help lower her stress in order to reduce any inflammatory cortisol and unbalanced estrogen levels. In fact, until recently, most of us didn't understand how both chronic stress and postmenopausal obesity harm our breast cells' mitochondria, too often leading to a breast cancer diagnosis.[87]

Although cortisol is able to enter almost every cell in the body, the combination of high cortisol levels, along with unbalanced estrogen levels creates a double whammy on breast cells. (Remember, estrogen can only enter a woman's breast, ovary and uterine cells, along with cells in a few other organs.) When a woman has too much cortisol, along with too much estrogen battering her cells every day, her breast cells' mitochondria can lose their ability to process oxygen, enabling the cells to suffocate; the first step in the cancer-creating process.[88]

Today we have a growing number of health practitioners and coaches who specialize in helping cancer patients (and others) lower their bodies' inflammation levels, to protect against all types of cancer, by lowering cortisol levels. This work can help us detoxify our minds along with our bodies. This unique cadre of individuals describes their work as *intuitive healing*. Two such practitioners are Adrea Brier[89] and Prajna Avalon.[90] Like many such healers, they are able to work with individuals in person or long-distance.[91]

Detox Task #10: Consider Cannabis—Saving the Best for Last

In 1991, Greg Munzi, a lanky 32-year-old antique dealer and native of Haverhill, Massachusetts, was diagnosed with renal cancer. After having his affected kidney removed, Munzi was considered cancer-free. By 1999, however, that same cancer had returned and had metastasized to Munzi's liver, bones, and lungs. During the next thirteen years, Munzi participated in at least six different clinical chemotherapy trials at Dana Farber Cancer Center in Boston, as doctors tried to shrink Munzi's existing tumors. Quietly, Munzi also continued to smoke large amounts of marijuana, use a variety of cannabis tinctures, and enjoy marijuana edibles each day. Munzi understood that the THC in the weed reduced his nausea, helped keep his stress levels low, and stimulated his appetite better than any prescription drugs being recommended. The cannabis products also had none of the nasty side effects of many of Dana Farber's standard cancer treatments and recommended prescription drugs. Meanwhile, this leading national cancer center, ignorant of Munzi's daily pot habit, continued to be overjoyed, but mystified, that Munzi's metastatic tumors weren't growing very rapidly in spite of the fact that additional tumors kept being diagnosed.

In the fall of 2014, Munzi politely said "goodbye" to Dana Farber's treatments; he had discovered a Canadian by the name of Rick Simpson. The Rick Simpson Protocol, as it is commonly called, uses heavy doses of cannabis oils or waxes to control the growth of tumors and help eliminate cancerous cells from a person's body.[92]

Within three months of ending Dana Farber's chemotherapy, while continuing to eat the standard glucose-filled American diet, and now using nothing but his homemade concentrated doses of cannabis tars and tinctures, Munzi's December 2014 MRI showed that most of his existing tumors had shrunk by half.

Excited by Munzi's personal experience with cannabis, I asked the question: If cannabis oils can continue to somehow manage Munzi's existing tumors in spite of his glucose-heavy eating habits, (think cereal like Wheaties, pasta, orange juice, rice, bananas, and lots of ice cream), can these tinctures, tars, edibles, and suppositories also be used to help stop cancer from developing in the first place? And how much more effective could cannabis products be in managing a cancer diagnosis when combined with a high-fat/very-low-glucose cancer-fighting diet?[93]

I quickly began looking for academic research on cannabis and breast cancer. I was delighted to find a rapidly expanding body of published, peer-reviewed papers from Israel, Spain, France, and even the US, with some of these studies published at least thirty years ago. All described how cannabis oils can help prevent and treat various stages of the disease.[94]

I then found peer-reviewed research detailing how the non-hallucinogenic oil, cannabidiol, or CBD (made from the marijuana plant's stem and leaves), along with THC, the hallucinogenic oil (made from the plant's female buds), were being used in laboratory research to help stop fast-growing, triple-negative breast cancer cells (and other types of breast cancer) in three different ways:[95]

1. Vacuum out or absorb toxic ROS (cellular exhaust) from breast cells.

2. Cut off the blood supply to any breast tumors that have begun to form (angiogenesis).

3. Stop the proliferation or duplication of any cancer cells, shrinking the existing tumors.

Given the pharmaceutical industry's continuing ability to finance the campaigns and gain apparent influence with US presidents and the majority of our senators and representatives, marijuana remains classified as a controlled substance under federal regulations. This means the National Cancer Institute and other agencies, with their hundreds of millions in annual taxpayer dollars, are not allowed to approve human-based clinical studies testing the effectiveness of CBD or THC oils in preventing and treating cancer. Meanwhile, Spain, Israel, China and other countries throughout the world are continuing to do more laboratory and clinical research, anxious to understand the ways that natural cannabis can prevent and treat cancer cells.[96]

A Detox Shopping List

Over the course of this chapter, we've seen ten simple ways that we can cleanse the insides of our minds and our bodies. These practices keep our mitochondria strong; helping prevent breast cancer (and other mitochondrial conditions).[97] So, here's a list of some tools that can help you cleanse the insides of your mind and body every day:

1. Shower filter and kitchen faucet filter, or a whole-house water filter

2. Dry skin brush

3. Massage oil for breast massage

4. Ambrotose glyconutritional powder (available from Mannatech, Inc.)

5. Chaga tea

6. Probiotic foods and/or supplements

7. Prebiotic foods

8. Near-infrared sauna

9. Meditation cushion, stool, or BackJack chair

10. Estrogen metabolite test

11. Hormone balancing test

12. CBD and/or THC tinctures and edibles

If there's one area where lifestyle-based prevention steps are proving particularly important, it's in dealing with the fast-growing type of cancer known as *triple-negative breast cancer*. That's why our next chapter looks at triple-negative breast cancer, a type of cancer cell that is currently developing disproportionately in obese, often impoverished, and highly stressed women of all races. This triple-negative disease also appears to be found disproportionally among the growing number of premenopausal women who are developing breast cancer. Recent (but little-publicized) laboratory, epidemiological, and clinical studies are helping identify unique, lifestyle-based prevention steps that can be used to help block the development of this often fast-growing type of breast cancer.

This next chapter also includes plenty of encouraging news about using metabolic therapies on one's own and in the clinic to mitigate early and metastatic stages of triple-negative breast cancer, including two case studies. The first describes a postmenopausal woman who has used only nontoxic metabolic therapies to achieve optimal health while successfully managing her early-stage triple-negative diagnosis since 2013. A second case study illustrates how a metabolic cancer clinic in Istanbul, Turkey, was able to successfully help a premenopausal woman manage her metastatic triple-negative diagnosis, also using only nontoxic metabolic therapies.

Read on and let's see how lifestyle changes and nontoxic therapies can help prevent triple-negative breast cancer and bring hope even to women facing this particularly frightening type of cancer.

⑥ CHAPTER ENDNOTES

1   Travis Christofferson, *Tripping Over the Truth: How the Metabolic Theory of Cancer is Overturning One of Medicine's Most Entrenched Paradigms* (White River Junction, VT: Chelsea Green Press, 2017).

2   National Cancer Institute, "Breast Cancer Risk in American Women," http://www.cancer.gov/types/breast/risk-fact-sheet.

3   P.S. Rosenberg, K.A. Barker and W.F. Anderson, "Estrogen Receptor Status and the Future Burden of Invasive and In-situ Breast Cancers in the United States," (Abstract # 1850), American Association of Cancer Research Annual Conference, Philadelphia, PA, April 15, 2015, https://mb.cision.com/Public/3069/9755232/81b414b4ec298479.pdf.

4   H. Y. Chung et al., "Redefining Chronic Inflammation in Aging and Age-Related Diseases: Proposal of the Senoinflammation Concept," *Aging and Disease* 10, no. 2 (April 2019): 367-82, https://doi.org/10.14336/AD.2018.0324.

5   See Chapter 1.

6   Philip Hunter, "The Inflammation Theory of Disease: The Growing Realization that Chronic Inflammation is Crucial in Many Diseases Opens New Avenues for Treatment," *EMBO Reports* 13, no. 11 (2012): 968–70, https://doi.org/10.1038/embor.2012.142; Marcelle Pick, "Causes of Inflammation," https://marcellepick.com/causes-inflammation/.

7   Lisa M. Coussens and Zena Werb, "Inflammation and Cancer," *Nature* 420, no. 6917 (December 2002): 860-67, https://doi.org/10.1038/nature01322.

8   Artemis, "Your Detoxification Pathway Explained," https://international.artemis.co.nz/your-detox-pathway-explained.

9   Joseph Mercola, "Fluoride Articles," mercola.com, https://fluoride.mercola.com; Paul Trayhurn, "Oxygen: The Forgotten Nutrient," *Journal of Nutritional Science* 6, no. e47 (September 4, 2017), https://doi.org/10.1017/jns.2017.53; Harvard Public Health, "Is Fluoridated Drinking Water Safe? Countries that Do Not Fluoridate their Water Have Also Seen Big Drops in the Rate of Cavities," (Spring 2016), https://www.hsph.harvard.edu/magazine/magazine_article/fluoridated-drinking-water/.

10 Paul Trayhurn, "Oxygen - The Forgotten Nutrient." *Journal of Nutritional Science* 6, no. e47 (Sep. 4, 2017), https://pubmed.ncbi.nlm.nih.gov/29152251/.

11 Muhammad Adeel et al., "Environmental Impact of Estrogens on Human, Animal and Plant Life: A Critical Review," *Environmental International*, 99 (February 2017): 107-19, https://doi.org/10.1016/j.envint.2016.12.010; A. M. Soto et al., "Androgenic and Estrogenic Activity in Water Bodies Receiving Cattle Feedlot Effluent in Eastern Nebraska, USA," *Environmental Health Perspectives* 112, no. 3 (2004): 346-52, https://doi.org/10.1289/ehp.6590; Silent Spring Institute, "Water Research," https://silentspring.org/research-area/water-research.

12 Silent Spring Institute, "Bisphenol A (BPA)," https://silentspring.org/glossary/bisphenol-bpa; Madisa B. Macon and Suzanne E. Fenton, "Endocrine Disruptors and the Breast: Early Life Effects and Later Life Disease," *Journal of Mammary Gland Biology and Neoplasia* 18, no. 1 (2013): 43-61, https://doi.org/10.1007/s10911-013-9275-7; Drew Thieman, "Scholar Feature: Dr. Katherine Reeves Studies Breast Cancer Link from BPA," University of Massachusetts at Amherst, Center for Research on Families, 2016, https://www.umass.edu/family/news/reeves-studies-breast-cancer-risk-from-BPA.

13 Janet Gray (editor), *State of the Evidence: The Connection Between Breast Cancer and the Environment*, (San Francisco: Breast Cancer Fund, 2008), https://doi.org/10.1186/s12940-017-0287-4.

14　Perry Santanachote, "Water Filter Pitcher Face-Off: Brit Stream Rapids vs. ZeroWater Ready-Pour," *Consumer Reports*, August 14, 2019, https://www.consumerreports.org/water-filter-pitchers/brita-stream-rapids-vs-zerowater-ready-pour-water-filter-pitcher-face-off/.

15　Joseph Mercola, "Dr. Mercola Discusses Water Filters," https://www.waterfilteradvisor.com/dr-mercola-discusses-water-filters/.

16　Lee Sutherland, "Why You Should Start Dry Body Brushing Today," http://www.mindbodygreen.com/0-7955/why-you-should-start-dry-body-brushing-today.html.

17　Susun S. Weed, *Breast Cancer? Breast Health! The Wise Woman Way: 10th Anniversary Edition* (Woodstock, NY: Ash Tree Publishing, 2006); The Women's Wellness Collective, "Dry Skin Brushing," https://thewomenswellnesscollective.com/journal/2018/3/1/the-benefits-of-dry-skin-brushing; Cheryl Chapman, *The Happy Breast Book*, 2003, http://www.cherylchapman.net/happbb.html; Khalid Mahmud, *Keeping Abreast: Ways to PREVENT Breast Cancer*, (Durham, CT: Strategic Book Publishing, 2008); Sat Dharam Kaur, *A Call to Women: The Healthy Breast Program and Workbook* (Beverly, MA: Quarry Press, 2000).

18　NCI Dictionary of Cancer Terms, "Interstitial Fluid," cancer.gov; https://www.cancer.gov/publications/dictionaries/cancer-terms/def/interstitial-fluid.

19　D. Bemben et al., "Relevance of Whole-Body Vibration Exercises on Muscle Power and Bone of Elderly Individuals," *Dose-Response*, (Dec 6, 2018):1-7, https://doi.org/10.1177/1559325818813066; Dave Asprey, "Whole Body Vibration Training with Bulletproof Vibe," https://blog.daveasprey.com/biohacking-fitness-upgrade-whole-body-vibration-training/.

20　Joseph Mercola, "Why Saunas are Ridiculously Good for You," June 29, 2018, https://fitness.mercola.com/sites/fitness/archive/2018/06/29/why-are-saunas-good-for-you.aspx.

21　"Human Nutrition, the Gut Microbiome and the Immune System," *Nature* 474, no. 7351 (June 2011): 327-36, https://doi.org/10.1038/nature10213; A.K. Simon, G.A. Hollander, and A. McMichael, "Evolution of the Immune System in Humans from Infancy to Old Age," *Proceedings: Biological Sciences* 282 (2015): 1821, https://doi.org/10.1098/rspb.2014.3085.

22　New England Biolabs, "Glycoproteomics: Understanding Protein Modifications," https://www.neb.com/~/media/NebUs/Files/Brochures/Glycobiology.pdf.

23　Stella Hurtly et al.,"Cinderella's Coach is Ready," *Scientific American* 287, no. 1 (July 2002): 40-47, https://doi.org/10.1126/science.291.5512.2337.

24　Ajit Varki, "Biological roles of glycans," *Glycobiology* 27, no. 1 (January 2017): 3-49, https://doi.org/10.1093/glycob/cww086; Also see: Ajit Varki et al., *Essentials of Glycobiology*, 2nd edition (Cold Spring Harbor, NY: Cold Spring Harbor Laboratory Press, 2009).

25　Victor S. Sierpina and Robert K. Murra, "Glyconutrients: The State of the Science and the Impact of Glycomics," *Explore* 2, no. 6, (November 2006): 488-94, https://doi.org/10.1016/j.explore.2006.08.016; "Front Matter." *Scientific American* 287, no. 1 (2002). Accessed March 7, 2020. https://www.jstor.org/stable/26059861?seq=1; Emil Mondoa, *Sugars That Heal* (New York: Random House, 2002); David Bird, "Natural Glyconutrients Recipe: How to Make Your Own Glyconutrient Powder & Jam," http://www.healingcancernaturally.com/glyconutrients-substitutes.html; Peter Smith, "Glyconutrients: The Missing Link?", http://www.positivehealth.com/article/nutraceuticals/glyconutrients-the-missing-link.

26　Andrea Lambert, "Why Cleanse? The Science Behind Increased Energy, Mental Clarity, Weight Loss, Disease Prevention, and Reversing the Aging Process," (Kindle, 2017), https://www.amazon.com/Why-Cleanse-increased-prevention-reversing-ebook/dp/B01MTAM9XR.

27　Melody Mischke, "The Importance of Agni: The Importance of Healthy Digestion," Banyan Botanicals, 2019, https://www.banyanbotanicals.com/info/ayurvedic-living/living-ayurveda/health-guides/understanding-agni/the-importance-of-agni/.

28   Orvida.com, "Chaga: The Facts: Medicinal Mushrooms–Backgrounds and Monographs: Reflections on Several Medicinal Mushrooms, Dosing and How to Get Your Money's Worth," July 5, 2016, https://oriveda.wordpress.com/chaga-the-facts/; "Chemical Characterization and Biological Activity of Chaga," *Journal of Ethnopharmacology* 13, no. 162 (March 2015): 323-32, https://doi.org/10.1016/j.jep.2014.12.069.

29   June L. Round and Sarkis K. Mazmanian, "The Gut Microbiota Shapes Intestinal Immune Responses During Health and Disease," *Nature Reviews: Immunology* 9, no. 5 (2009): 313–23, https://doi.org/10.1016/j.jep.2014.12.069; Vighi et al., "Allergy and the Gastrointestinal System," *Clinical and Experimental Immunology* 153, Suppl 1 (2008): 3–6, https://doi.org/10.1111/j.1365-2249.2008.03713.x.

30   Maria Kechagia et al., "Health Benefits of Probiotics: A Review," *ISRN Nutrition* 2013, no. 481651 (January 2, 2013), https://doi.org/10.5402/2013/481651.

31   Jillian Levy, "7 Reasons to Get Prebiotics in Your Diet: Plus, the Best Sources," August 4, 2019, https://draxe.com/nutrition/prebiotics/.

32   Michael Castleman, "Why?" *Mother Jones*, May/June 1994, https://www.motherjones.com/politics/1994/05/why/.

33   K. C. Jones and P. de Voogtb, "Persistent Organic Pollutants (POPs): State of the Science," *Environmental Pollution* 100, Issues 1-3, (1999): 209-22, https://doi.org/10.1016/S0269-7491(99)00098-6.

34   Carpenter Hire, et al., "Global Assessment of Organic Contaminants in Farmed Salmon," *Science* 303, no. 5655 (January 9, 2004): 226–29, https://doi.org/10.1126/science.1091447.

35   Lori Alton, "Is Organic Farmed Salmon Better for Us than Standard Farmed Salmon?" May 14, 2017, https://www.naturalhealth365.com/wild-salmon-2237.html.

36   J.B. Sass and A Colangelo, "European Union Bans Atrazine, While the United States Negotiates Continued Use," *International Journal of Occupational and Environmental Health* 12, no. 3 (July-September 2006): 260–67, https://doi.org/10.1179/oeh.2006.12.3.260.

37   Qian Liu et al., "Organochloride Pesticides Impaired Mitochondrial Function in Hepatocytes and Aggravated Disorders of Fatty Acid Metabolism" *Scientific Reports* 7, no. 4633 (April 11, 2017), https://doi.org/10.1038/srep46339.

38   Jane Kay, "Israelis Report Breast Cancer Deaths Drop After DDT Ban," writing for the *San Francisco Examiner*, https://www.chicagotribune.com/news/ct-xpm-1994-04-03-9404030054-story.html; Luita D. Spangler, "Xenoestrogens and Breast Cancer: Nowhere to Run," *WomanWise*, Winter 1996, Concord Feminist Health Center, https://www.fwhc.org/health/xeno.htm; Marion Moses, "Pesticides and Breast Cancer," Pesticide Action Network UK.

39   Mark Hay, "How Dangerous Are Dry-Cleaning Chemicals?" Vice.com, June 5, 2019, https://www.vice.com/en_us/article/kzmp7x/how-dangerous-are-dry-cleaning-chemicals.

40   P. Z. Ruckart et al., "Evaluation of Contaminated Drinking Water and Male Breast Cancer at Marine Corps Base Camp Lejeune, North Carolina: A Case Control Study," *Environmental Health* 14, no.74 (2015), https://doi.org/10.1186/s12940-015-0061-4.

41   Greenpeace, "Go PVC Free," https://www.greenpeace.org/usa/toxics/pvc-free/.

42   Florence Williams, *Breasts: A Natural and Unnatural History* (New York: W.W. Norton & Company, 2012).

43   Cleveland Clinic, "Should You Pay More for Cage-Free or Organic Eggs?" March 18, 2016, https://health.clevelandclinic.org/should-you-pay-extra-for-cage-free-or-organic-eggs/; Julia Calderone, "Here's Why Farmers Inject Hormones Into Beef But Never Into Poultry," March 31, 2016, https://www.businessinsider.com/no-hormones-chicken-poultry-usda-fda-2016-3.

44 Florence Williams, "The Wonder of Breasts," June 15, 2012, *The Guardian* online, accessed April 8, 2019, https://www.theguardian.com/lifeandstyle/2012/jun/16/breasts-breastfeeding-milk-florence-williams; Josh Harkinsson, "Turns Out Your 'Hormone-Free' Milk is Full of Sex Hormones," *Mother Jones*, April 10, 2014, https://www.motherjones.com/politics/2014/04/milk-hormones-cancer-pregnant-cows-estrogen/; Virginia Hopkins, "Xenohormones and Your Health," Virginiahopkinstestkits.com, https://www.virginiahopkinstestkits.com/xenohormoneI.html.

45 World Data Info, "Average Breast Size Worldwide," https://www.worlddata.info/average-breastsize.php.

46 Detritus is waste or debris of any kind.

47 M.G. Lorde, "Unnatural Women," review of Florence Williams, Breasts: *A Natural and Unnatural History* (New York: Norton & Norton, 2012), *The New York Times Book Review*, September 14, 2012, https://www.nytimes.com/2012/09/16/books/review/breasts-by-florence-williams.html.

48 Stacy Malkin, *Not Just A Pretty Face: The Ugly Side of the Beauty Industry* (British Columbia: New Society Publishers, 2007), https://newsociety.com/books/n/not-just-a-pretty-face. Malkin is also co-founder and co-director of the progressive nonprofit In the Public Interest. See Chapter 2.

49 C.E. Eberle et al., "Hair Dye and Chemical Straightener Use and Breast Cancer Risk in a Large US Population of Black and White Women," *International Journal of Cancer*, December 3, 2019 https://doi.org/10.1002/cam4.613; Laura Stiel et al., "A Review of Hair Product Use On Breast Cancer Risk in African American Women," *Cancer Medicine* 2016; 5(3): 597–604, https://doi.org/10.1002/cam4.613.

50 Janet Gray et al., "State of the Evidence 2017: An Update on the Connection Between Breast Cancer and the Environment," *Environmental Health* 16, no. 94 (September 2, 2017): 16–94, https://doi.org/10.1186/s12940-017-0287-4.

51 "Senator Decries 'Poisons' as Unregulated Chemical in Cosmetics Draw Scrutiny," April 15, 2019, CBSnews.com, https://www.cbsnews.com/news/cosmetics-unregulated-chemicals-lead-to-a-clean-beauty-movement/.

52 David Lazarus, "Cosmetics Industry Crushes Bill That Would Have Made Makeup and Hair Products Safer," *Los Angeles Times*, April 10, 2019, https://www.latimes.com/business/lazarus/la-fi-lazarus-california-cosmetics-regulation-20190410-story.html.

53 "Regulation (EC) No 1223/2009 of the European Parliament and of the Council of 30 November 2009 on cosmetic products," https://ec.europa.eu/health/sites/health/files/endocrine_disruptors/docs/cosmetic_1223_2009_regulation_en.pdf.

54 Environmental Working Group, "Toxic-Free Cosmetics Act Would Ban Cosmetics with Chemical Linked to Cancer or Reproductive Harm," press release, February 21, 2020, ewg.org, https://www.ewg.org/release/toxic-free-cosmetics-act-would-ban-cosmetics-chemicals-linked-cancer-or-reproductive-harm.

55 Campaign for Safe Cosmetics, "International Laws," safecosmetics.org, http://www.safecosmetics.org/get-the-facts/regulations/international-laws/.

56 Breast Cancer Prevention Partners, "Parabens at a Glance," https://www.bcpp.org/resource/parabens/; Silent Spring Institute, "Tips on How to Avoid Parabens," https://silentspring.org/resource/tips-how-avoid-parabens.

57 Environmental Working Group, "Skin Deep Cosmetics Database," http://www.ewg.org/skindeep/search.php.

58 In The Public Interest, https://www.inthepublicinterest.org.

59 Campaign for Safe Cosmetics, http://www.safecosmetics.org.

60 Angela Poff, personal correspondence with the author, June 13, 2019.

61 B. Seth, S. Arora and R. Singh, "Association of Obesity with Hormonal Imbalance in Infertility: A Cross-sectional Study in North Indian Women," *Indian Journal of Clinical Biochemistry* 4 (October 2013) :342-7, https://doi.org/10.1007/s12291-013-0301-8.

62 Elizabeth Siegel Watkins, "How the Pill Became a Lifestyle Drug: The Pharmaceutical Industry and Birth Control in the United States Since 1960," *American Journal of Public Health* 102, no.8 (June, 2012):1462-72, https://doi.org/10.2105/AJPH.2012.300706.

63 N. Hou et al., "Hormone Replacement Therapy and Breast Cancer: Heterogeneous Risks by Race, Weight, and Breast Density," *Journal of the National Cancer Institute* 105, no.18 (2013): 1365–, 72, https://doi.org/10.1093/jnci/djt207.

64 Daniel Schramek et al., "Osteoclast Differentiation Factor RANKL Controls Development of Progestin-Driven Mammary Cancer," Nature 468, no.7320, (2010): 98-102, https://doi.org/10.1038/nature09387.

65 Nasha Winters and Jesse Kelly, *The Metabolic Approach to Cancer*, 226-250.

66 Smoky Mountain Naturals, https://smnutrition.com/.

67 International Women's Pharmacy, https://www.womensinternational.com.

68 A. H. Eliassen et al., "Urinary Estrogens and Estrogen Metabolites and Subsequent Risk of Breast Cancer Among Premenopausal Women." *Cancer Research* 72, no.3 (2012): 696-706, https://doi.org/10.1158/0008-5472.CAN-11-2507.

69 Anna M. Cabeca, http://www.drannacabeca.com; M. N. Groves, "Why We Should Care About Estrogen Metabolites," zrtlab.com, https://www.zrtlab.com/blog/archive/why-we-care-about-estrogen-metabolites/.

70 Stephen Brewer, www.zrtlab.com;, "Understanding Cancer," https://www.canyonranch.com/blog/health/understanding-cancer/.

71 Women in Balance Institute, "Causes of Hormone Imbalance," https://womeninbalance.org/seventh-woman/causes/.

72 People's Health Movement et al., *Global Health Watch 5: An Alternative World Health Report*, (London: Zed Books Ltd., 2017 Kindle edition), https://tinyurl.com/GlobalHealthWatch.

73 Alliance for Natural Health, "FDA Rigs Process Against Estriol, Other Bioidenticals," https://anh-usa.org/fda-rigs-process-against-estriol-other-bioidenticals/.

74 Nick Mulcahy, "The Mystery of a Common Breast Cancer Statistic," *Medscape*, August 18, 2015, https://www.medscape.com/viewarticle/849644: Xiang H.-F. Zhang et al., "Metastasis Dormancy in Estrogen Receptor-Positive Breast Cancer," *Clinical Cancer Research* 19, no. 23 (2013): 6389-97, https://doi.org/10.1158/1078-0432.CCR-13-0838; J. O'Shaughnessy, "Extending Survival with Chemotherapy in MBC," *The Oncologist* 10 (2005); Musa Myers and Susan E. Grober, *Silent Voices: Living Beyond Breast Cancer*, Living Beyond Breast Cancer: 2006, https://www.lbbc.org/sites/default/files/LBBCsilentvoices.pdf; Noah Berkowitz, Sanjay Gupta and George Silberman, "Estimates of the Lifetime Direct Costs of Treatment for Metastatic Breast Cancer," *Value in Health* 3, no. 1 (2000):23-30, https://doi.org/10.1046/j.1524-4733.2000.31003.x.

75 M.C. van Maaren et al., "Ten-year Recurrence Rates for Breast Cancer Subtypes in the Netherlands: A Large Population-based Study." *International Journal of Cancer* 144, no. 2 (2019): 263-72, https://doi.org/10.1002/ijc.31914; Bernd Holleczek et al., "Risk of Loco-Regional Recurrence and Distant Metastases of Patients with Invasive Breast Cancer Up to Ten Years After Diagnosis-Results from a Registry-Based Study From Germany," *BMC Cancer* 19, no. 520,(2019), https://doi.org/10.1186/s12885-019-57-10-5.

76 Adjuvant definition, https://www.merriam-webster.com/dictionary/adjuvant.

77 Caroline Helwick, "More Data Show Small Benefit From Extended Endocrine Therapy," *The ASCO Post*, March 10, 2019, https://www.ascopost.com/issues/march-10-2019/more-data-show-small-benefit-from-extended-endocrine-therapy/; See Commission on Cancer, "Section Two: Instructions for Coding, Outcomes: (Recurrence Data), *FORDS: Facility Oncology Registry Data Standards*: 2016, i-3 & 321-333, https://www.facs.org/-/media/files/quality-programs/cancer/ncdb/fords-2016.ashx.

78 C. Li et al., "Adjuvant Hormonal Therapy for Breast Cancer and Risk of Hormone Receptor-specific Subtypes of Contralateral Breast Cancer," *Cancer Research* 69, no.1 (September 1, 2009): 6865-70, https://doi.org/10.1158/0008-5472.CAN-09-1355.

79 A. Awan and K. Esfahani, "Endocrine Therapy for Breast Cancer in the Primary Care Setting," *Current Oncology* 25, no. 4 (August 2018):285-89, https://doi.org/http:doi.org/10.3747/co.25.4139; Ofer Lavie et al., "The Risk of Developing Uterine Sarcoma after Tamoxifen Use," *International Journal of Gynecological Cancer* 18, no. 2 (February 2008): 352-56; Sherrill Sellman, "Tamoxifen: A Major Medical Mistake?" *Nexus Magazine* 5, no. 4 (June-July 1998), http://all-natural.com/womens-health/tamox/; C. Li et al., "Adjuvant Hormonal Therapy for Breast Cancer and Risk of Hormone Receptor-specific Subtypes of Contralateral Breast Cancer," *Cancer Research* 69, no.1 (September 1, 2009): 6865-70, https://doi.org/10.1158/0008-5472.CAN-09-1355.

80 P.A. Ganz and K. Van Dyk, "Cognitive Impairment in Patients With Breast Cancer: Understanding the Impact of Hemotherapy and Endocrine Therapy," Editorial, *Journal of Clinical Oncology*, April 24, 2020, https://doi.org/10.1200/JCO.20.00336.

81 Jake Halpern, "Amma's Multifaceted Empire, Built on Hugs," *The New York Times*, May 25, 2013, https://www.nytimes.com/2013/05/26/business/ammas-multifaceted-empire-built-on-hugs.html.

82 "What is Sakshi Bhava? "April 18, 2014, https://www.amritapuri.org/17513/14witness.aum.

83 Martin Picard and Bruce S. McEwen, "Psychological Stress and Mitochondria: A Systematic Review," *Psychosomatic Medicine* 80, no. 2 (2018): 141-53. https://doi.org/10.1097/PSY.0000000000000545.

84 Balakrishnan Vandana et al., "Impact of Integrated Amrita Meditation Technique on Adrenaline and Cortisol Levels in Healthy Volunteers," *Evidence-Based Complementary and Alternative Medicine* 2011, no. 379645 (2011): https://doi.org/10.1155/2011/379645; Yi-Yuan Tang et al., "Short-term Meditation Training Improves Attention and Self-regulation," *Proceedings of the National Academy of Sciences* 104, no.43 (October 23, 2007), https://doi.org/10.1073/pnas.0707678104; K. Sanada et al., "Effects of Mindfulness-Based Interventions on Salivary Cortisol in Healthy Adults: A Meta-Analytical Review," *Frontiers in Physiology* 7, no. 471 (October 2016), https://doi.org/10.3389/fphys.2016.00471.

85 Bruce Lipton, *The Biology of Belief: Unleashing the Power of Consciousness, Matter & Miracles* (New York: Hay House, 2005).

86 Elizabeth Edwards, *Saving Graces: Finding Solace and Strength from Friends and Strangers* (New York, Broadway, 2006); *Resilience: Reflections on the Burdens and Gifts of Facing Life Adversities* (New York, Broadway, 2009).

87 Sigrid Breit et al., "Vagus Nerve as Modulator of the Brain-Gut Axis in Psychiatric and Inflammatory Disorders." *Frontiers in Psychiatry* 9, no. 44. (March 13, 2018), https://doi.org/10.3389/fpsyt.2018.00044.

88 Martin Picard and Bruce S McEwen, "Psychological Stress and Mitochondria: A Systematic Review," *Psychosomatic Medicine* 80, no.2, (2018) 141-153, https://doi.org/10.1097/PSY.0000000000000545.

89 *Total Health Magazine*, "Adrea Brier Integrative Cancer Consultant," interview with Adrea Brier, March 22, 2018, https://www.youtube.com/watch?v=p6iQZS74ph; Adrea Brier, "Can We Really Be Healthier Living With Cancer?" *Total Health Magazine*, https://totalhealthmagazine.com/Lifestyle/Can-We-Really-Be-Healthier-Living-With-Cancer.html.

90 "Prajna Healing and Massage," prajnaavalon.com.

91 Phylameana Lila Desy, "Medical Intuitives: How Do They Know," May 19, 2019, https://www. learnreligions.com/medical-intuitives-1725021; Louise Hay, *Heal Your Body* (New York: Hay House, 1984).

92 Rick Simpson, Phoenix Tears- The Rick Simpson Story, www.phoenixtears.ca; Also see: Rick Simpson and Jindrich Bayer, *Cure for Cancer: The Rick Simpson Protocol*, https://jeffreydachmd. com/wp-content/uploads/2014/06/Cure-for-Cancer-The-Rick-Simpson-Protocol-e-book-2013.pdf.

93 See Chapter 1 and Chapter 2.

94 Manuel Guzmán, "Cannabis for the Management of Cancer Symptoms: THC Version 2.0?" *Cannabis and Cannabinoid Research* 3, no. 1 (May 2018): 117–19, https://doi.org/10.1089/ can.2018.0009.

95 S. S. Stith et al., "The Association Between Cannabis Product Characteristics and Symptom Relief," *Scientific Reports* 9, no. 2712 (2019), https://doi.org/10.1038/s41598-019-39462-1; Sean D. McAllister et al., "Pathways Mediating the Effects of Cannabidiol on the Reduction of Breast Cancer Cell Proliferation, Invasion, and Metastasis," *Breast Cancer Research and Treatment* 129, no.1 (2010): 37–47, https://doi.org/10.1007/s10549-010-1177-4; Mohamad Elbaz et al., "Modulation of the Tumor Microenvironment and Inhibition of EGF/EGFR Pathway: Novel Anti-tumor Mechanisms of Cannabidiol in Breast Cancer," *Molecular Oncology* 9, no. 4 https://doi.org/ (2015): 906–1910. https://doi.org/10.1016/j.molonc.2014.12.010.

96 Pawel Śledziński et al., "The Current State and Future Perspectives of Cannabinoids in Cancer Biology," *Cancer Medicine* 7, no. 3 (2018): 765–75, https://doi.org/10.1002/cam4.1312; Daniel A. Ladin et al., "Preclinical and Clinical Assessment of Cannabinoids as Anti-Cancer Agents," *Frontiers in Pharmacology* 7, no. 361. (October 7, 2016): https://doi.org/10.3389/fphar.2016.00361.

97 Anusha Angajala et al., "Diverse Roles of Mitochondria in Immune Responses: Novel Insights Into Immuno-Metabolism," Review Article, *Frontiers in Immunology* 1605 (July 12, 2018), https://doi. org/10.3389/fimmu.2018.01605.

PART III.
BREAST CANCER IN YOUNGER WOMEN

7 TRIPLE-NEGATIVE BREAST CANCER:
Young Women, Listen Up!

Robin Roberts, tall and sleek in a knockout floor-length, red sequined sheath, is walking bald-headed down the narrow runway. But the 5'10" forty-seven-year-old co-host of ABC's *Good Morning America* is not trying to start a fashion trend. It's 2007 and Roberts has just completed chemotherapy for an early-stage triple-negative breast cancer diagnosis. Four years later, it was reported, the same toxic chemotherapy treatments that temporarily took Roberts's hair also caused her to develop a dangerous blood disorder that required a lifesaving bone marrow transplant. The popular TV show host is clearly one of the "lucky ones." She's alive, more than a decade later. But for Roberts and many other women, today's mainstream toxic treatments for breast cancer, especially triple-negative breast cancer, can be worse than the disease itself.[1]

Jennifer Griffin, a correspondent for Fox News, was 39 and nursing her third child in 2009 when she was diagnosed with two fast-growing stage III triple-negative tumors. The larger of the two fast-growing primary tumors, found in her right breast, was already 9 cm—about 3.5 inches across,[2] the size of an orange. Griffin underwent 17 rounds of high-dosage chemotherapy. Doctors also added an experimental type of chemotherapy, ACT plus carboplatin, followed by a double mastectomy and six and a half weeks of radiation.[3]

With Fox since 1999, Griffin had spent her entire career, before and after joining Fox, covering war zones from Afghanistan to the Gaza Strip. During her early thirties, Griffin began having regular mammograms, prescribed because her mother and great-grandmother had both been diagnosed with breast cancer.[4]

Because of her challenging work, Griffin endured chronic stress for years. By also exposing her premenopausal breast cells to ionizing radiation from mammograms, she had unknowingly significantly increased her risk of developing breast cancer. Or, as oncologists might later say, "She was one of the unlucky ones."

The mainstream cancer industry and its investors now anticipate that the triple-negative drug market, especially in the US, will enjoy an expanding bull market for the foreseeable future. That's because the number of women being diagnosed with triple-negative breast cancer, and the cost of current treatment drugs, are both expected to steadily and dramatically rise in coming years.

Today, 10 to 20 percent of all invasive tumors diagnosed in the US are identified as triple-negative. This figure is expected to increase to 25 percent by 2026. Triple-negative cases however, comprise only 1 to 2 percent of all invasive breast cancer tumors diagnosed worldwide.

The value of the global triple-negative breast cancer treatment market is projected to grow at a compound annual growth rate (CAGR) of 4.7% throughout the forecast period (2018-2026). Valued at $293 million in 2015, it is expected to reach $720 million to $1 billion by 2026, with the greatest income growth and greatest ongoing revenues coming from women in the United States.[5] What's going on here?

Let's Turn Off the Triple-Negative Faucet

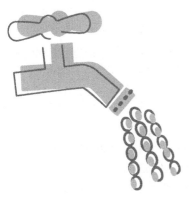

This puzzling name, "triple-negative," can be terrifying all by itself. And the name must be especially stress-producing to women who are given this diagnosis. The name *triple-negative* reflects the mainstream cancer industry's limited ability to treat this particular type of cancer cell. This is because the industry's current drug array used to slow the recurrence of the three more prevalent types of breast cancer (estrogen positive, progesterone positive, and HER2 positive[6]) once a woman's initial treatments have ended, doesn't affect the recurrence of triple-negative breast cancer (TNBC) cells. Since this type of breast cancer cell was first identified in 2005, oncologists continue to use this empty or default term, "triple-negative."[7]

In contrast to this depressing scenario, an effective approach to helping a woman eliminate triple-negative cells from her body is taking place today. This new approach is being practiced by both metabolic cancer clinicians and by self-motivated women diagnosed with TNBC. These are dramatic and hopeful stories. We'll see later in this chapter how metabolic cancer researchers, individual patients, and clinicians are now finding ways to work together, effectively eliminating early and metastatic triple-negative cells and managing their recurrence. But before we get into all that, what do we know about how a woman can best *prevent* the initial development of triple-negative breast cancer (TNBC) cells? What do published studies (although often ignored) tell us about the lifestyles and environmental assaults happening to women who are developing this type of cancer?

Not a Genetic-Based Disease

During the first decade of this century, Dr. Olufunmilayo "Funmi" Olopade, the Walter L. Palmer Distinguished Service Professor of Medicine and Human Genetics and the Director of the Center for Clinical Cancer Genetics at the University of Chicago Medical Center, was also a 2005 winner of a McArthur Foundation Genius Grant. It was her hope to one day be able to identify a gene that might be the cause of so many triple-negative diagnoses in younger African and African American women.[8] One of Dr. Olopade's initial research goals was funded with a $9.7 million grant from the National Institutes of Health. Her research team attempted to lay the groundwork for this gene identification project. They began by examining medical factors common to young, rural Nigerian women and to young, impoverished African American women from Chicago's South Side. All were facing a triple-negative diagnosis.[9] At this point in time, it was believed, and continues to be believed by some researchers, that premenopausal African American women and premenopausal African women are more susceptible to this disease than women of other racial groups and other age groups.[10]

With another multi-million-dollar federal grant, received in 2006, Dr. Olopade's research continued to explore how triple negative patients' genes, families and environmental exposure histories might be connected to their diagnoses.[11] "Why," I asked Dr. Olopade, in January 2009 as I was beginning my research into how best to prevent breast cancer, "Why don't you try and find those lifestyle habits, rather than just the medical factors, common to young African American, African, and Ashkenazi Jewish women today? These are the groups of young women that appear to be disproportionately affected. Wouldn't answers to such basic questions give us some real-life clues about what could be causing so many younger premenopausal women within these specific ethnic groups to develop this disease in such increasing numbers?"

Dr. Olopade, herself Nigerian-born, agreed. "We need to do more environmental sampling. But it is very expensive, and it is very difficult to find sources of funding for this type of research."[12]

Four years after that brief conversation with the eminent geneticist, I was introduced to the groundbreaking book, *Cancer As A Metabolic Disease*, by the eminent genetics-trained biologist, Dr Thomas N. Seyfried. Here, finally, was long-understood, but only recently uncovered, knowledge; pieced together into a coherent theory on the origin, management, and prevention of cancer. Here was a complete biological understanding of how cancer begins and continues forward, able finally to show biologists, physicians, and even nonscientists like myself, that breast cancer cells are not initiated by a damaged breast gene that decides to go rogue. Instead, every initial breast cancer cell, indeed every initial cancer cell that forms, has the same logical, biological origin. Cancer begins when the mitochondria within a cell or group of cells become damaged and begin to suffocate. This suffocation causes the oxygen-deprived mitochondria to transform into their own wildly duplicating, fermenting, prehistoric form.

Preventing Triple-Negative Breast Cancer

The late breast cancer prevention champion Dr. Samuel Epstein often spoke about the importance of using taxpayer dollars to design and fund research that can help women "turn off the breast cancer faucet."[13] Instead, the National Cancer Institute (NCI) and the National Breast Cancer Research Program (NBCRP) continue to try to simply "mop up the water" as they to use their annual budgets of billions or millions,[14] merely looking for ways to slow down the recurrence or the growth of cancerous tumors, ignoring the goal of prevention. The next part of this chapter tries to help achieve Dr. Epstein's lifelong goal: to turn off the faucet.

Beginning with a phone conversation with Dr. Epstein in 2008, I set out to find any published, peer-reviewed studies that could tell us something about the lifestyles of women who develop triple-negative breast cancer. If such studies existed, could they teach us how to then help women turn off the breast cancer faucet, specifically, the triple-negative breast cancer faucet? In 2009, I spoke with a leading triple-negative breast cancer oncologist. The clinician made a passing, but unforgettable, remark. "Triple-negative cancer cells are actually mature estrogen-positive breast cancer cells. All breast cells have estrogen receptors. All breast cancer cells start out with these receptors." Over the past decade, looking at the various lifestyle choices and environmental factors that are conducive to a woman's triple-negative diagnosis, his comment has been important for me to remember when it comes to understanding how to prevent the development of triple-negative breast cancer. Let's look at his statement in some more depth.

All healthy breast cells contain estrogen receptors. Estrogen, after all, is what enables a woman's breast to grow and develop milk ducts and lobes so she can nurse her offspring. The fact that triple-negative breast cancer cells no longer have these estrogen receptors means these cells have become so damaged or mutated along the way that even their estrogen receptors have now been "disappeared." This is why that oncologist called triple-negative breast cancer cells "mature" or "advanced" breast cancer cells.

With this knowledge tucked away in our minds, it also makes sense that a woman's breast cells' mitochondria could undergo a double or a triple whammy before and as they continue to suffocate. As we learned in Chapter 1, this is the moment when a woman's breast cells can begin to turn into a variety of "zombie" breast cancer cells, forming glucose-loving tumors, including, at some point, tumors filled with aggressive triple-negative cancer cells. Let's look at what a decade of statistical, laboratory, clinical and epidemiological studies can now tell us about some of these double or triple whammies that are causing so many women, including many premenopausal young mothers, to develop these triple-negative breast tumors. These studies also give us a clue about why so much triple-negative breast cancer is developing in US women, especially in certain sections of the country and within impoverished African American communities today.

Obesity and Stress: A Double Whammy

Some statistical studies tell us that women of all ages and races who are obese (with a BMI over 29) have an increased risk of developing triple-negative breast cancer.[15] The initial reason for this connection between obesity and an increased risk of all types of breast cancer, as we saw in Chapter 2, is because our excess body fat is alive. These fat cells produce excess or toxic estrogen, along with inflammatory enzymes. Both types of body fluids irritate the mitochondria of our breast cells, 24/7.[16]

Other researchers have also shown that being obese creates a huge amount of social stress in most women.[17] And stress, in turn, creates excess levels of cortisol, constantly flooding a woman's body—constantly irritating her breast cells' mitochondria.[18]

We also saw in Chapter 2 that the more excess body fat a woman has (no matter her age), the more leptin hormone her body fat produces. Like all hormones, a little is good. After all, hormones are critical to our sexual development, our brain's optimal functioning, our ability to regulate glucose levels, and other metabolic functions that create and maintain optimal health. But high levels of any hormone, from estrogen to cortisol to leptin, become toxic to our body.

In 2004, researchers in Japan found that excess amounts of leptin may be especially harmful to breast cancer patients, no matter their age. Laboratory experiments showed that excess leptin can accelerate the growth of early-stage breast-cancer tumors, causing cancer cells to metastasize fairly rapidly, spreading to other organs in the body. They concluded it was extremely important to lower the amount of an obese women's leptin as quickly as possible.[19] And of course, the optimal way to eliminate toxic levels of leptin from our bodies is to lose any excess body fat. Could leptin be a primary reason why triple-negative tumors often grow quickly and rapidly metastasize in both overweight and obese postmenopausal women and in premenopausal obese women?[20]

A few years later, Dr. Linda Vona-Davis studied a group of Euro-American women being treated for breast cancer at the University of West Virginia Medical Center. The researcher found that being impoverished, and obese put these white women at an equally high risk of developing triple-negative breast cancer cells as their African American peers. Dr. Vona-Davis also found that those patients who were under 50 years old had a much higher rate of triple-negative diagnoses than the older white breast cancer patients. Those patients under 40 years old had the highest rate of the triple-negative disease as a percentage of their age group.[21]

A few sociologists and biologists have also begun untangling the biology behind how the emotional triggers of impoverishment affect the growth of triple-negative cancer cells in younger women. Dr. Sarah Bollinger, while a PhD candidate at Washington University in St. Louis, interviewed a randomly selected group of younger African American women, each diagnosed with triple-negative cancer. Dr. Bollinger found, without exception, that each woman had experienced high stress from long-term chronic psychiatric conditions stemming from poverty-associated dysfunctional family lives.[22] Specifically, each of these women:

- had lived in highly stressful (often poverty-induced) environments from a young age, or was currently living in a highly stressful situation;
- was suffering from post-traumatic stress disorder (PSTD); and/or
- was suffering from other socially isolating factors.

Taking this knowledge a step further, Dr Suzanne Conzen, a Chicago biologist, questioned how and why this type of chronic stress was causing such rapidly growing triple-negative tumors in so many and in such young patients. Dr. Conzen first turned to that famous question asked by Bruce Lipton in his popular book, *The Biology of Belief*: "What specific biological connections are happening in a highly stressed patient's mind and body to cause these triple-negative tumors to grow so rapidly?"

Using a bunch of female Sprague Dawley rats, a highly social type of laboratory rodent, that had naturally occurring triple-negative tumors, Dr. Conzen's team divided the rodents into two groups. One group of rats was kept together, able to happily socialize. The rats in the second group were separated from one another—which, of course, created high stress levels among those sociable rodents. Dr. Conzen's group soon noticed that the highly stressed rats began to develop fast-growing tumors, while the triple-negative cells in the socially content rats' breast tumors duplicated at a much slower pace.[23]

In a later study, using mice, Conzen's team noticed that the fat cells within the stressed mice's breasts were pulling in much more glucose than the fat cells in the socializing mice's breasts. Dr. Conzen concluded that these fat cells must be secreting substances that caused those nearby precancerous epithelial cells to proliferate more rapidly, accelerating the development of the mice's breast cancer.[24]

"This local effect of fat cells in the breast was completely unanticipated," said Dr. Conzen about the study involving rats. "The occurrence of cancer in these isolated rats began early in their short lives...at 14 months of age. Those rats that lived in a happy social group setting did not develop tumors until they were much older...at 23 months of age, which in rats is the equivalent of 60–70 years of age in human beings."[25] Conzen's research with rats and mice helps us understand how a life history of both obesity and chronic stress, especially early on in life, often creates fast-growing triple-negative tumors in so many younger women, often before their fortieth birthdays. Commenting on the researchers' laboratory report about those mice, a University of Chicago publication said, "The mammary glands in both mice and humans include many cell types, but fat cells, the authors note, are arguably the most neglected and the least well understood component of the breast."[26]

Birth Control Drugs and Low Vitamin D3 Blood Levels: A Double Whammy

In Chapter 3 we saw the need for women to keep their vitamin D3 blood levels above 60 ng/ml to help their immune system block the development of breast cancer cells. Then, in Chapter 4, we saw the landmark 2010 discovery by the Penninger-Glimcher team of how the chemical progestin, found in all birth control drugs and in some hormone therapy drugs, causes and accelerates breast cancer. Five years later, researchers in Argentina discovered that the progestin chemical can also decrease the ability of a woman's immune system to recognize and eliminate highly metastatic triple-negative breast tumors. Yes, in their 2015 paper, "Progestin-Driven Regulatory T-Cells Directly Promote An Aggressive and Metastatic Phenotype In Triple-Negative Breast Cancer," the Argentine biologists described yet another metabolic reason why and how triple-negative tumors are able to grow at breakneck speed in so many women."[27]

Being Young and Using Birth Control Drugs for Multiple Years: A Double Whammy

We also learned in Chapter 5 and Chapter 6 that teens and very young women have a window of vulnerability; a specific time period when any type of assault to their fragile breast cells can cause extensive damage, leading to increased breast cancer rates early on, or later in their lives. *The timing of the attack*, not the dose, is the cause of this extensive damage.[28]

It is therefore no surprise that studies show how women between the ages of 20 and 44 who once used birth control drugs for more than fifteen years, and women who are currently and have been using these progestin contraceptives for more than five years, all experience a higher breast cancer risk than their peers who have never used and/or are not currently using these drugs. And younger women, those between the ages of 20 and 40, who are using birth control drugs when they are diagnosed with breast cancer, are most apt to find themselves facing triple-negative tumors.[29]

Using Placenta Hair Conditioners and Birth Control Drugs: A Double Whammy

Numerous statistical studies conducted by the Boston University epidemiologist Lynn Rosenberg also tell us that African American women who use birth control drugs have higher rates of triple-negative breast cancer than their Euro-American peers who also use these progestin-based contraceptives.[30] Meanwhile, recent studies tell us the majority of African American women (and African women) who frequently use placenta-based or other types of estrogenic hair straightening products can increase their breast cancer risk.[31] And the question remains; since both of these lifestyles assault a woman's breast cells' mitochondria, does this double-whammy attack from the contraceptive's toxic progestin and the hair conditioner's toxic estradiol create the well-known fact that a disproportionate number of black women continue to be diagnosed with triple-negative cells?

Over Age 65+ Treated for Hormone Positive Breast Cancer + Used Tamoxifen for Years = Increased Risk of Developing Triple Negative Tumor: A Triple Whammy

Dr. Christopher Li, one of the world's most respected breast cancer epidemiologists and a longtime staff member at the prestigious Fred Hutchinson Cancer Research Center in Seattle, noticed that increasing numbers of postmenopausal women, identified in various state cancer registries, were developing triple-negative breast cancer. Li also noticed that years earlier, these same women had been diagnosed with the more prevalent type of breast cancer, hormone positive or hormone receptor positive, also called HR positive or HR+.

Dr. Li wondered if this group of older triple-negative patients had anything else in common. In order to find out, he looked at the medical records of 1,000 women randomly drawn from a group of 16,000 women from the Pacific Northwest, all of whom had been diagnosed with some type of *second* primary breast tumor between 1990 and 2005. Dr. Li found that the women in this group who had chosen to use tamoxifen for a number of years, after being treated for their initial breast cancer diagnoses, developed four times more triple-negative breast tumors than their peers who had chosen *not* to use tamoxifen, and had also developed a second primary breast cancer diagnosis.[32] In other words, the women who had taken tamoxifen for a number of years, who went on to develop some type of invasive primary breast cancer for a second time (not a recurrence or a metastasis of their original breast tumor) had a *400 percent higher risk* of developing triple-negative tumors than women *who had not taken tamoxifen* after their initial diagnosis *and* who also went on to develop another primary breast tumor years later.[33]

This wasn't the first time tamoxifen had come under fire for increasing a woman's risk of later developing triple-negative breast cancer. Back in 1998, Dr. Sherrill Sellman wrote a comprehensive article on the numerous problems inherent in the use of this new endocrine suppressing drug. Her article remains important, especially today, when most anti-tamoxifen research, first published in the 1980s as the drug was first introduced, has been long forgotten. Sellman's extensive research on this subject is also found in her book, *Hormone Heresy, What Women Must Know About Their Hormones*, and through her ongoing interviews and talks today on the *Total Health Magazine* YouTube channel.[34]

The award-winning blog *Positives About Negative* reported on Dr. Li's 2009 study connecting tamoxifen with triple-negative breast cancer[35], as did Science Daily.[36] These were two of the very few publications to have ever reported on Dr Li's tamoxifen and triple-negative study. Written by Dr. Patricia Prijatel, the E.T. Meredith Distinguished Professor Emeritus at Drew University's School of Journalism and Mass Communication, her award-winning blog, *Positives About Negative*, can be depended upon to offer up-to-date, objective coverage of all significant research published about this triple-negative disease.

VERY Low Vitamin D3 Blood Levels = Triple Negative Breast Cancer

Today, we know (as we saw in <u>Chapter 3</u>) that it's important to maintain our vitamin D3 blood levels above 60 ng/ml in order to stop breast cancer cells from developing. But back in 2009, before Carole Baggerly and her GrassrootsHealth organization created today's worldwide D3 prevention movement,[37] a California oncologist did his own study. Glen Tisman had a hunch, but no studies had yet looked at the statistics. Was there a difference between the vitamin D3 blood levels of patients diagnosed with triple-negative breast cancer and the D3 blood levels of patients diagnosed with other types of breast cancer? Also, how did the D3 blood levels of all breast cancer patients compare with those of patients who had been diagnosed with other types of cancer? Using data from his own patient base, Dr. Tisman found that his breast cancer patients had a lower average D3 blood level than his other cancer patients. He also found that his triple-negative breast cancer patients had the lowest D3 blood levels of all![38] Who knew?

Obesity + Chronic Stress + Pesticide-Polluted Water = A Triple Whammy

For more than two decades, Professor Tyrone Hayes at the University of California-Berkeley has been sounding the alarm, along with other biologists and environmentally focused breast cancer prevention groups.[39]

The pesticide *atrazine* continues to poison both wildlife and people within communities exposed to the chemical's runoff from agricultural fields.[40] Atrazine is the most popular herbicide used by US agribusiness. It eliminates most weeds, and thus reduces labor costs where huge tracts of GMO soybeans, corn, and wheat are grown.

In 2014, atrazine's manufacturer, the Swiss pharmaceutical giant Syngenta, was forced to settle a federal lawsuit that required it to pay out $105 million to 1,000 affected Midwestern communities. The money was awarded to enable these communities to install water filtration systems in an effort to decrease the pesticide's contamination of their public water supplies.[41] Nevertheless, the US Congress has still not passed legislation equal to that of the European Union, banning the agricultural use of atrazine.[42] Although Syngenta is not allowed to sell atrazine within its home country of Switzerland, atrazine continues to be a big seller on the US market.[43]

According to the independent Natural Resources Defense Council, the 2010 US Geological Survey indicates that surface and drinking water in the Midwest and in Alabama, Mississippi, Kentucky, and Tennessee are "pervasively contaminated with atrazine."[44] Also, three of these states, all rural and impoverished, have the highest obesity rates in the nation.[45] In 2016, Yale University researchers reported that women living within these states, (known as the East South Central region of the US) currently develop *15 percent of all triple-negative tumors* nationwide, but represent only 5% of the US population.[46] Why such a disproportionate amount of triple-negative diagnoses? Is this simply more proof that obesity, impoverishment, *and* toxic water supplies together create yet another triple-negative cancer recipe? Is this the reason why so many triple-negative breast cancer diagnoses are happening throughout Alabama, Mississippi, Kentucky, and Tennessee?

This cluster of women in our East South Central states, struggling with such high numbers of triple-negative breast cancer diagnoses, is also a clear example of why the US needs to have well-funded state cancer boards. Often called *cancer registries* or *tumor registries*, these state agencies should all change their names to *Cancer Prevention Registries*. This is what their role needs to be today; a role we further describe in

Chapter 9. Once such cancer clusters are identified, environmental and health agencies can work to understand the causes behind them. Community health groups, guided by the statistics collected by these cancer prevention registries, can hopefully take action needed to try to protect the affected communities against the pollution, the polluters, and whatever other factors are causing these clusters.[47] We must never forget that Syngenta and their best-selling atrazine herbicide is a subsidiary of AstraZeneca...the pharmaceutical company that founded Breast Cancer Awareness Month and created tamoxifen.[48]

The Stop Triple-Negative Checklist

Do two or more of these situations apply to you?

Category #1: Lifestyles/Life Experience

- Currently obese (BMI over 29)

- Have chronic, long-term stress (often associated with poverty or with verbal/physical/domestic violence)

- Currently using a progestin drug, including:
  - Any type or brand of birth control drug

  - A progestin-laced IUD (US brand names include: Mirena, Liletta, Kyleena, or Skyla)

  - A "combination" menopausal relief drug (US brand names include: Activella, Angeliq, Femhrt, Jinteli, Mimvey, Prefest, Premphase, or Prempro)

  - Progestin drug (sometimes used before administering clomiphene citrate as part of some infertility workups)[49]

- Regularly use placenta-based hair straightening creams or placenta-based skin lightening creams

- Currently use tamoxifen, or recently used tamoxifen for a number of years

- Live in an area with an atrazine-polluted public water supply[50]

- Have experienced one or more mammograms (or other types of medical radiation) to your chest while still premenopausal.

Category #2: Immune System

- Have an extremely low vitamin D3 blood level (less than 30 ng/ml)
- Were born with a damaged or mutated BRCA1 or BRCA2 tumor-suppressor gene[51]

Pay attention: This is important! If you checked off two or more items from category #1 and at least one item in category #2, you have placed yourself in that group of women whom researchers indicate are most likely to develop triple-negative breast cancer. This can be a clear signal for you to begin implementing some or many of the simple prevention steps described throughout this book.

A New World: Successfully Managing Triple-Negative Breast Cancer

One third or more of women who are treated for an early-stage (stages I, II, or III) TNBC diagnosis go on to develop metastatic triple-negative breast cancer; most often during the first three years after their initial treatments.[52] Major drug companies, including Merck, openly tell us that today's mainstream cancer centers are not able to help women facing metastatic triple-negative breast cancer (mTNBC). Instead, new treatments must be found and used:

> *"Chemotherapies have limited effectiveness and are associated with unfavorable toxicity profiles, highlighting a considerable unmet medical need for improved therapeutic options in mTNBC. In addition to the recently approved combination of atezolizumab and nab-paclitaxel for PD-L1-positive mTNBC, new treatments resulting in durable clinical responses, prolonged survival, and manageable safety profile would greatly benefit patients with mTNBC."*[53]

With all of these projected increases in the incidence of triple-negative cases expected to take place, along with the death sentence this disease now brings to a significant percentage of those initially diagnosed, we certainly do need some new effective treatments that can offer us good news. And we have some—in the case studies and stories of women who choose to use only nontoxic metabolic therapies, instead of mainstream toxic treatments, when diagnosed with triple-negative breast cancer.

In both cases described below, each patient's choice of embracing only metabolic therapies enabled them to successfully manage their disease while also achieving optimal health.

Marissa: 2013

My friend Marissa was diagnosed with a tiny, pea-sized, 1.3-centimeter triple-negative breast tumor in August 2013. A 61-year-old African American woman who had long followed a vegetarian/high-sugar diet, Marissa had been obese for at least thirty years. She had also suffered from chronic stress, sometimes at debilitating levels, throughout much of her life. When diagnosed, Marissa's vitamin D3 blood level was at a "rickets' level," only 9 ng/ml.[54] She also often used a placenta-based skin cream. I mention all these lifestyle habits since, as described in this book, they are all possible risk factors for breast cancer, especially for triple-negative breast cancer.

In the summer of 2013, an annual mammogram found Marissa's small tumor. A needle aspiration biopsy then diagnosed triple-negative cells. Marissa immediately declined all additional treatment offered by mainstream cancer clinics. Just months after her diagnosis, she was introduced to Dr. Seyfried's metabolic understanding of cancer. She then began following a variety of metabolic protocols. This included a four-day, water-only fast and a long-term, high-fat, no-sugar, very-low-carb ketogenic diet. Marissa also increased her vitamin D3 blood level from 9 ng/ml to nearly 100 ng/ml, using high amounts of vitamin D3 supplements and a 1000 IU calcium supplement daily. Within a year, Marissa lost one hundred pounds, bringing her BMI from 30 to below 25.

Marissa also began having regular vitamin C infusions, and she participated in a three-week wellness program at the Hippocrates Institute in West Palm Beach, Florida. There she learned many detoxification practices to help further weaken any existing cancer cells and to strengthen her healthy mitochondria. In order to manage her ongoing stress, Marissa also expanded her daily meditation practice. She now understood that her lifelong chronic stress had probably been a major factor in her subsequent diagnosis.

It's now been more than seven years since Marissa's initial triple-negative diagnosis. Periodic ultrasound imaging, requested and read by the chief breast surgeon at a leading Boston clinic, continues to indicate that Marissa's triple-negative tumor has disappeared. Meanwhile, the surgeon continues to follow my friend's self-designed metabolic healing journey with great interest and respect. With Marissa's permission, I interviewed the doctor in late 2014, and asked why, unlike so many mainstream oncology practitioners, she is willing to support Marissa on her self-directed healing journey.

"I must have missed that course in medical school where they teach you how to think like God, how to override a woman's instinctive good sense when it comes to her own body," the surgeon said.

Azra: 2016

In October of 2016, twenty-nine-year-old Azra, nearly paralyzed with fear, arrived at Istanbul's only metabolic cancer clinic, Chemothermia, on Yeten Street in Turkey's capital. Chemothermia is the outpatient oncology clinic of Dr. Bulent Bernard (the first registered oncologist in Turkey), Dr. Mehmet Salih İyikesici (an assistant professor of oncology), and Dr. Abdul Kadir Slocum (an oncologist who is fluent in both Turkish and English).[55]

Azra, overweight, with a BMI of 28, had been diagnosed eleven months earlier with an early-stage, palpable, triple-negative breast tumor. When she finally sought treatment, metastasized cancer cells had formed tumors in her liver and lymph nodes.

In order to begin eliminating these triple-negative cells as quickly as possible, Azra was instructed to follow a no-sugar/no-starch/high-fat ketogenic therapeutic diet. This diet enabled her to switch her metabolism to a fat-burning operating system that strengthened her healthy cells and began to starve or weaken her cancer cells by denying them glucose, one of cancer cells' two fuels, glucose and glutamine.[56] Over the next four months, Azra was also given specific heat treatments, along with hyperbaric oxygen treatments (while remaining in metabolic ketosis),[57] to further weaken the cancer cells and strengthen the healthy cells in her body.[58] Meanwhile, she was also given the lowest dose of chemotherapy required by Turkish medical authorities, to help destroy her metastatic cells.

Azra received this minimal chemotherapy dose two days a week, every three weeks, during her initial four-month treatment period. In order to maximize the impact of these very low nontoxic doses of these drugs, Azra fasted for twelve hours prior to each treatment. This further weakened her already glucose-starved cancer cells.[59]

Table 7.1: Azra's Food Guidelines (Ketogenic Diet Recommendations)

DO EAT	DO NOT EAT
Eggs	Bread
Leafy greens	Pasta
Above-ground vegetables	Rice
High-fat dairy	Potatoes
Natural fats	Sugar
Meats	Honey
Nuts and seeds	Fruits

Azra: Healing and Managing her Stage IV recurrent metastatic triple negative (rMBC) diagnosis.

Iyikesici et al, "Efficacy of Metabolically Supported Chemotherapy Combined with Ketogenic Diet, Hyperthermia, and Hyperbaric Oxygen Therapy for Stage IV Triple-negative Breast Cancer," Cureus 9, no. 7 (2017): e1445, https://doi.org/doi:10.7759/cureus.1445.

After four months of following a ketogenic diet while continuing to receive these metabolic treatments, a PET scan of Azra's entire body did not detect a single cancer cell! In their 2017 case study documenting Azra's initial treatment and subsequent evaluation, her medical team described Azra as successfully managing her recurrent stage IV triple-negative cancer diagnosis. Since first arriving at the clinic ten months earlier, the young woman had also reached a healthy BMI of 21, continued to receive periodic metabolic treatments at the clinic, and maintained her vitamin D3 blood level at 50 ng/ml. In this same case study, published in July 2017, Azra reported she was now enjoying a higher quality of life than prior to her diagnosis.[60]

In early 2017, a PET scan indicated her metastatic cells had been eliminated from her body. A year later, against clinic instructions, Azra returned to a glucose-based lifestyle. She then stopped coming to the clinic for her other nontoxic therapies. The clinic subsequently learned that Azra had died. Dr. Abdul Slocum presented this September, 2018 follow-up to the Chemothermia team's original July 2017 case study:

As documented by PET-CT imaging in February 2017, the patient in our study was shown to have a complete response to our metabolic treatment. In April of 2017, she underwent a mastectomy and we were able to document a pathological complete response. After this outstanding result, the patient continued to receive maintenance treatment with the same protocols. Sadly, beginning in the spring of 2018, her adherence to the maintenance therapy diminished and she failed to appear for many of her scheduled treatments. When she did appear, she mentioned that she was no longer following the ketogenic diet. In May of 2018, the results of a PET-CT scan indicated a recurrence of her triple-negative breast cancer...The patient was distraught by this news and subsequently rejected any further treatment, effectively ending her contact with the clinic. As expected, her condition rapidly deteriorated and we learned that she was hospitalized for an infection in August 2018, which ultimately resulted in her death.

This is unfortunate, given that our experience shows that patients who have continued the metabolic therapies have had improved progression-free and (improved) overall survival when compared to standard of care treatments. As reported by Kassam et al., the median survival time for metastatic triple-negative breast cancer is just 13.3 months when treated with standard therapies.[61] Our patient fit into an (even) higher subgroup, with negative prognosis factors that included diagnosis at a younger age and the presence of visceral metastatic disease. Despite her generally poorer prognosis (when first diagnosed by the clinic) it is encouraging that she survived 21 months post-diagnosis of her advanced metastatic disease. However, her choice to discontinue treatment is distressing and underscores the urgent need for comprehensive patient support networks that may improve compliance of combined treatment strategies.[62]

Azra and Marissa are medical pioneers. Each woman's experience illustrates how these nontoxic and inexpensive metabolic treatments, when combined with ongoing dedicated compliance by the patient, can be effective. As more and more women are able to choose metabolic therapies alone, or in combination with limited mainstream therapies, additional triple-negative patients should be able to work with clinicians to successfully manage their triple-negative disease. Like Marissa and Azra, many women who are able to follow these metabolic therapies will also be able to experience a longer, higher-quality life than they could possibly have hoped for, even prior to their diagnoses. Alleluia!

In this chapter we've seen that a metabolic approach to cancer can bring hope to women facing the scary diagnosis of triple-negative breast cancer. We've also looked at those double and triple whammies that propel women into developing a triple-negative diagnosis. But what about women who are told that they're genetically predisposed to get breast cancer? The next chapter includes published (though not well-publicized) studies dealing with so-called *BRCA women*—those five percent of the world's female population who have been born with a damaged or mutated BRCA1 or BRCA2 tumor-suppressor gene. In these studies, we find startling statistics that illustrate how a BRCA woman's lifestyle choices and cultural environment can be much more important than the fact that she happened to be born with one of these defective 'tumor watchdog' genes in her breast cells. Read on!

CHAPTER ENDNOTES

1   The Triple-Negative Breast Cancer Forum, part of the TNBC Foundation's website, offers women who are undergoing and have experienced mainstream/genetics-based therapies, the opportunity to share their stories. See https://forum.tnbcfoundation.org.

2   Jennifer Griffin, "Jennifer Griffin's Blog: My War Against Triple Negative Breast Cancer," (November 9, 2011), https://jengriffinblog.blogspot.com/.

3   Ibid.

4   Everyday Health, "Jennifer Griffin's Fight Against Triple-Negative Breast Cancer," November 11, 2017, https://www.everydayhealth.com/cancer/breast-cancer/jennifer-griffins-fight-against-triple-negative-breast-cancer/; Lynn Okura, "Entering the Cancer War Zone," May 17, 2010, https://www.oprah.com/health/jennifer-griffins-battle-with-breast-cancer.

5   Transparency Market Research, "Triple-Negative Breast Cancer Treatment Market: Global Industry Analysis, Size, Share, Growth, Trends and Forecast, 2018-2026," press release, https://www.transparency marketresearch.com/triple-negative-breast-cancer-treatment-market.html; Persistence Market Research, "Global Triple-negative Breast Cancer Treatment Market Revenue to Cross US$ 720MN by 2026," October 3, 2018, http://www.prnewswire.com/news-releases/global-triple-negative-breast-cancer-treatment-market-revenue-to-cross-us-720-mn-by-2026-persistence-market-research-801093621.html.

6   The HER2 protein is sometimes called HER2/neu protein. A HER2 positive breast cancer diagnosis means tumor cells have a greater number of HER2 receptors (doors) on the cells, than normal breast cells. HER2 positive, like triple-negative breast cancer cells, are considered to be *hormone negative* types of breast cancer cells.

7   Zsuzsanna Suba, "Triple-negative Breast Cancer Risk in Women Is Defined by the Defect of Estrogen Signaling: Preventive and Therapeutic Implications," *OncoTargets and Therapy* 7 (January 23, 2014): 147-64, https://doi.org/10.2147/OTT.S52600; Carey Anders and Lisa A. Carey, "Understanding and Treating Triple-negative Breast Cancer," *Oncology* 22, no.11 (2008): 1233–39; discussions 1239–40, 1243, PMCID: PMC2868264.

8   Breast Cancer Research Foundation, "Meet the Researcher: Dr. Funmi Olopade, Part One: Dr. Olopade Talks Triple Negative Breast Cancer," March 2, 2015, https://www.bcrf.org/blog/meet-researcher-dr-funmi-olopade-part-one.

9   University of Chicago Medical Center, "University of Chicago Cancer Research Center Awarded $11.5 Million SPORE Grant for Breast Cancer Research, https://www.uchicagomedicine.org/forefront/news/university-of-chicago-cancer-research-center-awarded-115-million-spore-grant-for-breast-cancer-resea.

10 Sumit Siddarth and Dipali Sharma, "Racial Disparity and Triple-Negative Breast Cancer in African-American Women: A Multifaceted Affair Between Obesity, Biology, and Socioeconomic Determinants." *Cancers* 10, no.12 (December 2018), https://doi.org/10.3390/cancers10120514.

11 University of Chicago Medical Center, "University of Chicago Cancer Research Center awarded $11.5 Million SPORE grant...," https://www.uchicagomedicine.org/forefront/news/university-of-chicago-cancer-research-center-awarded-115-million-spore-grant-for-breast-cancer-resea.

12 Dr. Olufunmilayo Olopade, telephone interview with author, January 27, 2009.

13 Samuel Epstein, *The Breast Cancer Prevention Program* (New York: Wiley, 1998).

14 NCI spent $6.44 billion in 2019 and NBCRP spent $150 million in 2019 predominantly researching new toxic drug treatments and tumor diagnostic procedures. It is difficult to identify any non-toxic prevention studies or educational programs from their reports.

15 Heng Sun et al., "Triple-negative Breast Cancer and Its Association with Obesity," *Molecular and Clinical Oncology* 7, no. 6 (2017): 935–42, https://doi.org/10.3892/mco.2017.1429.

16 Ouissam Al Jarroudi et al., "Overweight: Is It a Prognostic Factor in Women with Triple-Negative Breast Cancer?" *Asian Pacific Journal of Cancer Prevention* 18, no. 6 (June 2017): 1519–23, https://doi.org/10.22034/APJCP.2017.18.6.1519.

17 Marja Koski and Hannu Naukkarinen, "The Relationship Between Stress and Severe Obesity: A Case-Control Study," *Biomed Hub* 2, no. 1, 458771 (2017); https://doi.org/10.1159/000458771.

18 See Chapter 1, Chapter 2 and Chapter 3.

19 M. Ishikawa, J. Kottayam, and H. Nagawa, "Enhanced Expression of Leptin and Leptin Receptor (OB-R) in Human Breast Cancer," *Clinical Cancer Research* 1, no.10 (July 2004): 4325–31, https://doi.org/10.1158/1078-0432.CCR-03-0749.

20 Ibid.

21 Linda Vona-Davis et al., "Triple Negative Breast Cancer and Obesity in a Rural Appalachian Population," *Cancer Epidemiology, Biomarkets and Prevention* 17, no.12 (December 2008): 3319–24, https://doi.org/10.1158/1055-9965.EPI-08-0544; Rajita Sinha and Ania M. Jastreboff, "Stress as a Common Risk Factor for Obesity and Addiction," *Biological Psychiatry* 73, no. 9 (2013): 827–35, https://doi.org/10.1016/j.biopsych.2013.01.032.

22 Sarah Bollinger, "An Exploration of the Lives of Young, African American Women with Triple-Negative Breast Cancer," PhD dissertation, Washington University, St. Louis, MO (September 2013), https://openscholarship.wustl.edu/cgi/viewcontent.cgi?article=2120&context=etd.

23 Gretchen L Hermes et al., "Social Isolation Dysregulates Endocrine and Behavioral Stress While Increasing Malignant Burden of Spontaneous Mammary Tumors," *Proceedings of the National Academy of Sciences of the United States of America* 106, no.52 (2009): 22393–8, https://doi.org/10.1073/pnas.0910753106.

24 Paul A. Volden et al., "Chronic Social Isolation Is Associated with Metabolic Gene Expression Changes Specific to Mammary Adipose Tissue," *Cancer Prevention Research* 6, no.7 (June 18, 2013): 634–46, https://doi.org/10.1158/1940-6207.CAPR-12-0458.

25 John Easton, "Fat Cells in Breast May Connect Social Stress to Triple-negative Breast Cancer," June 18, 2013, https://sciencelife.uchospitals.edu/2013/06/18/fat-cells-in-breast-may-connect-social-stress-to-triple-negative-breast-cancer-2/.

26 Ibid.

27 Tomas Dalotte Moreno, B.A. Rabinovich and Mariana Salatino, "Abstract 1573: The Progesterone Analogue, Norgestre, Impairs Tumor Immunity and Promotes Metastatic Breast Cancer Progression," *Cancer Research*, July 2016, https://doi.org/10.1158/1538-7445.AM2016-1573; Tomas Dalotto Moreno et al., "Abstract 465: Progestin-driven Regulatory T Cells Directly Promote an Aggressive and Metastatic Phenotype in Triple-negative Breast Cancer," *Proceedings: AACR 106th Annual Meeting* 75, No. 15 Sup (August 2015), https://doi.org/10.1158/1538-7445.AM2015-465; Judith A Malmgren et al., "Differential Presentation and Survival of de novo and Recurrent Metastatic Breast Cancer Over Time: 1990-2010," *Breast Cancer Research and Treatment* 167, no.2 (2018): 579-590, https://doi.org/10.1007/s10549-017-4529-5.

28 Silent Spring Institute, "Hair Products for Black Women Contain Mix of Hazardous Ingredients, "April 10, 2018, https://silentspring.org/news/hair-products-black-women-contain-mix-hazardous-ingredients.

29 E.F. Beaber et al., "Oral Contraceptive and Breast Cancer Risk Overall and by Molecular Subtype Among Young Women," *Cancer, Epidemiology, Biomarkers & Prevention* 23, no. 5 (May 2014), https://doi.org/10.1158/1055-9965.EPI-13-0944.

30 Lynn Rosenberg et al., "Oral Contraceptive Use and Estrogen Progesterone Receptor-Negative Breast Cancer Among African American Women," *Cancer Epidemiology, Biomarkers & Prevention* 19, no. 8 (August 2010): 2073–79, https://doi.org/10.1158/1055-9965.EPI-10-0428.

31 J.S. Helm et al., "Measurement of Endocrine Disrupting and Asthma-associated Chemicals in Hair Products Used by Black Women," *Environmental Research*, (August 9, 2018): 448-58, https://doi.org/10.1016/j.envres.2018.03.030; L.A. Brinton et al., "Skin Lighteners and Hair Relaxers as Risk Factors for Breast Cancer: Results from the Ghana Breast Health Study," *Carcinogenesis* 39, no.4 (2018): 571-79, https://doi.org/10.1093/carcin/bgy002.

32 Anywhere from 7% to 20% of women treated for an early-stage primary breast tumor go on to develop a second primary breast tumor. The risk of developing a second primary tumor increases over time. See: Dan Li et al., "Risk of Second Primary Cancers Among Long-Term Survivors of Breast Cancer," *Frontiers in Oncology* (January 13, 2020), https://doi.org/10.3389/fonc.2019.01426.

33 Christopher Li et al., "Adjuvant Hormonal Therapy for Breast Cancer and Risk of Hormone Receptor-specific Subtypes of Contralateral Breast Cancer," *Cancer Research* 69, no. 17 (2009): 6865–70, https://doi.org/10.1158/0008-5472.CAN-09-1355.

34 Sherrill Sellman, "Tamoxifen: A Major Medial Mistake?" *Nexus Magazine* 5, no. 4 (June–July 1998):43-8, https://nexusmagazine.com/product/tamoxifen-a-major-medical-mistake/?v=7516fd43adaa; Sherrill Sellman, *Hormone Heresy; What Women Must Know About Their Hormones* (GetWell International: 2000); *Total Health Magazine*, https://www.youtube.com/channel/UC1XVahfBic9XkbEPm5oA3DA.

35 Patricia Prijatel, "Positives About Negative," http://hormonenegative.blogspot.com/.

36 Science Daily, "Long-term Tamoxifen Use Increases Risk of An Aggressive, Hard To Treat Type Of Second Breast Cancer, "August 26, 2009, https://www.sciencedaily.com/releases/2009/08/090825150954.htm.

37 See Chapter 3.

38 Christa Rainville, Yasir Khan, and Glenn Tisman, "Triple Negative Breast Cancer Patients Presenting with Low Serum Vitamin D Levels: A Case Series," *Cases Journal* 2 (2009): 8390, https://doi.org/10.4076/1757-1626-2-8390.

39 Rachel Aviv, "A Valuable Reputation: After Tyrone Hayes Said That a Chemical was Harmful, Its Maker Pursued Him," *The New Yorker*, February 10, 2014, https://www.newyorker.com/magazine/2014/02/10/a-valuable-reputation.

40 Olga Naidenko and Sydney Evans, "Hormone-Disrupting Weed Killer Taints Drinking Water for Millions of Americans, Water Utility Tests Commonly Underreport Atrazine Contamination Spikes," Environmental Working Group, November 14, 2018, https://www.ewg.org/research/hormone-disrupting-weed-killer-taints-drinking-water-millions-americans.

41 Associated Press, "Sygenta Pays Millions in Settlements to Farming States," *The Topeka Capital-Journal*, January 25, 2013, https://www.cjonline.com/article/20130125/news/301259667.

42 Environmental Working Group, "Congress Fails on PFAS, Trump's EPS Bear Hug for Hormone-Disrupting Pesticide," https://www.ewg.org/news-and-analysis/2019/12/ewg-news-roundup-1220-congress-fails-pfas-trump-epa-s-bear-hug-hormone.

43 Janet M. Gray et al., "State of the Evidence 2017: An Update on the Connection Between Breast Cancer and the Environment," *Environmental Health* 16, no. 94 (September 2, 2017), https://doi.org/10.1186/s12940-017-0287-4.

44 Mae Wu, Jennifer Sass and Andrew Wetzler, "Atrazine: Poisoning the Well, Atrazine Continues to Contaminate Surface Water and Drinking Water in the United States," April 30, 2010, https://www.nrdc.org/resources/atrazine-poisoning-well.

45 World Population Review, "Most Obese States 2019," http://worldpopulationreview.com/states/most-obese-states/.

46 Magdalena L Plasilova et al., "Features of Triple-negative Breast Cancer: Analysis of 38,813 Cases from the National Cancer Database," *Medicine* 95, no. 35 (2016): e4614, https://doi.org/10.1097/MD.0000000000004614.

47 T.E. Aldrich and T. Sinks, "Things to Know and Do About Cancer Clusters," *Cancer Investigation* 20, no. 5–6 (July 17, 2002): 810–16. https://doi.org/10.1081/CNV-120003546.

48 Emma Smith, "Tamoxifen-the start of something big," *Science Blog,* Cancer Research-UK, https://scienceblog.cancerresearchuk.org/2012/10/15/high-impact-science-tamoxifen-the-start-of-something-big/.

49 ClinicalTrials.gov, "Effect of Progestin-Induced Withdrawal Bleed on Ovulation Induction Cycles with Clomiphene Citrate," https://clinicaltrials.gov/ct2/show/NCT01966575.

50 Naidenko and Evans, "Hormone-Disrupting Weed Killer," 2; Jane A. McElroy et al., "Risk of Breast Cancer for Women Living in Rural Areas from Adult Exposure to Atrazine from Well Water in Wisconsin," *Journal of Exposure, Science and Environmental Epidemiology* 17 (2007): 207–14, https://doi.org/10.1038/sj.jes.7500511.

51 See Chapter 8.

52 Katarzyna Pogoda, "Analysis of Pattern, Time and Risk Factors Influencing Recurrence in Triple-Negative Breast Cancer Patients," *Medical Oncology* 30, no.388 (2013), https://doi.org/10.1007/s12032-012-0388-4.

53 C.H. Li et al., "Current Treatment Landscape for Patients with Locally Recurrent Inoperable or Metastatic Triple-negative Breast Cancer: A Systematic Literature Review," *Breast Cancer Research* 21, no.143 (2019), https://doi.org/10.1186/s13058-019-1210-4.

54 Manisha Sahay and Rakesh Sahay, "Rickets: Vitamin D Deficiency and Dependency," *Indian Journal of Endocrinology and Metabolism* 16, no. 2 (2012): 64-76, https://doi.org/10.4103/2230-8210.93732.

55 David Eigen, "Integrative Oncology with Optimal Results" (transcript of interview with Dr Abdul Slocum, January 14, 2018), P5 Health Ventures, https://p5hv.com/dr-abdul-slocum/.

56 Iyikesici et al, "Efficacy of Metabolically Supported Chemotherapy Combined with Ketogenic Diet, Hyperthermia, and Hyperbaric Oxygen Therapy for Stage IV Triple-negative Breast Cancer" *Cureus* 9, no. 7 (2017): e1445, https://doi.org/10.7759/cureus.1445.

57 Daniela D. Weber et al., "Ketogenic Diet in Cancer Therapy," *Aging* 10, no. ,2 (2018): 164-165. https://doi.org/10.18632/aging.101382.

58 Ibid.

59 A.M. Poff, N. Ward, T. Seyfried, et al., "Non-toxic Metabolic Management of Metastatic Cancer in VM Mice: Novel Combination of Ketogenic Diet, Ketone Supplementation, and Hyperbaric Oxygen Therapy" *PLoS One* 10 (2015): 127407, https://doi.org/10.1371/journal.pone.0127407; Thomas Seyfried and Leanne C. Huysentruyt, "On the Origin of Cancer Metastasis," *Critical Reviews in Oncogenesis* 18, no. 1–2 (2013): 43–73, https://doi.org/10.1615/critrevoncog.v18.i1-2.40.

60 Ibid.

61 F. Kassam et al., "Survival Outcomes for Patients with Metastatic Triple-negative Breast Cancer: Implications for Clinical Practice and Trial Design," *Clinical Breast Cancer* 9, no.1 (February 2009): 29-33, https://doi.org/10.3816/CBC.2009.n.005.

62 Dr. Abdul Slocum, Chemothermia Clinic, Istanbul, 2018, "Follow-Up Report to Iyikesici et al., 'Efficacy of Metabolically Supported Chemotherapy Combined with Ketogenic Diet, Hyperthermia, and Hyperbaric Oxygen Therapy for Stage IV Triple-negative Breast Cancer," *Cureus* 9, no. 7 (2017): e1445 (September 24, 2018), https://doi.org/10.7759/cureus.1445; Email correspondence to author from Thomas N Seyfried, February 5, 2019.

8 BORN WITH A BROKEN BRCA GENE? TRY THE POLISH SOLUTION:

Nurture Your Breasts—Don't Amputate Them!

Angelina Jolie, the American actress, director, and film producer, lost her 56-year-old mother to ovarian cancer in 2007. Jolie's mother, Marcheline Bertrand, also an actress and film producer, had been born with a damaged BRCA1 tumor-suppressor gene.

In 2013, once Jolie, then 38 years old, found that she also had inherited this damaged gene, she was counseled by oncologists to have her healthy breasts surgically amputated in order to prevent being diagnosed with breast cancer. Writing in a *New York Times* op-ed piece in April of that year, Jolie said doctors estimate that all women born with a BRCA1 mutated gene have a 65 percent breast cancer risk,[1] while Jolie was told she personally faced an 87 percent risk of developing invasive breast cancer unless her breasts were immediately removed.[2]

This high risk of 87% may have been based on the fact that the majority of premenopausal "BRCA women" such as Jolie, if they go on to develop breast cancer, are diagnosed early in their lives, often before they reach age 50. Such younger women and, in fact, all BRCA women who develop breast cancer, are also disproportionally diagnosed with triple-negative breast cancer tumors, discussed in Chapter 7.[3]

Today's mainstream cancer industry still follows the genetic theory of cancer; a theory that cannot fully explain how that first breast cancer cell develops, let alone how or why a woman born with a mutated BRCA gene develops triple-negative or any other type of cancer cells. Therefore, this seemingly draconian preventive option of double breast amputation, Jolie wrote, loomed as her only effective protection against her reported, astronomically high breast cancer risk.[4]

But what is actually behind these high-risk levels for BRCA women? How helpful are such statistics? Long-term population studies calculating risk numbers for BRCA women have never been done.[5] Back in 2000, the most definitive study on the subject to date reflected an average BRCA1 and BRCA2 risk level (called "penetrance" by biologists) of about 40 percent.[6] This means that two decades ago, epidemiologists estimated that 40 percent of women, worldwide—not 65 or 87 percent, as Jolie wrote in her *New York Times* piece—born with either of these genetic defects could expect to develop breast cancer before their eightieth birthday.

Today, recent studies of North American and British BRCA women tell us that BRCA penetrance is about 65 percent, but similar studies of Polish[7] and Colombian[8] BRCA women indicate 49 percent and 14 percent penetrance, respectively. Why do studies of BRCA women in North America indicate a breast cancer risk that is two or three times higher than the risks BRCA women face in other countries, where these rates have been studied?

What Is "Penetrance"?

Penetrance refers to the proportion of people with a particular genetic change (such as a mutation in a specific gene) who exhibit signs and symptoms of a genetic disorder. If some people with the mutation do not develop features of the disorder, the condition is said to have reduced (or incomplete) penetrance. For example, many people with a mutation in the BRCA1 or BRCA2 gene will develop cancer during their lifetime, but some people will not. Reduced penetrance probably results from a combination of genetic, environmental, and lifestyle factors.

"What Are Reduced Penetrance and Variable Expressivity?" US National Library of Medicine, https://ghr.nlm.nih.gov/primer/inheritance/penetranceexpressivity.

How BRCA Genes Protect Women's Breasts

Before I try to answer this startling question about why a BRCA woman's country of residence significantly affects her risk of developing breast cancer, let's first look at some known benefits given to the 95 percent of us who have been born with two perfectly healthy (i.e., undamaged) BRCA genes. According to recent studies, there are at least three different ways our BRCA (BReast CAncer) genes are helpful in preventing breast cancer:

1. Block Tumor Development

Both of our BRCA genes, known as BRCA1 and BRCA2, are called tumor-suppressor genes. This is because when either is activated, they express or bring forth a tumor-killing or tumor-blocking protein that can often help stop the development of cancer cells in their tracks.[9]

2. Maintain Adequate Vitamin D3 Blood Level

A recent study also shows that the BRCA1 gene helps a woman increase and maintain sufficient levels of vitamin D3 in her blood. As we saw in Chapter 3, maintaining certain levels of vitamin D3 in your body helps create and maintain an immune system that is able to also help block cancer cells or help evolving cancer cells to self-destruct.[10] In one of these researcher's words, "Here we report for the first time that a fully-functioning BRCA1 is critical for vitamin D3-mediated growth inhibition of breast cancer cells via co-regulation of cell cycle progression and p21waf1 expression."[11] This means that the BRCA1 gene, when fully functioning, enables breast cells to utilize vitamin D3 in order to help stop the development or slow the growth of cancer cells.

3. Help Eliminate Toxic Estrogen

The BRCA1 gene, we recently learned, also helps efficiently eliminate any used-up or processed estrogen in our bodies. As we saw in Chapter 6, when you have an overabundance of this useless *hormonal residue* or metabolite in your body, you have created a toxic environment inside your breast cells. These toxic estrogen metabolites end up assaulting your breast cells' mitochondria—the first step in the development of that first cancer cell.[12] According to one of the researchers who first published this finding in 2014, "We found that BRCA1 also regulates estrogen metabolism...by repressing the transcription of estrogen-metabolizing enzymes...in breast cells."[13]

Transcription is a process in which information is rewritten. Transcription is something we do in our everyday lives, and it's also something our cells must do, in a more specialized and narrowly defined way. In biology, **transcription** is the process of copying out the DNA sequence of a gene in the similar alphabet of RNA.

BRCA Penetrance: US and Ashkenazi BRCA Women Have Highest Risk in World

About 8 to 10 percent of women of Ashkenazi descent, worldwide, are born with either a damaged BRCA1 or BRCA2 gene.[14] This is probably a significant reason why this group of Jewish women develops a disproportionate amount of breast cancer, compared to other women in whatever countries they reside. Meanwhile, at least one major study of Ashkenazi women finds that breast cancer risk for younger Ashkenazi BRCA women is higher than risk levels for older Ashkenazi BRCA women. This same study mentions that obesity and lack of exercise during adolescence and obesity at menarche and before age 21 also increase the group's premenopausal breast cancer risk.[15]

As mentioned earlier, once I began to delve into cross-cultural epidemiological studies on BRCA women, I was startled to discover that BRCA penetrance seems to differ widely from country to country. North American women appear to have the highest penetrance, around 70 percent.[16] Meanwhile, a small study of Colombian BRCA1 women indicates they have a 14 percent penetrance,[17] while a large study of Polish women indicates a 49 percent penetrance. Similar studies out of Great Britain, France, and other Western European nations report BRCA women's penetrance between 48 and 60 percent.[18] Are these differences based on merely imperfect studies, or are these differences based on actual environmental causes and lifestyle choices that continue to affect all women in the US?

Clearly, as we have seen throughout this book, all American women are stuck in the same "high-risk boat." Today's statistics (as we'll see in Chapter 9) tell us that women living in the United States have the highest breast cancer rates, as compared to women of the same age, racial, and/or ethnic group, living in other major nations. Why should a cross-cultural comparison of breast cancer rates among BRCA women look any different?

Table 8.1: Much Ado About Very Few: Estimated Prevalence of US Women Born with a BRCA1 Mutation

	BRCA1
Asian American	0.5%
African American	1.3%
Caucasian (non-Ashkenazi Jewish)	2.2%
Hispanic	3.5%
Ashkenazi Jewish	8.3%

Percentage of non-Ashkenazi women in the US population who are born with a BRCA1 gene mutation is estimated at less than 2 percent.

EM John et al., "Prevalence of Pathogenic BRCA1 Mutation Carriers in 5 US Racial/Ethnic Groups," JAMA 298, no.24 (December, 2007):2869-2876, doi:10.1001/jama.298.24.2869.

The causes of American women's record-breaking breast cancer rates today are the things we've already seen in this book. They include high obesity rates, low vitamin D3 levels, high use of birth control drugs, progestin-laced IUDs, and progestin menopausal drugs, along with the fact that the majority of American women over forty continue to subject their bodies to regular radiation from mammograms. Add to that the continuing use of mostly unregulated carcinogens in pesticides, public water supplies, personal care products, fresh and processed food, and cleaning supplies, and you've got a toxic mix. Given these enormous obstacles to breast health that all American women face, it's especially important that BRCA women in the US make the many lifestyle changes that are necessary to protect the mitochondria in their vulnerable breast cells.[19]

Seven Prevention Guidelines for BRCA Women

1. Eliminate All of Your Excess Body Fat: Lower Toxic Estrogen Levels and Strengthen the Mitochondria in Your Breast Cells

In Chapter 2 we learned that obese women often double their breast cancer risk, due in part to the constant damage that excess fat cells inflict on their breast cells' mitochondria.[20] This is because those inflammatory enzymes and toxic estrogen metabolites, generated by a woman's adipose tissue or excess body fat, keep assaulting breast cells' fragile mitochondria 24/7. Statistical research shows us that obese BRCA women have a demonstrably higher incidence of breast cancer than BRCA women who enjoy a healthy BMI of less than 25.[21] A five-year study funded by the National Cancer Institute is currently underway to establish this exact increased risk level for BRCA women who remain significantly overweight or obese.[22]

2. Keep Vitamin D3 Blood Levels Above 60/ng/ml Throughout the Entire Year

Studies described in Chapter 3 show that keeping your vitamin D3 blood level above 60 ng/ml year-round significantly reduces even BRCA women's higher breast cancer risk. A few years ago, US and Israeli researchers found that a damaged or mutated BRCA gene can make it difficult for a BRCA woman to raise and maintain her vitamin D3 levels. The study begins by telling us, "The incomplete penetrance of BRCA1 suggests that environmental and/or genetic factors modify the risk and incidence among mutation carriers."[23] This could include obese postmenopausal BRCA women whom, we found in Chapter 3, have an even greater difficulty maintaining a protective level of D3 in their blood *any time* during the year.

3. Use Thermograms to Measure Precancerous Inflammation in Breasts

In order to block the development of slow- or fast-growing cancerous tumors in your breasts, it is especially important for BRCA women to stay up to date on the level of inflammation now existing within their breast tissue and within their entire body. After all, breast cancer cannot develop if your breast tissue is not inflamed. It is this inflammation from so many chronic causes, described throughout this book, that can suffocate your breast cells' mitochondria. This is why having regular thermograms, using whole body regulation thermography or infrared breast imaging, is critical for every BRCA woman, and for other women who feel they may be at high risk for developing this disease. Your thermogram can be that clear wake-up call to change your ways and begin to follow *Busting Breast Cancer*'s five simple prevention steps or these specific BRCA guidelines.

4. Use Only Breast Self-Exams, Clinical Breast Exams, Ultrasound Diagnostic Tests and MRIs to Detect and Diagnose Fast-Growing Cancerous Tumors

Many oncologists in the US, along with the industry-funded American Cancer Society, appear determined to have young BRCA women, and other premenopausal women with a family history of breast cancer, undergo regular mammograms at younger and younger ages. In 2009, however, Johns Hopkins University epidemiologist Dr. Amy Berrington de Gonzalez sounded an alarm over this practice. Her research showed that mammograms are especially harmful to BRCA women under 35 years old. The researcher showed how just *a single mammogram* can significantly increase a young BRCA woman's risk of developing invasive breast cancer later in life.[24]

Biophysicists at the University of California's Berkeley Labs, along with those at New York University, have also looked at how medical radiation affects the breast cancer risk of all premenopausal BRCA women. This national team has developed a detailed picture of how any amount of ionizing radiation—even RADS from a single mammogram—can increase a young woman's breast cancer risk later in life.[25] "Essentially, exposure of the breast to ionizing radiation generates an overall biochemical signal that tells the system that something bad happened," said Dr. Sylvane Costes, one of the study's authors.[26]

"This groundbreaking work shows how breasts that have been radiated develop a much larger-than-normal pool of stem cells, which increases the risk of developing triple-negative breast cancer later in life," said Costes' co-researcher, Dr. Jonathan Tang.[27] No wonder statistical studies have always shown that any number of mammograms are risky for BRCA women, especially for premenopausal BRCA women.[28] Meanwhile, as mentioned, statistics also tell us this group of women is predisposed to develop triple-negative breast cancer, should they develop breast cancer at all.[29] As mentioned in Chapter 5, along with regular breast self-exams and clinical breast exams, Dr. Nasha Winters, co-author of *The Metabolic Approach to Cancer*, offers this guidance for all premenopausal women who want to use only radiation-free and effective breast diagnostic exams: "What we *do* favor is a combination of screening approaches. I use—and love—thermography, but know it is a tiny piece of the equation. I use things like SonoCiné, high-definition ultrasound,[30] Prenuvo (the next-generation nontoxic MRI),[31] and if someone has had breast cancer, then breast MRI is the gold standard for follow-up screening."[32]

Automated whole breast diagnostic technologies, such as SonoCiné and the ABUS system (Automated Breast Ultrasonography), both FDA-approved, use safe ultrasound technology. Sure Touch, a handheld device, also FDA-approved, uses the new elastography technology that measure hardness rather than density to provide a through, safe and inexpensive screening of the tissue throughout each breast, as part of every clinical breast exam.[33] All of these tests are able to replace the need for BRCA women, of any age, to be exposed to damaging radiation from even a single mammogram.[34] Alleluia.

5. Measure Your Body's Ability to Balance Estrogen and to Eliminate Toxic Estrogen

Described in Chapter 6, Dr. Heather Eliassen, an epidemiologist at Harvard Medical School and researcher at Brigham and Women's Hospital's Channing Center, found that premenopausal women who have trouble eliminating processed toxic estrogen have higher breast cancer rates than other women.[35] Just a year later, Dr. Martin Widschwendter, head of University College London's Women's Cancer department, found that women born with a BRCA1 mutation have higher than normal levels of circulating estrogen in their bodies, no matter what their body weight. In other words, at least some BRCA women have difficulty naturally eliminating these toxic or processed estrogen metabolites.

"We have shown for the first time that cancer risk in BRCA1 and BRCA2 carriers is not just caused by local defects in the ability of [breast] cells to repair themselves," Dr. Widschwendter announced.[36] Together, Dr. Widschwendter's and Dr. Eliassen's studies show us that BRCA women of all ages can have additional issues, such as this hormone-cleansing defect that can increase their breast cancer risk. Thankfully, it is possible to help the body clear itself of this toxic hormone on a regular basis. If ignored, however, this condition can increase any woman's breast cancer risk.

How does a woman know if she is effectively balancing the natural and chemical estrogens and the natural progesterone and any chemical progestin in her body? Also, how does a woman know if her body is efficiently eliminating her processed hormones? As also mentioned in Chapter 6, functional medicine practitioners use two different tests to assess these two questions: a saliva-based hormone balancing test and a urine-based estrogen metabolite test. The urine-based test compares the amount of "good" (or "non-irritating") estrogen to the amount of "bad" (or "irritating") estrogen circulating in a woman's body. ZRT Labs, founded by Dr. David Zava, a co-author of the forever popular *What Your Doctor May Not Tell You About Breast Cancer*,[37] has offered both tests for many years.[38]

Canyon Ranch, a holistic health spa with facilities in Lenox, Massachusetts and Tucson, Arizona, and the Hippocrates Institute in West Palm Beach, Florida, both offer women a residential, integrative health assessment and learning program that can include both of these tests. The results can then be used to help develop personalized breast-cancer prevention plans.[39]

6. Be Aware that Pregnancies Can Increase BRCA Women's Breast Cancer Risk

Statistical studies tell us that women born with a BRCA1 or BRCA2 mutation who then go on to give birth in their teens, twenties, or thirties are significantly more likely to develop breast cancer by age 40, when compared to BRCA women who have never given birth. Each additional pregnancy for a BRCA woman, it appears, becomes directly associated with an increased breast cancer risk.[40] This same phenomenon is true for many young women who do not have a BRCA mutation, but who go on to develop triple-negative cancer soon after having one or multiple births, as was the situation with Fox News correspondent Jen Griffin, mentioned in Chapter 7.[41]

Interestingly, this finding is the direct opposite of a well-known risk factor for hormone-positive breast cancer. For decades, researchers have shown that women who have never given birth (null parous women) have a statistically greater risk of developing hormone-positive breast cancer than women who have experienced even a single full-term pregnancy.[42] The opposite finding applies, however, to women who develop hormone-negative breast cancers.[43]

What is going on here? What is the biological or metabolic process that can increase the rate of BRCA women's and others' triple-negative diagnoses when they experience one or multiple pregnancies when very young? Some researchers have shown that high levels of natural estrogen produced during a pregnancy, *in combination with high pre-pregnancy estrogen levels,* may be the culprits. Is this a part of the "double whammy" for some young mothers that results in developing triple-negative cancer cells as described in Chapter 7?

From a metabolic perspective, experiencing very high levels of unbalanced chemical, animal, and natural estrogens for years can mean that the mitochondria in the young woman's breast cells have already been damaged prior to her first pregnancy. Successive pregnancies, when huge surges of natural estrogen are released, can then exacerbate existing mitochondrial damage and accelerate the development of existing tumors.[44] This information, again, should not discourage a woman from becoming pregnant. Instead, this knowledge can encourage younger BRCA women to carefully monitor their estrogen and progesterone balance, and their breasts' inflammation levels using thermography, while remaining at a healthy body weight prior to and during each pregnancy.

7. Avoid Progestin Drugs for Birth Control, Hormonal Imbalance and/or for Menopausal Relief

Little-publicized epidemiological research from University of Toronto epidemiologists tells us that North American BRCA women who use birth control drugs increase their already high risk of developing invasive breast cancer by an additional 33 percent, as compared with their non-BRCA peers.[45] Another study by the Italian epidemiologist Dr. Patrizia Pasanisi found that very young BRCA1 women who begin birth control drugs while in their teens experience higher breast cancer rates than BRCA women who begin birth control drugs later in life.[46] In other words, there's a developing consensus that the younger a BRCA woman is when she begins using birth control drugs, the greater her risk of developing breast cancer while continuing to use these drugs.[47]

These findings make so much sense, now that the Penninger-Glimcher team's 2010 study has been published. As we saw in Chapter 4, their study showed the specific biological events that take place when a woman is using a progestin drug. Their research clearly describes how the progestin chemical in birth control drugs can initiate and accelerate breast cancer. As earlier described, in 2012, the Congressionally Directed Breast Cancer Research Program honored the importance of this finding by awarding Dr Penninger their annual $7.4 million Innovator Award.[48] Penninger's Vienna-based research center jubilantly announced this honor in an October 29, 2012 press release, distributed to thousands of media outlets worldwide:

"The innovator award recognizes Josef Penninger's work in identifying a key molecular pathway (re) how hormone replacement therapies and contraceptive pills can lead to breast cancer...Penninger's group went on to show that RANKL is indeed a missing link between sex hormones...in particular progestin, and breast cancer, leading to the hypothesis that RANKL is a key driver of breast cancer initiation."[49]

2018 Update from the BCRP on their 2012 $7.4 million Innovator's Award to Dr. Josef Penninger for "Novel Approach to Breast Cancer Prevention for BRCA Women."

With a Fiscal Year 2011 Breast Cancer Research Program Innovator Award, Dr. Penninger sought to assess the role of RANK/RANKL in BRCA1 mutation-driven breast cancers and determine whether inhibition of RANK/RANKL signaling would provide a protection against the development of tumors. In a *Cell Research* publication, Dr. Penninger showed that high RANK and RANKL protein expression could be found in 70.4% and 59.1% of BRCA1 mutation carrier

---

breast cancer tumor samples, respectively. Moreover, high levels of RANK could be found in the earliest tumor lesions detectable in BRCA1 mutation carriers.

To determine whether inhibition of RANK/RANKL would influence the development of BRCA1 mutation-driven breast cancer, Dr. Penninger genomically and pharmacologically inhibited RANK/RANKL. Using BRCA1 mutation carrier mouse models, genomic inhibition of RANK in mammary epithelial cells was found to not only delay the onset of breast cancer, but it also reduced the incidence and attenuated the progression of tumorigenesis. Using the US Food and Drug Administration (FDA) approved RANKL inhibitor, denosumab, to pharmacologically inhibit RANKL, the number of pre-neoplastic lesions that developed were dramatically reduced in BRCA1-mutant mice. After 1 year of treatment, remarkably, only 7% (1 out of 13) of BRCA1-mutant mice showed evidence of tumors, whereas 82% (9 out of 11) of control-treated mice developed breast tumors.

...Results from Dr. Penninger's study supported the initiation of a randomized, double-blind, placebo-controlled Phase III clinical trial set to open in November 2018 aimed at determining whether the preventative effects of denosumab (XGEVA) are effective in preventing breast cancer in BRCA1 mutation carrier women.[49]

Author's Note: The XGEVA clinical trial, made possible by the 2012 $7.4 million in taxpayers' funds, given to Dr. Penninger, was considered successful. Women born with a BRCA mutation can now purchase XGEVA for the list price of $2,352.25 per dose, or approximately $31,000/year. XGEVA is dosed once every four weeks. The drug carries significant adverse side effects.[50]

Federal Breast Cancer Research Program: $150m a year

For the past few decades, the Breast Cancer Research Program (BCRP) has funded what they describe as innovative research to help prevent and manage breast cancer. As mentioned in 2012 the BCRP awarded $7.4 million from their $150 million annual budget to Dr. Josef Penninger to understand whether the osteoporosis drug (denosumab) that he developed years earlier could also be used by BRCA women to help prevent the development of breast cancer. Dr. Penninger's multi-million-dollar award focused on a small, but significant portion of his international team's 2010 published findings. *At the same time, the team's major finding, connecting the progestin chemical to the onset and acceleration of breast cancer in current users, continues to be ignored.*

Women throughout the US still do not know that the Penninger/ Glimcher Team uncovered the key ingredient and the first step in the biological mechanism that now explains *how birth control drugs, progestin-laced IUDs and progestin-based HRT drugs can initiate and accelerate breast cancer in current users so quickly.*

The Polish Cancer Prevention Goulash Recipe

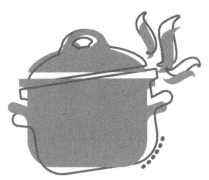

Here's that astounding statistic again: Polish women born with a BRCA1 mutation develop 32 percent less breast cancer during their lives than their North American peers. Meanwhile, all Polish women, no matter their BRCA status, have much lower breast cancer incidence than women in North America. Specifically, 49 out of 100,000 Polish women develop breast cancer each year, compared to 126 out of 100,000 women in the US.[51] No matter how you describe these data, Polish women, knowingly or unknowingly, practice more effective breast cancer prevention compared to North American women. Here are some epidemiological data for these jaw-dropping statistics.[52]

In 2012, University of Toronto breast cancer epidemiologist Dr. Steven Narod and Dr. Jan Lubinski of the International Hereditary Cancer Center at Pomeranian Medical University in Szczecin, Poland, along with researchers at Creighton University School of Functional Medicine in Nebraska and numerous Canadian medical research centers, co-published a stunning statistical study that compared breast cancer rates between Polish BRCA1 women and North American BRCA1 women.[53] They uncovered this big surprise.

It turns out that 72 percent of the North American BRCA women in the study developed breast cancer before their seventieth birthdays. Pretty scary! In contrast, the epidemiologists found that 49 percent of the BRCA women in Poland developed breast cancer before their seventieth birthdays. Not a good number, but significantly better than the North American BRCA women's penetrance[54] of 72 percent.

The study went on to mention that Poland's national breast cancer rate—for all women—is also much lower than the North American rate; actually, it's about 60 percent lower! This Polish–North American study clearly tells us, in no uncertain terms, that today's risk of developing breast cancer has a great deal more to do with where a woman lives, than with the presence of a damaged or healthy BRCA gene within her breast cells. Instead, a woman's geographic location in the world, her cultural and chosen lifestyles, and lifetime exposure to environmental toxins, all play a role. Without underplaying the extra threat that BRCA women face, there's clearly more at work here than genetics. Put simply, *where you live and how you live, matter more than whether you were born with a damaged BRCA gene.*

If North American women could "become Polish"—and reduce the US national breast cancer incidence by 60 percent each year—we could see about 145,000 fewer breast cancer diagnoses, including 12,000 fewer BRCA women being diagnosed annually.[55] Such potentially good news is amazing to even consider!

In order to take this hopeful idea of helping American women become "more Polish," I've created a highly unorthodox Polish prevention "recipe." This recipe is based on four "ingredients," each derived from some of the lifestyle choices of the 840 Polish women described in the Lubinski/Narod BRCA study, compared to the documented lifestyle choices made by the North American women who participated in this same 2012 cross-cultural study. I also folded in some scattered, basic knowledge of contemporary Polish culture, along with Polish lifestyle choices that commonly differ from North American habits. Finally, I "cooked" all this information within the metabolic theory of cancer and *Busting Breast Cancer*'s five prevention steps. Now, I don't claim that my "Polish Prevention Goulash" is scientifically proven to have all the elements needed to successfully prevent breast cancer. But might it help if North American women would take such commonsense steps that could reduce US breast cancer risks to Polish rates? Let's hope so.

Polish Prevention Goulash Ingredients

More Vitamin D3

Average D3 levels for many Poles reach 42 ng/ml in summer months.[56] Meanwhile, most studies report that the average vitamin D3 level for most Americans continues to be less than 25 ng/ml, with only 30 percent of Euro-Americans and 5 percent of African-Americans testing above 25 ng/ml throughout the year.[57] What causes this difference in Polish versus North American D3 blood levels? Here are some possible factors:

> Many more Americans have cars than Poles, so the average Polish woman probably spends more time walking or bike riding in the sunshine than the average North American woman.[58] Meanwhile, market research studies tell us that Eastern European women do not like to use high-SPF sunscreen, if they use sunscreen at all. Here's how one study describes the Poles' pro-tan cultural preference: "Also holding back the growth of higher SPF creams is the ongoing love affair of the Eastern European with a bronze glow. Tans are synonymous with holidays, and holidays are synonymous with success and wealth. It is little wonder Eastern Europeans continue to flock to beaches and lakes during the summer holidays in search of a bit of color to show off, when they return. Tanning oils with a very low SPF continue to be popular."[59] Meanwhile, solariums and tanning salons are also very popular throughout Eastern Europe during the winter months.

Fewer Progestin Drugs

Birth control drugs are not used widely in Poland. In the 2012 Lubinski/Narod study, only 34 percent of the Polish women reported they had ever used contraceptive drugs in their lives, compared to 85 percent of their North American counterparts.[60] Hormone replacement therapy (HRT) is also not used widely by Poles. Only 8 percent of the Polish women in the 2012 study had ever used Prempro, Premarin, or other HRT drugs, compared to more than a quarter of the North American women.[61]

Fewer Mammograms

Polish women are instructed to never have a mammogram until they are postmenopausal, usually over 50 years old. This same policy is followed throughout much of the European Union, with Switzerland (as we saw in Chapter 5) now considering a ban on all mammography clinics nationwide. In contrast, almost 70 percent of American women age 40 and over report having a mammogram every year, or every few years.

Figure 8.1: In the US, No Cabbage or Broccoli in Sight!

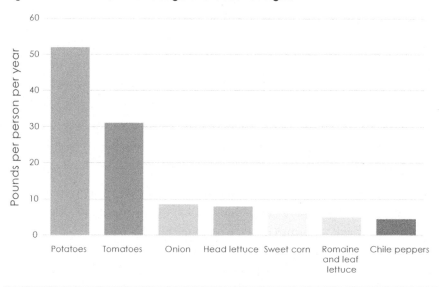

Most commonly consumed vegetables in the US.

–Source: Data from US Department of Agriculture Economic Research; "The Most-Eaten Vegetable in the US Is the Potato," The Atlantic, June 11, 2014; https://www.theatlantic.com/health/archive/2014/06/the-most-popular-vegetable-in-america-is-the-potato/372502/.

More Cabbage

Ever enjoyed a pierogi or two? Some popular dishes in Poland include fermented cabbage (sauerkraut), steamed cabbage, gołąbki (cabbage leaves stuffed with meat and rice), and those pierogis (dumplings), often stuffed with sauerkraut. As we saw earlier, the diindolylmethane (DIM) found only in cruciferous vegetables (like cabbage, broccoli, Brussels sprouts, cauliflower, kale, and bok choy) helps clean out any toxic (or "used") estrogen metabolites. Cabbage and broccoli also contain the wonder nutrient *sulforaphane*. This is an enzyme-stimulating substance that increases our body's ability to absorb vitamin D3. Eating lots of cabbage (or broccoli) therefore becomes incredibly important for BRCA women, given their difficulty raising and maintaining their D3 levels above 60 ng/ml.[62] For women born without the full protection of one of their BRCA genes, eating daily amounts of cruciferous veggies, especially cabbage and broccoli, while also taking DIM supplements, seems a smart and easy-to-adopt lifestyle choice.

A Final Word to BRCA Women

Researchers are continuing to uncover the fact that not all BRCA mutations are the same. Some types of BRCA1 and BRCA2 mutations apparently cause more havoc in a woman's body than others.[63] Meanwhile, we always need to remember that most women throughout the world who are born with a damaged BRCA1 or BRCA2 mutation *never* develop breast cancer during their lives. Unfortunately, though, this fact doesn't yet apply to North American BRCA women as a group.[64]

Thanks to the metabolic approach to cancer, we now understand that it is not just a woman's mutated or damaged BRCA gene that causes that first breast cancer cell to form. This catastrophe called breast cancer is always at least a two-part event for every BRCA woman. Being born with a damaged BRCA tumor suppressor gene means a woman faces at least three disadvantages when it comes to her body's natural breast cancer prevention tools. But it still requires subsequent damage to the mitochondria of a BRCA woman's breast cells before a cancer cell will form. And that damage can come from any number of lifestyle and environmental assaults—which our Polish Prevention Goulash could help you avoid.

In order to compare the experience of Polish BRCA women with their North American counterparts, I relied on the landmark cross-cultural study carried out by Doctors Lubinski and Narod and many others. But shouldn't it be easier to compare cancer data in one place with cancer data in another place—especially within our own country? Sadly, such data is surprisingly hard to come by in the United States. Chapter 9 takes a look at the chaotic, outdated, and often misleading national cancer-tracking system used throughout our country, where the focus is on better understanding the breast tumors diagnosed, not on the women who have developed them. Demographic data about the individuals who continue to develop this deadly disease, it would appear, are of secondary concern to the agencies that track cancer tumor data. If we're going to change that, we need to know how state and federal cancer registries currently collect their data. So, let's take a look.

CHAPTER ENDNOTES

1 J.T. Casaubon, U.S. Grewal, J. Regan, "BRCA 1 and 2," NCBI Bookshelf (Washington, National Library of Medicine, NIH, January 29, 2020), PMID: 29262038; A. Antoniou et al., "Average Risks of Breast and Ovarian Cancer Associated with BRCA1 or BRCA2 Mutations Detected in Case Series Unselected for Family History: A Combined Analysis of 22 Studies." *American Journal of Human Genetics* 72, no.5 (2003): 1117-30. https://doi.org/10.1086/375033.

2 Angelina Jolie "My Medical Choice," *The New York Times*, May 14, 2013, Section A, 25, https://www.nytimes.com/2013/05/14/opinion/my-medical-choice.html; Rachael Rettner, "Breast Cancer Genes: How Much Risk Do BRCA Mutations Bring?," https://www.livescience.com/50404-brca-mutations-cancer-risk.html; T.R. Rebbeck et al., "Association of Type and Location of BRCA1 and BRCA2 Mutations with Risk of Breast and Ovarian Cancer," *JAMA* 313, no.13 (2015):1347-61, https://doi.org/10.1001/jama.2014.5985.

3 Haxia Chen et al., "Association Between *BRCA* Status and Triple-Negative Breast Cancer: A Meta-Analysis," *Frontiers in Pharmacology* 9, no. 909 (August 21, 2018), https//:doi.org/10.3389/fphar.2018.00909; Yong Tao Li et al., "The Prevalence of BRCA1/2 Mutations of Triple-negative Breast Cancer Patients in Xinjiang Multiple Ethnic Region of China," *European Journal of Medical Research* 19, no. 135 (June 25, 2014), https://pubmed.ncbi.nlm.nih.gov/24961674/.

4 Jolie, 25.

5 G.M. Findlay et al., "Accurate Classification of BRCA1 Variants with Saturation Genome Editing," *Nature* 562 (2018): 217-22, https://doi.org/10.1038/s41586-018-0461; Sharon Begley, "Study Cracks Open the Secrets of the Cancer Causing BRCA1 Gene," September 12 2018, https://www.scientificamerican.com/article/study-cracks-open-the-secrets-of-genetic-mutations-that-boost-breast-and-ovarian-cancer-risk/; Veronique Desaulniers, "What Angeline Jolie's Doctors Didn't Tell Her about the BRCA Gene Before Her Double Mastectomy," October 26, 2015, https://thetruthaboutcancer.com/angelina-jolie-brca-gene/.

6 Anglian Breast Cancer Study Group, "Prevalence and Penetrance of BRCA1 and BRCA2 Mutations in a Population-based Series of Breast Cancer Cases," *British Journal of Cancer* 83, no. 10 (2000): 301-8, https://pubmed.ncbi.nlm.nih.gov/11044354/.

7 Jan Lubinski et al., "The Risk of Breast Cancer in Women with a BRCA1 Mutation from North America and Poland," *International Journal of Cancer* 31, no.1 (2012): 229-34, w https://doi.org/10.1002/ijc.26369.

8 D. Torres et al., "Prevalence and Penetrance of BRCA1 and BRCA2 Germline Mutations in Colombian Breast Cancer Patients," *Scientific Reports* 7, 4713 (2017), https://doi.org/10.1038/s41598-017-05056-y.

9 Chu-Xia Deng, "BRCA1: Cell Cycle Checkpoint, Genetic Instability, DNA Damage Response and Cancer Evolution," *Nucleic Acids Research* 34, no. 5 (March 6, 2006): 1416-26, https://doi.org/10.1093/nar/gkl010.

10 Itay Pickholtz et al., "Cooperation Between BRCA1 and Vitamin D is Critical for Histone Acetylation of the p21waf1 Promoter and Growth Inhibition of Breast Cancer Cells and Cancer Stem-like Cells," *Oncotarget* 5, no. 23 (2014): 11827-46, https://doi.org/10.18632/oncotarget.2582.

11 Ibid, p. 11839.

12 K.I. Savage et al., "BRCA1 Deficiency Exacerbates Estrogen-induced DNA Damage and Genomic Instability," *Cancer Research* 74, no. 10 (2014): 2773-2784, https://doi.org/10.1158/0008-5472.CAN-13-2611.

13 Ibid, 2773.

14 M.C. King, J.H. Marks and J.B. Mandell (for the New York Breast Cancer Study Group), "Breast and Ovarian Cancer Risks Due to Inherited Mutations in BRCA1 and BRCA2," *Science* 203, no. 5645, (October 24, 2003):643-46, doi:10.1126/science.1088759.

15 Ibid, 645.

16 Lubinski et al., 229.

17 D. Torres et al., "Prevalence and Penetrance of BRCA1 and BRCA2 Germline Mutations in Colombian Breast Cancer Patients," *Scientific Reports* 7, 4713 (2017), https://doi.org/10.1038/s41598-017-05056-y.

18 Anglian Breast Cancer Study Group, "Prevalence and Penetrance of BRCA1 and BRCA2 Mutations in a Population-based Series of Breast Cancer Cases: Anglian Breast Cancer Study Group," *British Journal of Cancer* 83, no. 10 (2000):1301-08, https://doi.org/10.1054/bjoc.2000.1407; Li et al., "The Prevalence of BRCA1/2 Mutations…; Ramūnas Janavicius, "Founder BRCA1/2 Mutations in Europe: Implications for Hereditary Breast-Ovarian Cancer Prevention and Control," *The EPMA Journal* 1, no. 3 (2010): 397–412, https://doi.org/10.1007/s13167-010-0037-y.

19 J Lammert, S Grill, and M Kiechle, "Modifiable Lifestyle Factors: Opportunities for (Hereditary) Breast Cancer Prevention-a Narrative Review," *Breast Care (Basel)* 13, no2 (2018):109-114. doi:10.1159/000488995.

20 Priya Bhardwaj et al., "Estrogen and Breast Cancer: Mechanism Involved in Obesity-related Development, Growth and Progression," *The Journal of Steroid Biochemistry and Molecular Biology* 189 (May 2019): 161–70. https://doi.org/10.1016/j.jsbmb.2019.03.002.

21 Priya Bhardwaj et al., "In BRCA Mutation Carriers, Obesity is Linked with Increased DNA Damage in Normal Breast Gland Cells," presentation to The Endocrine Society, March 18, 2018, Chicago, https://www.endocrine.org/news-and-advocacy/news-room/2018/in-brca-mutation-carriers-obesity-is-linked-with-increased-dna-damage-in-normal-breast-gland-cells.

22 Andrea Jess Dannenberg and Kristy Brown, "Obesity Increases Breast Cancer Penetrance in BRCA Mutation Carriers: A Role for Local and Systemic Factors," NCI Project #1R01CA215797-01, https://grantome.com/grant/NIH/R01-CA215797-01.

23 Pickholtz et al., "Cooperation Between BRCA1 and Vitamin D…," 11827.

24 Jonathan Tang et al., "Irradiation of Juvenile, but not Adult, Mammary Gland Increases Stem Cell Self-Renewal and Estrogen Receptor Negative Tumors," *Stem Cells* 32, no.3, (March 2014): 649-6, https://doi.org/10.1002/stem.1533; Amy Bennington de Gonzalez et al., "Estimated Risk of Radiation-induced Breast Cancer from Mammographic Screening for Young BRCA Mutation Carriers," *Journal of the National Cancer Institute* 101 (2009): 205–09, https://doi.org/10.1093/jnci/djn440; Jeffrey Norris, "Mammograms Bad for Young Women with (Mutated) Breast Cancer Genes?" *University of California: San Francisco News*, March 17, 2009, https://www.ucsf.edu/news/2009/03/8163/mammograms-bad-young-women-breast-cancer-genes.

25 Lynn Yarris, "Radiotherapy in Girls and the Risk of Breast Cancer Later in Life," September 11, 2013, DOE, Lawrence Berkeley National Laboratory, https://www.eurekalert.org/pub_releases/2013-09/dbnl-rig091113.php; Jonathan Tang et al., "Irradiation of Juvenile, but not Adult, Mammary Gland Increases Stem Cell Self-Renewal and Estrogen Receptor Negative Tumors," *Stem Cells* 32, no.3 (March 2014):649-61, https://doi.org/10.1002/stem.1533.

26 Mark Tan, "U.C. Berkeley Researchers Find Correlation Between Radiotherapy and Breast Cancer in Young Girls," *The Daily Californian*, September 17, 2013, https://www.dailycal.org/2013/09/17/uc-berkeley-researchers-find-correlation-between-radiotherapy-and-breast-cancer-in-young-girls/. Also see Gilbert Welch and Honor Passow, "How Cancer Stem Cells Drive Triple-negative Breast Cancer," *Science Daily*, February 8, 2018, https://www.sciencedaily.com/releases/2018/02/180208084816.htm.

27 Mary Helen Barcellos-Hoff and Jian-Hua Mao, "HZE Radiation Non-targeted Effects on the Microenvironment that Mediate Mammary Carcinogenesis," *Frontiers in Oncology* (March 11, 2016), https://doi.org/10.3389/fonc.2016.00057; Irineu Illa-Bochaca et al., "Densely Ionizing Radiation Acts Via the Microenvironment to Promote Aggressive Trp53-Null Mammary Carcinomas," *Tumor and Stem Cell Biology* (October 10, 2014), https://doi.org/10.1158/0008-5472. CAN-14-1212, published December 2014.

28 Amy Berrington de Gonzalez, "Estimated Risk of Radiation-induced Breast Cancer from Mammographic Screening for Young BRCA Mutation Carriers," p. 205, https://doi.org/10.1093/jnci/djn440.

29 Haxia Chen et al., "Association Between *BRCA* Status and Triple-Negative Breast Cancer: A Meta-Analysis," *Frontiers in Pharmacology* 9, no. 909 (August 21, 2018), https://doi.org/10.3389/fphar.2018.00909.

30 See http://www.sonocine.com/.

31 See https://www.prenuvo.com/.

32 Dr. Nasha Winters, personal email correspondence with the author, October 15, 2019.

33 Suretouch, "High Resolution Elastography," https://suretouch.global/.

34 Hee Jung Shin, Hak Hee Kim, and Joo Hee Cha, "Current Status of Automated Breast Ultrasonography," *Ultrasonography* 34, no.3 (July 2015), 165-72, https://doi.org/10.14366/usg.15002.

35 A. Heather Eliassen et al., "Urinary Estrogen and Estrogen Metabolites and Subsequent Risk of Breast Cancer Among Premenopausal Women," *Cancer Research* 72, no. 3 (February 2012), https://doi.org/10.1158/0008-5472.CAN-11-2507.

36 Science Daily, "Female Hormones Key to Breast, Ovarian Cancer in BRCA Gene Carriers," October 16, 2013, https://www.sciencedaily.com/releases/2013/10/131016212603.htm; Martin Widschwendter et al., "The Sex Hormone System in Carriers of BRCA1/2 Mutations: A Case Control Study," *The Lancet Oncology* 10, no. 12, (November 2013): 1226-32, https://doi.org/10.1016/S1470-2045(13)70448-0.

37 John Lee, David Zava, and Virginia Hopkins, *What Your Doctor May Not Tell You About Breast Cancer* (New York: Grand Central Publishing, 2002).

38 ZBT Laboratory, "Estrogen Metabolites & Their Relevance to Breast Cancer Risk," https://www.zrtlab.com/resources.

39 Canyon Ranch.com, "What Is Ultraprevention?" https://www.canyonranch.com/blog/health/what-is-ultraprevention/; Hippocrates Institute, "Cancer and Chronic Immune Disease Program," https://hippocratesinst.org/comprehensive-cancer-wellness-program.

40 H. Jernstrom et al., "Pregnancy and the Risk of Early Breast Cancer in Carriers of BRCA1 and BRCA2," *The Lancet* 354, no. 9193 (November 1999): 1846-50, https://www.thelancet.com/journals/lancet/article/PIIS0140-6736(99)04336-6/fulltext.

41 Amanda I. Phipps et al., "Reproductive History and Oral Contraceptive Use in Relation to Risk of Triple-negative Breast Cancer," *Journal of the National Cancer Institute* 103, no. 6 (2011): 470-77, https://doi.org/10.1093/jnci/djr030.

42 Amanda I. Phipps et al., "Reproductive History and Risk of Three Breast Cancer Subtypes Defined by Three Biomarkers," *Cancer Causes & Control* 22, No. 3 (2011): 399-405, https://doi.org/10.1007/s10552-010-9709-0.

43 The issue of parous vs nonparous in determining a woman's breast cancer risk is virtually a nonstarter for postmenopausal women. Also, the metabolic theory of cancer tells us that it is *damage to the mitochondria within breast cells* that initiates that first cancer cell; not because one's breast cells are nonparous. See: Chapter 1.

44 L. Hilakivi-Clarke, S. de Assis, and Luoto R. Warri, "Pregnancy Hormonal Environment and Mother's Breast Cancer Risk," *Hormonal Molecular Biology and Clinical Investigation* 1, no. 9 (April 2012): 11–23, https://doi.org/10.1515/hmbci-2012-0019; Sonia de Assis et al., "Exposure to Excess Estradiol or Leptin During Pregnancy Increases Mammary Cancer Risk and Prevents Parity-induced Protective Genomic Changes in Rats," *Cancer Prevention Research* 6, no. 11 (2013): 1194–211., https://doi.org/10.1158/1940-6207.CAPR-13-0207.

45 Steven Narod et al., "Oral Contraceptives and the Risk of Breast Cancer in BRCA1 and BRCA2 Mutation Carriers," *Journal of the National Cancer Institute* 94 (2002): 1773–79, https://doi.org/10.1093/jnci/94.23.1773.

46 Patrizia Pasanisi, "Oral Contraceptive Use and *BRCA* Penetrance: A Case-Only Study," *Cancer Epidemiol Biomarkers Prevention* 18, no. 7, (July 1, 2009): 2107-2113; https://pubmed.ncbi.nlm.nih.gov/19549808/.

47 Pasanisi has done a number of other excellent prevention studies, also helpful to BRCA women. See Patrizia Pasanisi: "Fondazione IRCCS Istituto Nazionale dei Tumori," https://moh-it.pure.elsevier.com/en/persons/patrizia-pasanisi/publications/. See also Patrizia Pasanisi et al., "A Randomized Controlled Trial of Diet and Physical Activity in BRCA Mutation Carriers," Short Communication, *Familial Cancer* (October 27, 2013), https://doi.org/10.1007/s10689-013-9691-2.

48 Congressionally Directed Medical Research Program, "Innovator Award: Josef Penninger was given the Innovator Award for his project 'Novel Approaches to Breast Cancer Prevention and Inhibition of Metastases,' (contract number W81XWH-12-1-0093)," http://cdmrp.army.mil/bcrp/.

49 IMBA, "Breast Cancer Advance Wins IMBA $7.4 M US Award," October 10, 2012, https://www.imba.oeaw.ac.at/about-imba/general-news-press/breast-cancer-advance-wins-imba-74m-us-award/.

50 CDMRP, "RANKL/RANK Control BRCA1 Mutation-Driven Mammary Tumors," Breast Cancer, Oct 29, 2018, https://cdmrp.army.mil/bcrp/research_highlights/18josef_penninger_highlight. See also: EU Clinical Trials Register, https://www.clinicaltrialsregister.eu/ctr-search/trial/2017-002505-35/AT.

51 Lubinski et al., 230.

52 Lubinski et al., 2012, 231-233.

53 Lubinski, et al., 229-34.

54 Penetrance: The frequency or rate of occurrence, typically in percentage, of a particular trait or condition (e.g., disease) expressed among individuals carrying the same deleterious (or disease-causing) gene. From https://www.biologyonline.com/dictionary/penetrance.

55 Based on the American Cancer Society's 2016 estimate: 242,000 invasive breast cancer diagnoses in the US in 2017. Breast Cancer Facts & Figures 2015-2016, 1; breast-cancer-facts-and-figures-2015-2016 pdf; BRCA figure based on 5% of 242,000.

56 Pudowski et al., "Vitamin D Status in Central Europe," *International Journal of Endocrinology* (2014), article ID 589587, https://doi.org/10.1155/2014/589587.

57 K.A. Kennel, M.T. Drake, and D.L. Hurley, "Vitamin D Deficiency in Adults: When to Test and How to Treat," *Mayo Clinic Proceedings* 85, no. 8 (2010): 752–58, https://doi.org/10.4065/mcp.2010.0138.

58 Chartsbin.com, "Worldwide Total Motor Vehicle," According to World Bank data, there are 809 cars per 1,000 people in the US compared to 537 cars per 1,000 people in Poland, http://chartsbin.com/view/1114.

59 Cosmetics Design USA, "Eastern Europe: The Great Hope for Sunscreen," April 14, 2005, https://www.cosmeticsdesign.com/Article/2005/04/14/Eastern-Europe-the-great-hope-for-sunscreen.

60 Lubinski, 231.

61 Only Prempro and other "combination menopausal drugs" contain progestin. It is the progestin that raises breast cancer risk. Estrogen-only menopausal drugs, such as Premarin, do not increase these rates; see Chapter 4.

62 USDA Research, Education & Economics Information System, "Use of Bioactive Food Components to Modulate Vitamin D Receptor," September 30, 2015, https://portal.nifa.usda.gov/web/crisprojectpages/0223609-use-of-bioactive-food-components-to-modulate-vitamin-d-receptor-function.html.

63 Chu-Xia Deng, "BRCA1: Cell Cycle Checkpoint, Genetic Instability, DNA Damage Response and Cancer evolution," *Nucleic Acids Research* 34, no. 5 (2006): 1416–26, https://doi.org/10.1093/nar/gkl010; Karen Kaplan, "For Cancer Risk, Some BRCA Mutations are More Dangerous than Others," *Los Angeles Times*, April 8, 2015, https://www.latimes.com/science/sciencenow/la-sci-sn-brca1-brca2-mutations-cancer-risk-not-same-20150408-story.html; Timothy Rebbeck et al., "Association of Type and Location of BRCA1 and BRCA2 Mutations with Risk of Breast and Ovarian Cancer," *JAMA: Journal of the American Medical Association*, April 7, 2015; 313(13): 1347–1361, https://doi.org/10.1001/jama.2014.5985; K.B. Kuchenbaecker et al., "Risks of Breast, Ovarian, and Contralateral Breast Cancer for BRCA1 and BRCA2 Mutation Carriers," *JAMA: Journal of the American Medical Association* 317, no. 23 (June 20, 2017): 2402–16, https://doi.org/10.1001/jama.2017.7112.

64 LingJiao Zhang et al., "Breast and Ovarian Cancer Penetrance of BRCA1/2 Mutations Among Hong Kong Women," *Oncotarget* 9, no. 38 (February 2018): 25025–33, https://doi.org/10.18632/oncotarget.24382.

PART IV.
RECURRENT METASTATIC BREAST CANCER

9 OUR HUSH-HUSH EPIDEMIC

"The global Breast Cancer Diagnostic and Drug Therapy Market was valued at $20.9 billion in 2019 and is expected to reach $28.2 billion by the year 2024, at a compound annual growth rate (CAGR) of 6.2%."[1] "...By region, North America dominated the global breast cancer drugs market with a market share of about 43% in 2018 and is projected to retain its leading position over the forecast time period as well."[2] "...the global metastatic breast cancer treatment market is projected to grow at a CAGR of 9.4% over the forecast period of 2019-2025...North-America accounts for the largest revenue followed by Europe due to increased diagnosis of disease...".[3]

—Various market research reports

"You girls have discovered a national cover-up that nobody, outside of these cancer registries, knows anything about."

—Dr. Timothy Aldrich, former director,
North Carolina Central Cancer Registry

How many women under the age of 40, over the age of 50, or in between, were diagnosed with breast cancer in the US last year? How many were diagnosed ten years ago? No one seems to have these numbers. That's right: No single federal agency appears to be counting the actual number of women diagnosed or rediagnosed with breast cancer each year. Instead, each state's cancer board counts each primary tumor, not each person; and each federal agency involved uses its own unique formula, coming up with *estimates of cases*, always applying three- or four-year-old tumor data from a variety of different states, never just a current or total headcount of all women diagnosed with breast cancer, and *never* sharing data on the thousands or tens of thousands of women who are rediagnosed each year with terminal recurrent metastatic breast cancer. These rediagnosed women, we are told, comprise the vast majority of women within today's metastatic breast cancer population, the basis for today's expanding US metastatic breast cancer drug market. "North America accounts for the largest revenue followed by Europe due to increased diagnosis of disease," a 2019 market research report announced to its investors.[4] Yet the US public is never told how many women are being diagnosed with this deadly condition each year. Does all of this sound strange? It is.

Back in 2011, while working on my slowly evolving *Busting Breast Cancer* manuscript, a literary agent became interested in the project. "Susan, could you include some basic statistics in your overview? It would be helpful to show how much breast cancer has increased in American women over the past twenty years. Also, how much is breast cancer increasing in just younger women these days? Are all age groups experiencing similar trends? And, how do our breast cancer rates compare to other countries?"

I laughed in exasperation. "It's unbelievable," I said, "but I have yet to find those numbers, and I've been looking for a few years now. The federal government doesn't seem to have a centralized, up-to-date annual database of every woman diagnosed with breast cancer."

All I could find at the time were different estimates from different agencies, each using different population samples and formulas. And, as mentioned, these estimates were based on three- to four-year-old state-based data, but never included all fifty states. In fact, no federal agency ever shows us any five-, ten-, or twenty-year trends. Federal sources just tell us that breast cancer is unusual in women under 40 or 50, or that breast cancer hasn't been increasing in younger or older women in the US in recent years—with no transparent data to back up any of these claims.[5] Yet, some small studies from government registries outside the US, have indicated that for at least a decade, the number of women under 40, who are being diagnosed, is increasing; sometimes doubling their rate of invasive breast cancer in a matter of a few years.[6]

Strangely, in the US, a small private organization jointly funded by the cancer industry and government cancer agencies is the only public or private group apparently allowed access to the raw data from all 50 states. Technically, this means the US government does not have a federal agency in charge of tracking and reporting out our national cancer statistics.[7] Instead, the small staff of the private North American Association of Central Cancer Registries (NAACCR), based in Springfield, Illinois, receives, compiles and publishes all of our state-based national cancer data, as directed by the group's industry and government-based funders.

After this frustrating conversation with the literary agent, I became determined to look a little closer. To date, almost a decade later, the best long-term trend or historical information I've ever been able to find on the growth of our breast cancer epidemic is a graph created for a 2016 *Forbes* magazine article by a determined physician journalist who is also a former breast cancer patient. She compiled this long-term view of the development of our national epidemic using annual estimates from the National Cancer Institute (NCI), creating an Excel spreadsheet.[8]

Figure 9.1: US Breast Cancer Cases and Mortality Trends, 1975–2013

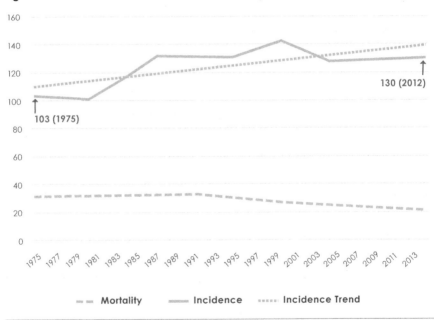

Invasive breast cancer incidence, and deaths (mortality). Rates are per 100,000 women. Incidence source is SEER 9 data accessed from the SEER website on October 20, 2016. A trend line generated with Microsoft Excel software (dots) demonstrates the upward pattern since 1975.

Elaine Schattner, "The Unfortunate Reality of a Rising Rate of Breast Cancer," Forbes.com, October 21, 2016, https://www.forbes.com/sites/elaineschattner/2016/10/21/the-unfortunate-reality-of-a-rising-rate-of-breast-cancer/#455008dfea10. American College of Surgeons' National Cancer Database, "Female Breast Cancer: Diagnosis Year: 2017," facs.org. Database represents 70 percent of all female breast cancer patients.

Her graph shows that breast cancer rates for women of all ages reflected an estimated 103 cases diagnosed per 100,000 women in 1975, increasing to 130 cases diagnosed per 100,000 women in 2013. That's an average one-percent annual increase of cases over a span of forty years among all age groups. Some would call that an ongoing and steadily increasing epidemic. But remember, these numbers don't show the actual picture. As mentioned, the terms "cases," "incidences," and "rates" that are being counted by NAACCR and by NCI are based on the number of primary *invasive tumors* initially diagnosed in women; not on the number of individual women diagnosed or rediagnosed. Also, the annual estimates in the graph have been calculated from a currently outdated sample of just nine percent of the US population—a sampling called the SEER 9 database[9]

Today's data collection practices also appear to be fairly useless when it comes to helping public health agencies identify and create cancer prevention programs. Here, then, are a few questions that women's health networks, breast cancer support groups, and concerned individuals can begin asking the National Cancer Institute. These same questions should also be shared with our elected officials on both the state and national levels. Hopefully, this combination of grassroots and bi-partisan legislative pressure, can help reform and improve today's questionable and incomplete official national breast cancer statistics.

1. Why doesn't the US government fund our state cancer registries to track and publish the actual number of *women* who are being diagnosed each year?[10] Why are most state cancer registries only sharing the types, sizes and numbers of primary tumors being diagnosed each year?

2. Why doesn't the US government have a single computerized federal agency that collects, calculates, produces, and publishes user-friendly, transparent, up to date, state-based, person-based breast cancer statistics at the end of each calendar year, along with multi-year trends?

3. Why is our profit-driven cancer industry allowed a hand in developing the only state-based national cancer statistics the public

gets to see, using three-year-old state-based data, produced and published by the private/public North American Association of Central Cancer Registries (NAACCR)?

4. Why don't our state cancer registries, or the NAACCR, share the annual state-based reported number and demographics of individual women who are diagnosed with recurrent early stage breast cancer and with recurrent metastatic breast cancer?

5. Who benefits by keeping the American public ignorant— "barefoot and pregnant," as the saying goes —when it comes to knowing the actual size, shape, and ongoing growth of today's hush-hush recurrent metastatic breast cancer epidemic?

6. What other recurrent metastatic cancer epidemics are now being hidden from the US public?

Another private cancer database, created by the American College of Surgeons (ACS),[11] also shares some of its own statistics with the public. Since 2008, the surgeons' National Cancer Database has offered the public user-friendly charts and graphs describing the national tumor statistics submitted by the hospitals that have been certified by US medical associations' Commission on Cancer (CoC).[12] The CoC's hospital data is helpful because it shows us the stage of each tumor when first diagnosed, as well as the number of primary tumors that are annually diagnosed within various age groups.[13]

Meanwhile, cancer industry executives, venture capitalists, and investment groups appear to ignore all of these publicly available data sources. Instead, they willingly prefer to pay five or six thousand dollars apiece for numerous privately developed market research reports that focus either on the current and anticipated breast cancer treatment market or cover just the metastatic breast cancer drug market. These high-priced items are filled with data, reportedly obtained from both cancer industry and government insiders.

I can only assume these $6,000 reports include specific estimates or the actual numbers, or close approximations of the number of women who are being treated for breast cancer, and those who are expected to be treated in the next few years for recurrent metastatic breast cancer.[14]

Table 9.1: Breast Cancer Tumors Diagnosed by Stage in 2017

BREAST CANCER DIAGNOSED IN 2017 BY AGE GROUP & STAGE

Estimates cover 100% primary tumors & 100% dnMBC diagnoses

Age Group	Stage 0	I	II	III	IV	NA	UNK	Totals N	%
Under 20		1 4.5%	11 50%	1 4.5%	2 9.1%	5 22.7%	2 9.1%	22 100%	0.01%
20–29	183 11.6%	446 28.2%	626 39.5%	183 11.6%	117 7.4%	5 0.3%	24 1.5%	1,584 100%	0.52%
30–39	1,584 14%	3,553 37%	4,208 27%	1,483 13%	706 6%	21 0.2%	107 0.9%	11,662 100%	3.84%
40–49	10,577 24%	16,109 37%	12,007 27%	3,469 8%	1,434 3%	25 0.1%	433 1%	44,054 100%	14.5%
50–59	15,666 22%	29,845 42%	17,027 24%	4970 6%	2,832 4%	46 0.1%	732 1%	71,118 100%	23.4%
60–69	17,551 20%	42,262 48%	19,314 22%	4,955 6%	3,651 4%	44 0.05%	861 1%	88,638 100%	29.17%
70–79	10,724 17%	31,111 50%	13,393 22%	3,183 5%	2,563 4%	43 0.1%	704 1%	61,721 100%	20.31%
80–89	2,544 12%	9,425 44%	6,012 28%	1,682 8%	1,429 7%	29 0.1%	470 2%	21,591 100%	7.11%
90 and over	208 6%	1,052 30%	1,292 37%	416 12%	327 9%	9 0.3%	166 5%	3,470 100%	1.14%
Total	59,037	133,804	73,890	20,342	13,061	227	3,499	303,860	100%
%	19.4%	44.0%	24.3%	6.7%	4.3%	0.1%	1.2%		100%

American College of Surgeons' data (70% of total US female primary breast cancer tumor diagnoses) used as basis to calculate 100% estimates.

American College of Surgeons' National Cancer Database, "Female Breast Cancer: Diagnosis Year: 2017" http://oliver.facs.org/BMPub/.

Metastatic breast cancer drugs, we are told, create an especially vibrant market in the US today. All of these toxic drugs, including immunotherapies, are used to try to extend metastatic patients' lives, and are considered the largest and most profitable segment of today's entire breast cancer drug market.[15] None of these drugs are described as resolving the disease. A press release announcing the publication of one recent market research report tells us, "As stated by the World Health Organization, the rate of death by breast cancer is increasing in number and predicted that it will continue to increase in [the] near future. This [is] expected to increase the market share for [the] Metastatic Breast Cancer Industry."[16]

The Busting Breast Cancer Study: If You Want to Get the Job Done, Sometimes You Just Have to Do It Yourself

In 2011, a few months after talking with that literary agent about my inability to find historic, up-to-date, complete, transparent, representative and trustworthy national breast cancer statistics that traced the growth of this apparent, but hush-hush, epidemic, I attended a spiritual retreat in Michigan. On our last day there, I found myself talking with the woman next to me, a statistics professor from Colorado Springs who was also a meditation instructor. Sitting in that crowded Hyatt Regency Hotel ballroom, where whatever gift you need is often given, I described my breast cancer prevention research, and my utter frustration at the lack of any current or past verifiable national statistical trends of those women who have been diagnosed with breast cancer in recent years or in recent decades.

My newfound friend, Jacquie Ostrom, was shocked and intrigued. She had taught introductory college statistics for decades. She agreed to formulate a plan to ask some state cancer boards for their original data, going back to the mid-1980s. This would allow us to compile at least a state-based snapshot of partial, possibly representative, raw data telling us if, and by how much, breast cancer was increasing among various age groups within some areas of the United States. Returning home to Colorado, and in spite of our limited funding, Jacquie got to work calling and emailing eight state cancer registries scattered across various sections of the country. Unlike most state registries that were created in the mid-1990s, each of our chosen registries were known by their peers to have consistently produced the highest quality data, having existed for many decades.[17] Jacquie was asking each of these state boards to send us their most recent data on the number of women diagnosed with breast cancer, broken down by various age groups and by year. She was looking for data covering the past five, ten, or fifteen years, and wanted it to include any trend data they had compiled on their state's epidemic. And so, it began: the *Busting Breast Cancer Study.*

Around this same time, I discovered a 1995 article by Dr. Timothy E. Aldrich, then a professor of epidemiology at Eastern Tennessee State University. The article's research, conducted in the early 1990s when Dr. Aldrich was director of the long-established North Carolina Central Cancer Registry, described a new procedure to speed up breast cancer reporting from seven months to just a few weeks.[18] After next researching many of Dr. Aldrich's other papers on cancer registry operations and geographic cancer clusters, my intuition told me this well-respected researcher would be able (and, I hoped, willing) to give Jacquie and me an insider's view of our current, seemingly Paleolithic, national cancer reporting system.[19]

Professor Aldrich agreed to a conference call. But his first words suggested that our quest for clear and accurate data would not be an easy one. "You girls have discovered a national cover-up that nobody outside of these cancer registries knows anything about," he said, a cynical chuckle rippling through his Southern drawl.

Tumors, Not People

The epidemiologist then told us that all the annual cancer "incidence" information reported to the public through state registries does not actually refer to how many *people* are diagnosed with cancer. Instead, all these estimates refer to the number of *primary tumors* radiologists diagnosed that year.[20] Jacquie and I were stunned, to say the least. This was the first time we learned this startling fact. But then the epidemiology professor's story got even more bizarre.

"State cancer registry personnel have been sworn to secrecy. I was there when it happened," said Dr. Aldrich. "Since Bernie Sanders's law calling for an up-to-date, transparent, person-based national cancer registry was passed in 1992, the state registries have all been instructed instead to implement this statutory law, as interpreted by the National Cancer Institute; to only publish the number of separate or primary invasive tumors diagnosed each year, not the number of individual women and men newly diagnosed with invasive cancer." Dr. Aldrich also explained that an original (or "primary") tumor is one that has not been spawned by another tumor; it is not a metastasized tumor.[21]

"This means that unless a researcher like Jacquie specifically asks each state registry, 'How many women were diagnosed with at least one invasive primary breast cancer tumor last year,' the registries will give Jacquie their standard *incidence reporting number*, which is how many distinct or primary breast tumors (or 'cases') were diagnosed by radiologists and oncologists in all women in their state during any single year."[22] And state personnel must give the feds this same tumor data, if the agency expects to receive its federal funding each year—funding that apparently pays for most state registries' operations.[23]

Why count primary tumors instead of women, I wondered? Don't our public health programs need to know the number and demographics of the individuals who develop invasive breast cancers within their state each year? Why focus on primary tumors? Prevention programs, after all, are about helping people prevent the development of *any* tumors. Shouldn't state cancer registries be collecting data that focuses on the number, age, and occupations of those being diagnosed? Shouldn't this data then try to identify any geographic, economic or vocational clusters of women being diagnosed within each state or region? This is the data public health offices need to design, implement and measure their so-called "cancer-control" programs.[24]

What Do National Incidence and Mortality Rates Actually Represent?

Are today's national breast cancer incidence and mortality rates meaningful or useful? Do we care if 60,000 women in the US were diagnosed with a total of 180,000 primary breast tumors last year, or if 180,000 women developed a single primary breast tumor last year? Which figures are of more concern to women: the 180,000 primary breast tumors or the 60,00 and 180,000 women?

A few statistical studies tell us that "Overall, the frequency of multiple primaries is reported in the range of 2-17 percent...In patients with breast cancer, the incidence of multiple primaries has been reported in the range of 4.1 percent."[25] Also, the NCI's SEER office and the International Association of Cancer Registries have two different definitions of primary tumors, with comparisons causing a difference of a few percentage points.[26] This means that the number of women who are being diagnosed with breast cancer in the US each year is hidden somewhere in the midst of these varying tumor incidence numbers.

This focus on diagnosed primary tumors, instead of on the individual women being diagnosed, makes the National Cancer Institute's formula for calculating our annual national breast cancer incidence unique among other major countries. The US formula seems to compare apples (primary tumors) to oranges (all women in the US population). Unbelievably, the number of women diagnosed with breast cancer in any year is always left out of this equation!

Breast Cancer Incidence

Incidence Rate=(Primary Tumors Diagnosed)/(Female Population)×100,000[27]

Regarding breast cancer mortality numbers, the American public is sometimes triumphantly told that "breast cancer mortality rates are declining." This is seen as the single piece of good news the industry can offer women as national breast cancer tumor rates continue to increase, or remain unimaginably high, compared to the rest of the world.[28] What does this official term, breast cancer "mortality rate," actually mean? Here is the National Cancer Institute's formula for calculating this rate:

Mortality Rate=(Cancer Deaths/Population)×100,000[29]

Today, the vast majority of women who die from breast cancer are those who have been diagnosed with metastatic breast cancer. Given this fact, shouldn't our national breast cancer mortality rate be based on this segment of our national population? Instead, today's tumor incidence rates and our breast cancer mortality rates don't appear to actually connect with one another in any meaningful way. I'm not a mathematician by any stretch of the imagination, but I do know that while a woman can be diagnosed with multiple primary tumors, we each only die once.

Also, untold thousands more women treated for a breast cancer diagnosis, under today's toxic "standard of care" therapies, die an early death each year of complications from, or directly from, chronic medical conditions stemming from their breast cancer treatments. The cancer industry calls this new field of treatment *cancer survivor medicine*.[30] Such potentially lethal complications can range from an early heart attack, to liver failure and suicide. Today, 44 percent of US women who are "cancer survivors" are breast cancer survivors.[31] How much would our current breast cancer mortality rates increase, if deaths from treatment complications were included in these rates?

During Dr. Aldrich's lengthy interview with Jacquie and me, the epidemiologist also understood my frustration over the lack of transparency in the estimates published by the American Cancer Society. "Most epidemiologists ignore numbers produced by the American Cancer Society, as one can never be clear what data they use, or how they use the data to come up with their estimates," he told us. Is this why the American Cancer Society never offers the public any breast cancer incidence information, going back multiple years?[32]

Meanwhile, according to Dr. Aldrich, the National Cancer Institute's SEER R9 database—the NCI's oldest estimating database—is still seen as the premier source for calculating national statistical trends. The SEER R9 is a formula-based sample of six state and two urban registries, along with a single rural regional cancer registry. It is the only consistent US cancer database going back three decades. As mentioned, this sample covers about nine percent of the US population. However, according to Dr. Aldrich, this 50-year-old slice of the US population doesn't take into account any of the following:

- **Chief geographic differences**, such as the fact that women in northern states develop 20 percent more invasive breast cancer each year than women who live in southern states.[33]

- **Significant regional issues**, such as the growing reality that individuals living in the Ohio River Valley have higher cancer rates than anywhere else in the US.[34]

- **Significant local issues**, such as the existence of clusters of children, women, or men in specific communities who have been (or are currently being) hard-hit with specific types of cancer because of possible economic, environmental or occupational hazards.[35]

Dr. Aldrich also told us that the surgeons and the oncologists, fascinated with the tumor data, "run the show." This is the reason the NCI's focus continues to be on *tumor data* and not on *people data*. This is the reason tumors continue to be the only information state cancer boards are ordered to supply to their federal bosses each year. Finally, Dr. Aldrich explained, the National Cancer Institute serves as the chief agency over the Centers for Disease Control, dictating what and how all states' cancer data are reported out. He also mentioned, that unlike all other federal agencies within the National Institutes of Health, the director of the NCI is a political appointee, chosen by the president.

The NCI chief oversees the distribution of more than $6 billion each year for new treatment protocols, drug development and prevention programs. All of these funds are spent today on the mistaken belief that all cancer is controlled by mutating genes, not by the cancer cell's fermenting mitochondria. What a waste of money. As described in Chapter 1, if the mitochondria in cancer cells run out of their two fuels, they can no longer keep the cancer cell alive. Those mutating genes, along with the entire mitochondria-powered cancer cell, simply die.

The NCI also receives additional millions of dollars in funding each year from drug companies to conduct joint research on new drugs that might be better at killing these mutating genes than current drugs.[36] The results of these studies can carry the endorsement of the NCI, while the drug manufacturers enjoy any resulting profits.[37] The NCI and today's cancer industry have become the same organism, or at least members of the same exclusive genetics-focused family.

Having concluded our eye-opening interview with Dr Aldrich, Jacquie and I changed our data request to those state cancer registries. Armed with this new information about tumor-counting versus person-counting, Jacquie reworded our data application, and then contacted each of the eight state registries on our list once again. Now we were specifically asking for the number of *women* (not the number of primary tumors) diagnosed over the past twenty years—and would the agencies be kind enough to send us their information, sorted out by year and by age groups?

NCI Directors: Chosen for their Affinity to the Mainstream Cancer Industry

Norman E. Sharpless, the current NCI director within the Trump Administration, was director of the University of North Carolina's Lineberger Cancer Center, until his appointment to the NCI in 2017. He is also a co-founder and current principal of a privately held drug company, G1 Therapeutics, that views cancer as a genetic disease.

Harold Varmus, NCI director during the Obama administration, is the quintessential hybrid industry/university/government leader promoting the genetic theory of cancer in each of these roles. Prior to directing NCI, he was Director of Sloan Kettering Memorial Cancer Center; served as head of the National Institutes of Health, and was a university research professor in genetics-based cancer research. He and colleague Michael Bishop shared the Nobel Prize in Medicine or Physiology in 1989 for proposing a theory of how specific viruses may initiate genetic changes that cause cancer.

It's probably no surprise that Jacquie was unsuccessful in obtaining this person-based statistical information. Still, we were astounded. Well-intentioned as the state cancer statisticians may have been, our requests were genuinely foreign to all but one of these state cancer boards.[38] Unfortunately, Dr. Aldrich had been right.

Most of these state employees were simply unable to handle Jacquie's people-centered data request. It was true. The focus of state cancer boards is to report the number of primary tumors diagnosed in a given year, along with the size, shape, and types of cells found within each diagnosed mass.[39]

"The reason we count tumors is because some patients will have more than one tumor, and these tumors can be diagnosed many years apart. To count only people and not a second tumor would underestimate the rate," according to Dr. Sandra Kwong, then acting chief of the Cancer Surveillance Research Unit in the California Department of Public Health.[40] As we read and then re-read Dr. Kwong's email, Jacquie and I shook our heads in disbelief. Why couldn't you count that same woman again in later years, since she has now been diagnosed with a second primary tumor, or rediagnosed with metastatic tumors, or with a recurrence of her original primary tumor? Why is only understanding the numbers and types of unique primary tumors more important than understanding the number and the demographics of the individual women who continue to develop a new cancer diagnosis each year? None of these tumor-counting procedures seemed to make much sense, especially if state cancer agencies want to help public health agencies identify and help mitigate unexpected clusters of cancer patients who now face unique environmental, economic or occupational hazards.[41]

Busting Breast Cancer's Three-State Study

In the end, three state cancer boards—Massachusetts, Colorado and Florida—were willing and able to send us their annual tumor-based data, divided by age groups, for a fifteen to twenty year period, running between 1984 and 2008. By sheer coincidence, these three states represented geographic diversity. Each also happened to fall into three groupings of states: those with ongoing low, medium, and high annual breast cancer tumor rates.

According to the CDC, Massachusetts is among the states that traditionally have the highest rates of diagnosed breast cancer tumors, while Colorado is among the states traditionally with moderate rates, and Florida is among the states where traditionally women develop the lowest numbers of these invasive primary tumors.[42] These two coincidental factors, different regional locations and historically different breast cancer rates, would hopefully help make our simplistic three-state data sample more representative of the entire country's unofficial epidemic. Maybe it would be possible to create at least a blurry snapshot of today's breast cancer epidemic. Maybe Jacquie and I could at least begin to understand the pace of the epidemic's development over the past few decades in younger and in older women.

Once Jacquie plotted out the received tumor data from these three states, our *Busting Breast Cancer* study confirmed the existence of a new type of breast cancer epidemic. Our three-state data snapshot showed that young women being diagnosed with breast cancer (those under fifty years old) had experienced about a one-to-two percent *annual* increase in the rate of primary tumors diagnosed from at least the mid-1980s through 2008. For example, in Florida, in 1984, 53 primary tumors were diagnosed per 100,000 women under 50 years old. By 2008, Florida's annual breast cancer tumor rate for this group of younger women had increased by 40 percent, to 74 primary tumors per 100,000 women. This meant the number of breast cancer tumors in younger Florida women had continued to increase by an average of 1.7 percent a year between 1984 and 2008. Although we do not know the number of women who developed all of these tumors, it would appear that these increasing tumor numbers might somehow mean an increasing number of women were being diagnosed with breast cancer.

Figure 9.2: Breast Cancer Rates by State, indicating high to low levels during 2017

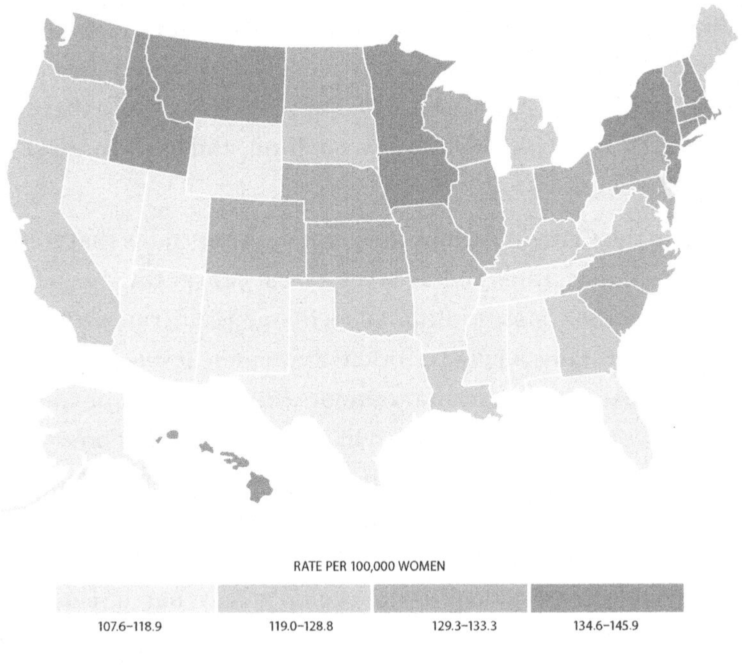

RATE PER 100,000 WOMEN

| 107.6–118.9 | 119.0–128.8 | 129.3–133.3 | 134.6–145.9 |

Each state has a different rate of breast cancer based on days of sunshine, levels of water pollution, rates of mammograms, etc.

Centers for Disease Control and Prevention, US Cancer Statistics Visualization, https://gis.cdc.gov/Cancer/USCS/DataViz.html.

In Massachusetts, women under 50 years old had developed almost double the rate of tumors than younger women in Colorado or Florida. These Massachusetts women had struggled with a 2.34% average annual increase in invasive breast cancer tumors, up from 55 tumors per 100,000 younger women in 1985, to 83 tumors per 100,000 younger women in 2008. Meanwhile, women under 50 years old in Colorado had faced about a 1% annual increase, up from 60 primary tumors per 100,000 women in 1985, reaching 70 primary tumors per 100,000 women in 2008.

Back in the 1970s, the breast tumor rate for US *women of all ages*, according to various federal reports, was about 70 per 100,000 women.[43] American Cancer Society sources tell us there were an estimated 68,000 new cases of breast cancer each year during the 1970s. By 2014 there had been a 242 percent increase (232,670) in new cases of female breast cancer. This means that while the US population increased by 56.8 percent, the US women's breast cancer rate quadrupled.[44] Comparing this number with the increase in population over this period of time indicates that the increase in female breast cancer has been four times the population increase.[45] Our *Busting Breast Cancer Study* found that by 2008, younger women's rate, alone, was now 70 primary tumors per 100,000. Meanwhile all three states' data showed that older women, those over 50 years of age, had continued to develop between 260-420 primary tumors (per 100,000), as far back as 1984, continuing on to 2008!

The 2012 *Busting Breast Cancer* Study, in my mind, identifies the clear existence of a continuing breast cancer epidemic among older women and an accelerating epidemic among premenopausal women, that had begun at least by the mid-1980s. What role had the increasing popularity of birth control drugs played in these rising statistics? What about the increasing role of the plastics, pesticides and chemical estrogens that continue to engulf the US population? What about the stress from the increasing economic impoverishment that most younger and older women in the US have faced since the mid-1980s, as the nation's wealth has been redistributed to the top one percent of the population?[46] What's the impact of the introduction of progestin-laced IUDs, our rising obesity rates, and the overuse of high-SPF sunscreens that lower a person's Vitamin D3-powered immune system? And how has the overdiagnosis and overtreatment of DCIS (stage 0 breast cancer) and tiny indolent stage I tumors, most identified by mammograms, increased today's hidden recurrent breast cancer rates?

The Epidemic Rise of Breast Cancer in Our Younger Women (those below 50 years old)

Table 9.2: The *Busting Breast Cancer* Study

STATE	YEAR	# OF TUMORS PER 100,000	ANNUAL INCREASE	TOTAL % INCREASE
Massachusetts	1985	55	1.2%	51%
	2007	83		
Florida	1984	53	1.7%	40%
	2008	74		
Colorado	1990	60	0.9%	17%
	2008	70		

©*Busting Breast Cancer 2012 (tumor data submitted to Busting Breast Cancer by state cancer boards in Massachusetts, Florida, and Colorado). Credit: Jacquie Ostrom.*

In 2015, hoping to validate or correct our 2012 three-state snapshot, I decided to see if the North American Association of Central Cancer Registries (NAACCR) might share their state-based tumor information with me. I contacted Dr. Recinda Sherman, data manager at NAACCR. This is the joint industry/government national cancer registry group mentioned earlier. NAACCR's database had now become available to the public, beginning with their 2008 numbers. As mentioned, their database is unique, insofar as this is the only group, inside or outside of the US government, that the National Cancer Institute allows to collect raw tumor data from all fifty state cancer registries, the District of Columbia, Puerto Rico and US territories.

Under the control of their cancer industry/government funders, some NAACCR data, while not offered in a user-friendly format, is available to the public. The group also issues a short and fairly academic summary report to the public each year.[47]

I asked Dr. Sherman if she would give me her group's breast cancer rates for women under fifty years old and for women age fifty years and older, beginning with her agency's oldest 50-state data, from 2008 up to 2012. Dr Sherman was kind enough to generate graphs mapping out my request.

Figure 9.3: The *Busting Breast Cancer Study*: Three-state study 1984–2009 combined with NAACCR's 50 state tumor data 2008–2016 (women below 50 years old)

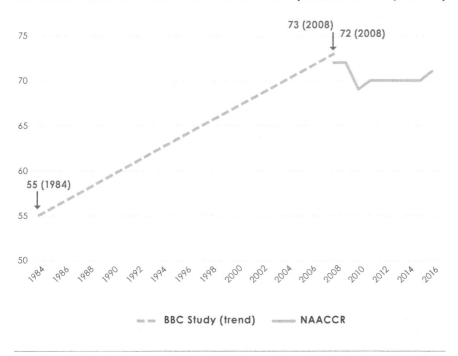

Breast cancer primary tumor rates in young women began to rise with the increase in birth control drug use, progestin IUDs, pesticide runoff in public water supplies & increasing poverty among majority of population. Chapters 2 through 8 describe all the causes mentioned behind this national increase.

Busting Breast Cancer © 2012 (tumor data submitted to Busting Breast Cancer by state cancer boards in Massachusetts, Florida, and Colorado)

I was pleasantly surprised...actually shocked. The NAACCR's official 2008 national data were virtually the same as the 2008 tumor data uncovered by *Busting Breast Cancer's* 3-state study. Our joint statistical picture, tracking national tumor rates beginning in the mid-1980s, up to 2008, illustrated that premenopausal women (those under 50 years old) began to experience a steady upsurge in primary breast cancer diagnoses beginning as early as the mid-1980s. This level of diagnosed invasive primary tumors for those 20-49 years old continued to increase, reaching about 72 primary tumors per 100,000 continuing through 2012. Our three-state *Busting Breast Cancer* Study had also been able to connect with the NAACCR's official data, illustrating the existence of a postmenopausal breast cancer epidemic facing women over 50 years old in 2008. Postmenopausal women experienced average tumor rates of 340 primary tumors per 100,000 women from at least the mid-1980s through 2016. The accuracy of our three-state *Busting Breast Cancer* Study had exceeded our wildest dreams.

In 2019, Dr Sherman was again kind enough to send me NAACR's latest figures. Their state-based numbers between 2008-2016 indicated that breast cancer rates in younger women under 50 years old was still creeping up. The average rate between 2008 and 2016 for these younger women had now become 72.47 tumors per 100,000 women. Meanwhile, rates for postmenopausal women between age 50 and 65 also continued to creep up, moving from, 262.11 to a five-year average of 265.43 tumors per 100,000 women. Between 2012 and 2016, NAACCR's rates for women over 65 years old did not seem to change much. However, this group' average of 422.45 tumors per 100,000 women, probably continues to reflect a world-record high.[48]

There Are Two Types of Metastatic Breast Cancer: De novo and Recurrent

Very rarely does a woman die from an early-stage breast cancer. Breast cancer mortality rates reflect the number of women who have been diagnosed with stage IV (metastatic) breast cancer.[49] There is no stage V breast cancer. A metastatic diagnosis is considered a terminal diagnosis assuring an early death sentence, by today's cancer industry.

There are two types of metastatic breast cancer diagnoses: *de novo metastatic breast cancer (dnMBC) and recurrent metastatic breast cancer (rMBC)*. This Latin term, "de novo," means "from new" or "at first." This is an apt name as it describes this stage IV diagnosis as being *the first time* a woman receives a diagnosis of any type of breast cancer. In the case of a de novo metastatic diagnosis, a cancer cell from a woman's existing, but undiscovered, primary breast tumor has broken away, entered her blood or lymph system, and invaded her bone, liver, brain and/or lungs by the time this initial diagnosis of dnMBC is made. We are told that only 3 to 4 percent of women initially diagnosed with breast cancer each year are facing the stage IV terminal diagnosis of de novo metastatic breast cancer (dnMBC).[50] Since any type of metastatic diagnosis, by definition, identifies an individual woman, not an individual primary tumor, each reported dnMBC diagnosis, unlike other published US breast cancer statistics, actually represents an individual woman!

Metastasis: The spread of cancer cells from the place where they first formed to another part of the body. In metastasis, cancer cells break away from the original (primary) tumor, travel through the blood or lymph system, and form a new tumor in other organs or tissues of the body.

National Cancer Institute Dictionary of Cancer Terms

De novo Metastatic Breast Cancer (dnMBC)

In 2011, Dr. Rebecca Johnson, a young Seattle pediatrician, was diagnosed and treated for a stage I breast tumor and underwent a mastectomy. She was just a year out of medical school. Johnson soon heard that a few of her classmates and other peers had also recently been treated for breast cancer. The young doctor wondered if breast cancer had somehow suddenly increased among premenopausal women. Breast cancer, as presented in her recent medical school classes, was described as a disease affecting menopausal and post-menopausal women; a disease rarely faced by women in their twenties and thirties. Medical journals were also silent on this phenomenon. Just as Jacquie and I had discovered, data-based trend data on this subject, going back even a few years or decades, is not readily available. Dr Johnson soon discovered that she too, would have to do her own data collection and computations.[51]

Assembling a team of three, including Dr. Archie Bleyer, a well-known research professor of radiation medicine,[52] the trio used NCI population samples, which covered 9 to 18 percent of the national population over various decades. Data from these small samples showed no increase in invasive breast cancer in premenopausal women over the past few decades, with one small, although statistically significant, exception. The researchers found that the number of very young premenopausal women, ages 25-39 years old, diagnosed with stage IV *de novo metastatic breast cancer*, had increased from 1.53 women/100,000 to 2.90 women/100,000, between 1976 and 2009.[53]

The Johnson-Blyer peer-reviewed study, published in the November 22, 2012 issue of the *Journal of the American Medical Association*, marked the first time a major medical journal had ever published any specific government data documenting that breast cancer was increasing in premenopausal women.[54] The buzz from the subsequent press coverage from the US corporate media, although short-lived, was enormous.[55] In my mind, however, the full significance of the Johnson-Blyer team's finding was that they had identified the emerging tip of a growing de novo metastatic iceberg, now developing in US women of all ages. I call this an iceberg, since it is still somewhat undercover news, never described as a national problem by major news media.

Here is the data to back up my statement about our growing de novo breast cancer epidemic. Using the American College of Surgeons' National Cancer Database, (representing about 70% of breast cancer patients), I compared the surgeons' 2008 data with the group's most recent 2017 de novo metastatic data. This same group of very young premenopausal women (those 20–39 years old) identified in the Johnson-Blyer study, went on to experience an estimated 56% increase in de novo metastatic breast cancer (dnMBC) diagnoses over the following decade, 2008–2017.[56] Also alarming, the surgeons' data for this recent decade indicates that women of all ages experienced a 48 percent increase in dnMBC diagnoses between 2008 and 2017.[57]

Recurrent Metastatic Breast Cancer

Here is another iceberg of unknown proportions. The number of women who are being rediagnosed each year with metastatic cancer or rMBC are never released to the public. Numerous clinical studies tell us, however, that 20-40 percent or more of women, treated for an early stage (I,II or III) breast tumor, will later be diagnosed with stage IV, also called recurrent metastatic breast cancer (rMBC).[58] Take a moment and let this statement sink into your mind. This means the initial treatments these women received for their early-stage (non-metastatic) primary breast cancer diagnoses were "not adequate" or "not successful." Their mainstream breast cancer treatments failed; so now an undisclosed number, possibly tens of thousands, of women each year in the US alone find themselves facing another breast cancer diagnosis, along with an early death sentence.[59] This number must be very embarrassing to cancer centers throughout the US.

As described in Chapter 1, metabolic biologists, epidemiologists and some clinical researchers have shown or understand how a rMBC diagnosis can be set in motion, be initiated, or can originate, during a fine needle or core breast biopsy.[60] Do sentinel node biopsies also play a role in this huge number of women developing rMBC?[61] Since mainstream cancer centers insist on doing one or more breast biopsies, and often lymph node biopsies as their first steps in diagnosing DCIS or a primary tumor, women who choose to be treated by mainstream cancer clinics are put at an immediate risk of developing rMBC. Again, I do not mention this fact lightly. In fact, the studies indicating how, and by how much, biopsies can initiate rMBC are probably the most controversial research in this entire book.

In 2017, epidemiologists at the NCI and the Fred Hutchinson Cancer Center in Seattle, published a study, based on a variety of suppositions and estimates, that created an estimate of the possible number of women currently being treated for metastatic breast cancer in the US. They calculated this number to be 155,000.[62] But why guess at such a critical number? This is silly, or plain irresponsible to every woman who has ever been treated for an early-stage breast cancer diagnosis, and to those now living with an early death sentence from their rMBC diagnoses.

The Commission on Cancer requires US physicians to report each patient's new breast cancer diagnosis or rediagnosis within six months, to the appropriate state cancer board. To maintain their state medical licenses, physicians must also answer a variety of questions describing each of their patients' cancer diagnoses/rediagnoses, including the molecular type (hormone positive, triple-negative, etc.) and describing this particular diagnosis (first time, first recurrence, second recurrence), type or stage of each rediagnosis, and which organs have now been invaded by the woman's primary breast cancer tumor's cells.[63]

State cancer boards must then undergo a quality control review every three years by the College of Surgeons' Commission on Cancer (CoC). Failure to include all of these details for each patient diagnosed and rediagnosed in any one year, can result in the state cancer board losing its much-coveted "high quality" certification by the NAACCR, or the reporting cancer center losing their coveted CoC accreditation, and/or the physician losing her or his state medical license, effectively terminating their medical career.

Industry leaders and investors in the metastatic drug market also have an excellent understanding of the current and changing number of women who are being diagnosed with rMBC each year. As mentioned, these numbers are required to develop a full understanding of the size of their client base, so that current and anticipated research, development, manufacturing and marketing costs can be projected, in order to calculate anticipated drug revenues and future net income. Without current rMBC data, investors have no sound information on which to invest billions of dollars each year. Every woman must ask, what are the rMBC numbers behind the 9% CAGR (compound annual growth rate) now being promised investors in today's worldwide metastatic breast cancer drug market? Why is the US expected to continue to lead this booming worldwide industry? Why are US women expected to continue to contribute over 40% of the metastatic breast cancer drug companies' income each year? How large is today's population of women diagnosed with rMBC? How quickly can women get hold of these critical rMBC statistics? How can women work to shut this booming industry down?

A 2000 study estimating lifetime costs of metastatic breast cancer treatment by industry researchers states that "more than 40% of women diagnosed with breast cancer will progress to metastatic disease.[64] Another study about chemotherapy and metastatic breast cancer by Baylor University Cancer Center oncologist Joyce O'Shaughnessy was published in the peer-reviewed journal *The Oncologist* in October 2005. Describing the current metastatic breast cancer landscape in which she worked, the oncologist needed to include the size of her client base. How many metastatic breast cancer patients might be able to benefit from her treatment review? In a matter-of-fact manner, the oncologist tells us, "Despite advances in the treatment of breast cancer, approximately 30% of women initially diagnosed with earlier stage of breast cancer eventually develop recurrent advanced or metastatic disease."[65]

Dr. O'Shaughnessy did not feel the need to describe how she calculated this apparently known or obvious number, nor does she offer a citation that could indicate where or how this number had been derived. Since then a number of other clinicians and researchers, writing in their own journal articles, continue to piggyback on Dr. O'Shaughnessy's presumably honest and useful 30 percent rMBC rate, citing her study as their data source.[66] To my knowledge, a retraction of this 30 percent figure has never been published.[67]

Did Dr. O'Shaughnessy forget and let a well-known cancer industry insider statistic accidentally slip out into the public eye? Did her peer review panel of fellow metastatic breast cancer clinicians, also quite familiar with this statistic, also let this secretive or hush-hush 30 percent figure slip by their eyes?

I recently found two straightforward, transparent studies that offer raw data on actual rMBC rates in Germany and in The Netherlands. Researchers in both studies were able to use their national or state cancer registries and individual patients' hospital records to track the rMBC rates for their selected groups of breast cancer patients, post-treatment, for five- or ten-year periods.

The Netherlands

Using their national cancer registry that records each woman's initial diagnosis and using individuals' hospital records that record subsequent types of recurrent diagnoses, this 2019 study looked at all women diagnosed with an early-stage breast cancer (I-III) in The Netherlands during 2005. Researchers tracked this group of 8,062 early breast cancer patients, for any and all types of recurrent diagnoses during the following decade, from 2005 to 2015.

The Dutch data show that overall, 15 percent of the 8,062 women within the study group developed rMBC within the ten years following their 2005 early-stage breast cancer diagnosis. However, recurrence rates for different groups of women by type of tumor cells diagnosed were radically different.

The Dutch women who had been diagnosed with a hormone negative triple-negative primary tumor experienced a much higher recurrence rate of 23.2 percent. Women diagnosed with HER2-positive, another type of hormone negative primary breast tumor, experienced an even higher rMBC recurrent rate: 25.6 percent. Women who had been diagnosed with different types of hormone positive primary tumors had significantly lower rMBC rates of 7 to 10 percent. This study also found that women who had been initially diagnosed with a hormone positive lobular tumor, rather than the more prevalent hormone positive ductal tumors, experienced a higher rMBC rate.[68]

Germany

Using data from the population-based cancer registry of the small state of Saarland in western Germany, researchers identified all women diagnosed with a primary breast tumor between 1999-2009. Each woman was tracked for a ten-year period, again using hospital records to follow their diagnosis and identify any type of disease recurrence.[69] Again, women who had originally been diagnosed with hormone negative primary tumors (HER2/positive or triple negative) experienced higher rMBC rates than women who had been diagnosed with a hormone positive primary tumor. The HER2/positive group experienced a 28 percent recurrence, while those who had been treated for a triple-negative tumor (TNBC) experienced a 23 percent recurrence. The overall ten-year rMBC recurrence rate for the entire group, however, was 11 percent, given that the largest group of patients in the study had been diagnosed with hormone positive primary tumors.

US studies of women diagnosed with hormone-negative triple-negative primary tumors (TNBC) are also available. These studies consistently tell us that a disproportionate number of younger premenopausal women, often diagnosed with very large, fast-growing primary triple-negative tumors, face a 30% to 33% rMBC rate. Here is one sobering quote on the subject. "After six years of observation, metastatic disease occurred in 35% of all TNBC patients."[69]

Figure 9.4: Metastatic Breast Cancer Market Value, 2016–2021 ($Million)

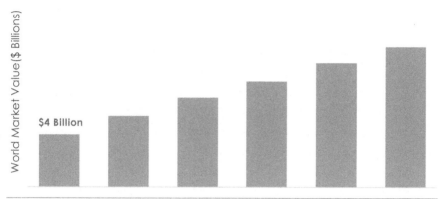

US women comprise about 4.3% of the world's female population. They have the highest rate of breast cancer of any major country in the world. US women and their insurance companies are currently expected to contribute over 40% of the metastatic drug industry's worldwide revenues for the coming five years.

Industry ARC, "Metastatic Breast Cancer Market Forecast (2020-2025)," Report Code: HCR 0340, https://www.industryarc.com/Report/16161/metastatic-breast-cancer-market.html.

These same studies report that these younger women usually experience their rMBC diagnosis within the first two years following their initial breast cancer treatment.[70] Recent studies show that women with large TNBC tumors who choose breast-conserving surgery instead of breast amputation or mastectomy have similar recurrence rates.[71] Following the threads of conversation by caregivers and patients alike in the Triple-Negative Breast Cancer Foundation's online chat room can be a horrifying and heartbreaking experience.[72] Their stories, backed by a growing number of epidemiological studies, describe metastatic TNBC tumors usually forming in these young women's brains, lungs and liver.[73]

Meanwhile, US women continue to represent only 4.3% of the world's female population, but US women and their families continue to finance more than fifty percent of the worldwide breast cancer drug market's annual income. As mentioned, those piles of $6,000 research reports, sold each year to breast cancer drug investors, continue to jubilantly announce that tens of thousands more US women will develop dnMBC and rMBC next year.

Figure 9.5: What is Actual Size of US Breast Cancer Epidemic?

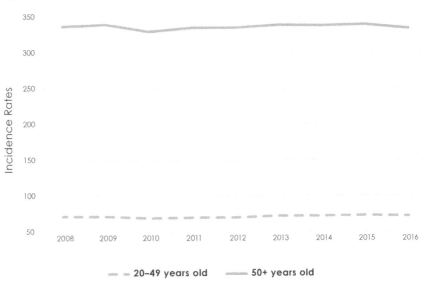

Initial breast cancer diagnoses by two age groups (2008-2016). Numbers do not include additional 20 to 40 percent of women re-diagnosed with metastatic breast cancer after receiving standard of care treatment for early stage breast cancer. Actual size of today's breast cancer epidemic is exponentially larger than shown.

NAACCR Age-Adjusted Incidence Rates, 2000 US Standard Population By Cancer Site, 2015; updated 2019.

The National Cancer Registries Act

The size of today's rMBC population is apparently dependent on how many women are treated for an early-stage breast cancer diagnosis each year. As described in Chapter 5, this means the entire breast cancer drug market's growth is also dependent on the mammography industry and its recent track record of being able to overdiagnose and overtreat increasing numbers of women each year.

The National Cancer Institute, led by its presidentially appointed director, could easily institute a national, centralized, computerized and federally funded cancer registry that receives, records and publishes up-to-date, anonymous, individual patient-based and demographically organized statistics from all state cancer registries. Such a system would be able to tell us the number of women diagnosed and those rediagnosed each year with which type of invasive breast cancer.[74]

Congress can also pass a law that requires the establishment of a centralized database, and insures complete and immediate public access to such data. But, believe it or not, we already have a law that says we should! This is the law that Dr. Aldrich had first described to us as "Bernie Sanders' Law," when we spoke to the epidemiology professor back in 2011.

In the early 1990s, Vermont state statistics indicated women were experiencing increased rates of breast cancer, along with increasing deaths from the invasive disease. A concerned group of women asked their freshman congressman, Bernie Sanders, to help them compare Vermont's breast cancer statistics with those of other states. Was Vermont experiencing a unique phenomenon, or was this uptick in breast cancer diagnoses and deaths also happening around New England—and around the country?

Sanders agreed to look into their concerns. He was shocked at his discovery: "[W]e found that only ten states in the country had effective cancer registries. And while some national statistics were being tabulated by the National Cancer Institute, they ignored 90 percent of the population," Sanders wrote in his 1997 political biography.[75]

Having learned that most states didn't have cancer registries, Sanders realized it was impossible for state health boards to identify, let alone address, any local cancer clusters. That's what led the rookie congressman to draft his 1992 Cancer Registries Amendment Act.[76] Essentially, the law created and funded registries in each state; it also created the National Program of Cancer Registries within the CDC. To this day, however, only *some* of these fifty state cancer boards report their annual data to the national office. Instead, annual data from all state cancer boards is sent to the North American Association of Central Cancer Registries, the previously mentioned independent organization supported by funding from the cancer industry and the federal government. The cancer industry's control over our national cancer statistics was not what this 1992 law was meant to achieve.

In his 1997 biography, Senator Sanders describes his thinking behind his 1992 Cancer Registries Amendment Act:

> *What does it mean that certain types of cancer are more prevalent in Vermont than in California? What is the relationship between environmental degradation and cancer? Are people working at certain types of jobs more likely to come down with particular types of cancer than people working at other jobs?*
>
> *Are people living near landfills or incinerators more likely to develop cancer? If we had uniform national statistics, would we learn more about the connection between diet and cancer, and lifestyle and cancer? Would we discover more geographical "clusters" of certain types of cancer?...This country spends $1 trillion a year on healthcare, almost all of it goes into...treatment. In the long run we can eliminate much human suffering, and great cost, if we better understand the causation of disease.*[77]

Senator Sanders clearly hoped to create fifty cancer registries, each reporting out the number of women diagnosed each year, to a single federal board—a group that would become our federal cancer watchdog. It would be able to generate people-based data, useful in designing, monitoring, and evaluating cancer prevention, treatment and support programs at the regional, state, and community levels. It's interesting that the opening statement in this 1992 law says, "cancer control efforts, including prevention, and early detection, are best addressed locally by state health departments that can identify unique needs."[78]

Today, American women remain stuck with a government that refuses to fully implement the 1992 Cancer Registry Amendment Act. Instead, our government appears to allow our for-profit cancer treatment industry to run the show. US treatment centers' staff now stand by help-lessly as at least 118 women continue to die each day from metastatic breast cancer, while more than 1600 people continue to die each day from all types of cancer.

Figure 9.6: Where in the World is Breast Cancer?

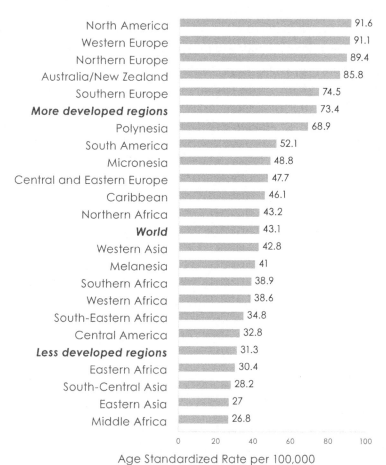

Age Standardized Rate per 100,000

According to the World Health Organization, the US has the highest rate of breast cancer in the world.

"Where in the World is Breast Cancer?" December 9, 2016, http://humagna.com/article_where_in_the_world_is_breast_cancer.html.

More individual women and health groups must begin to openly question why the US continues to have the world's highest rates of breast cancer among younger women, among older women, among "BRCA women," and quite possibly among those women who continue to develop recurrent metastatic breast cancer each year.

The late Beth Caldwell, metastatic breast cancer activist, patient, civil rights attorney, wife, and mother of two, understood. "The idea that we don't know how many people are living with a particular disease in this country seems pretty backward. Especially in an era where Amazon can predict that I'm going to like a particular cell phone case," Caldwell told a reporter in May of 2017.[79] Beth Caldwell died from de novo metastatic breast cancer on November 2, 2017, at the age of 41.[80]

CHAPTER ENDNOTES

1   BCC Research, "Breast Cancer Diagnostic and Drug Technologies: Global Markets," December 2019, https://www.bccresearch.com/market-research/healthcare/breast-cancer-diagnostic-and-drug-technologies-global-markets-report.html.

2   Zion Market Research, "Global Breast Cancer Drugs Market Will Reach USD 38.3 Billion by 2025," March 18, 2019, https://www.globenewswire.com/news-release/2019/03/18/1756033/0/en/Global-Breast-Cancer-Drugs-Market-Will-Reach-USD-38-3-Billion-By-2025-Zion-Market-Research.html.

3   Infinium, "Metastatic Breast Cancer Treatment Market," May, 2019, https://www.infiniumglobalresearch.com/healthcare-medical-devices/global-metastatic-breast-cancer-treatment-market.

4   Ibid.

5   Louise Brinton et al., "Recent Trends in Breast Cancer Among Younger Women in the United States." *Journal of the National Cancer Institute* 100, no. 22, (2008):1643-8, https://doi.org/10.1093/jnci/djn344.

6   C. Bouchardy, et al., "Recent Increase of Breast Cancer Incidence Among Women Under the Age of Forty," *British Journal of Cancer* 96, (2007):1743-46, https://doi.org/10.1038/sj.bjc.6603783; A Bodmer et al., "Breast Cancer in Younger Women in Switzerland 1996-2009: A Longitudinal Population-based Study. *Breast* 24, no.2 (2015):112-117, https://doi.org/10.1016/j.breast.2014.11.004Swiss.

7   North American Association of Central Cancer Registries, "Annual Report to the Nation on The Status on Cancer," https://www.naaccr.org/annual-report-to-the-nation/.

8   Elaine Schattner, "The Unfortunate Reality of a Rising Rate of Breast Cancer," Forbes.com, October 21, 2016, https://www.forbes.com/sites/elaineschattner/2016/10/21/the-unfortunate-reality-of-a-rising-rate-of-breast-cancer/#455008dfea10.

9   National Cancer Institute, "Cancer Stat Facts: Female Breast Cancer," https://seer.cancer.gov/statfacts/html/breast.html.

10 Centers for Disease Control, "Contact a Local Registry," Program Contacts by Funding Status," https://nccd.cdc.gov/dcpc_Programs/index.aspx#/3.

11 The ACS mentioned in this chapter refers to the American College of Surgeons. In previous chapters ACS refers to the American Cancer Society. They are two distinct organizations with different methods of collecting and calculating national cancer statistics. They are both private organizations that receive all or most of their funding from the cancer industry. We have no transparent,up-to-date, or complete government sources of national cancer statistics.

12 The Commission on Cancer (CoC) is comprised of 56 national medical organizations. It is the medical industry's governing body over cancer diagnostic and treatment procedures that licensed physicians in the US are mandated to use for every cancer patient. Not adhering to these standard of care treatments can jeopardize the physician's medical license and leaves the practitioner open to medical malpractice suits. The CoC continues to strictly adhere to and enforce the view that cancer is a genetic disease. Federal cancer agencies also adhere to CoC's direction. Clinical trials that do not first use standard of care procedures are neither allowed nor funded by government sources.

13 American College of Surgeons, National Cancer Database, https://www.facs.org/quality-programs/cancer/ncdb.

14 Global Breast Cancer Treatment Market, https://www.businesswire.com/news/home/20170928005543/en/Global-Breast-Cancer-Treatment-Market-2017-2025; MarketWatch,

"Breast Cancer Treatment Market 2020 Global Share, Growth, Size, Opportunities, Trends, Regional Overview, Leading Company Analysis, And Key Country Forecast To 2025," May 28, 2020, https://www.marketwatch.com/press-release/breast-cancer-treatment-market-2020-global-share-growth-size-opportunities-trends-regional-overview-leading-company-analysis-and-key-country-forecast-to-2025-2020-05-28.

15   MarketWatch, "Metastatic Breast Cancer Treatment Market 2020: Global Countries Data, Global Analysis, Market Size, Growth, Definition, Business Opportunities and Forecast To 2026, "April 13, 2020, https://www.marketwatch.com/press-release/metastatic-breast-cancer-treatment-market-2020-global-countries-data-global-analysis-market-size-growth-defination-business-opportunities-and-forecast-to-2026-2020-04-13.

16   Industry ARC, "Metastatic Breast Cancer Market Forecast (2020-2025), Report Code: HCR 0340, https://www.industryarc.com/Report/16161/metastatic-breast-cancer-market.html.

17   Massachusetts, California, North Carolina, Florida, New Mexico, Colorado, Connecticut, and Minnesota were the only states with cancer registries or boards prior to 1992. See: William Haenszel and Mary G. McCrea Curnen, "The First Fifty Years of the Connecticut Tumor Registry: Reminiscences and Prospects," *The Yale Journal of Biology and Medicine* 59, no. 5, (1986): 475-84, PMCID: PMC2590186.

18   T.E. Aldrich et al., "Rapid Reporting of Cancer Incidence in a Population-based Study of Breast Cancer: One Constructive Use of a Central Cancer Registry," *Breast Cancer Research and Treatment* 35, no. 1 (1995): 61–64; https://doi.org/10.1007/BF00694746.

19   Steven Benowitz, "Busting Cancer Clusters: Realities Often Differ from Perceptions," *Journal of the National Cancer Institute* 100, no. 9 (May 7, 2008) 614-21, https://doi.org/10.1093/jnci/djn144.

20   Jorge N. Izquierdo and Victor J. Schoenbach, "The Potential and Limitations of Data from Population-Based State Cancer Registries," *American Journal of Public Health* 90, no. 5 (May 2000), https://ajph.aphapublications.org/doi/pdf/10.2105/AJPH.90.5.695.

21   Ibid.

22   Tim Aldrich, telephone interview with author and Jacquie Ostrom, February 7, 2011.

23   Florence K L Tangka, et al. "Cost of Operating Central Cancer Registries and Factors That Affect Cost: Findings from an Economic Evaluation of Centers for Disease Control and Prevention National Program of Cancer Registries." *Journal of Public Health Management and Practice: JPHMP* 22, no.5,(2016): 452-60. https://doi.org/10.1097/PHH.0000000000000349; cancer.gov, "About the SEER Registries, "https://seer.cancer.gov/registries/.

24   M. Padek et al., "Toward optimal implementation of cancer prevention and control programs in public health: a study protocol on mis-implementation," *Implementation Sci* 13, no. 49, (2018), https://doi.org/10.1186/s13012-018-0742-9.

25   A. Vogt et al., "Multiple Primary Tumors: Challenges and Approaches: A Review," *European Society for Medical Oncology Open* (2017): e000172,. https://doi.org/10.1136/esmoopen-2017-000172; A. Coyte, D.S. Morrison, and P. McLoone, "Second Primary Cancer Risk: The Impact of Applying Different Definitions of Multiple Primaries: Results from a Retrospective Population-based Cancer Registry Study," *BioMed Central: Cancer* 14, no. 272 (2014): https://doi.org/10.1186/1471-2407-14-272; B. Perez-Nevot, "Cumulative Risk of Second Primary Contralateral Breast Cancer in BRCA1/BRCA2 Mutation Carriers with a First Breast Cancer: A Systematic Review and Meta-analysis," *Breast* 23 (2014): 721–42, https://doi.org/10.1016/j.breast.2014.10.005. https://seer.cancer.gov/statistics/types/incidence.html.

26   Alexia Vogt et al., 2.

27   Cancer.gov, "Cancer Incidence Statistics," https://surveillance.cancer.gov/statistics/types/incidence.html.

28 American Cancer Society, "Decades-Long Drop in Breast Cancer Death Rate Continues," October 2, 2019 https://www.sciencedaily.com/releases/2019/10/191002102757.htm.

29 National Cancer Institute, "Cancer Mortality Rates," https://seer.cancer.gov/statistics/types/mortality.html BC mortality formula.

30 Larissa Nekhlyudov et al., "Integrating Primary Care Providers in the Care of Cancer Survivors: Gaps in Evidence and Future Opportunities," *The Lancet. Oncology* 18, no. 1 (2017): e30-e38, https://doi.org/10.1016/S1470-2045(16)30570-8.

31 Larissa Nekhlyudov, "Overview of Cancer Survivorship Care for Primary Care and Oncology Providers," https://www.uptodate.com/contents/overview-of-cancer-survivorship-care-for-primary-care-and-oncology-providers.

32 Nancy Knoche, "Is the American Cancer Society Putting Money Ahead of Mission?" March 28, 2011, https://nonprofitquarterly.org/is-the-american-cancer-society-putting-money-ahead-of-mission/; Samuel Epstein, *Cancer-Gate: How to Win the Losing Cancer War* (Amityville, NY: Baywood Publishing, 2005).

33 Esther M. John, et al., "Sun Exposure, Vitamin D Receptor Gene Polymorphism, and Breast Cancer Risk in a Multiethnic Population," *American Journal of Epidemiology* 166, no.12 (2007):1409-19, https://doi.org/10.1093/aje/kwm259; Also see Chapter 3.

34 Robert Herrick et al., "Polyfluoroalkyl Substance Exposure in the Mid-Ohio River Valley, 1991-2012," *Environmental Pollution* 228, (2017): 50-60, https://doi.org/10.1016/j.envpol.2017.04.092; Eva C. Bonefeld-Jørgensen et al., "Breast Cancer Risk After Exposure to Perfluorinated Compounds in Danish Women: A Case-control Study Nested in the Danish National Birth Cohort," *Cancer Causes & Control* 25, no. 11 (2014): 1439–48, https://doi.org/10.1007/s10552-014-0446-7.

35 Perri Zeitz Ruckart et al., "Evaluation of Contaminated Drinking Water and Male Breast Cancer at Marine Corps Base Camp Lejeune, North Carolina: A Case Control Study," *Environmental Health* 14, no. 74 (September 16 2015): https://doi.org/10.1186/s12940-015-0061-4; D. Hopey and D. Templeton, "Region at Risk: Can Higher Rates of Death Be Linked to Air Pollution?" *Pittsburgh Post-Gazette*, December 12, 2010, https://www.post-gazette.com/news/health/2010/12/12/Region-at-risk-Can-higher-rates-of-death-be-linked-to-air-pollution/stories/201012120161.

36 National Cancer Institute, "NCI — Cooperative Group — Industry Relationship Guidelines", https://ctep.cancer.gov/industryCollaborations2/guidelines.htm. Last updated: 09/08/17.

37 Patients For Affordable Drugs, "Taxpayer-Funded Drugs and a Pricing Crisis," July 23, 2019, https://www.patientsforaffordabledrugs.org/2019/07/23/nam-comments/.

38 The Massachusetts Cancer Registry collects and shares both tumor- and person-based data from physicians and hospital reports. They were able to send us two charts, each based on these different parameters. The tumor chart showed about a two percent increase in rates over the person-based data.

39 See: Commission on Cancer, "Cancer Registry Quality Control," *Optimal Resources for Cancer Care: 2020 Standards, Effective January 2020,* 57, https://www.facs.org/-/media/files/quality-programs/cancer/coc/optimal_resources_for_cancer_care_2020_standards.ashx; Also see: Commission on Cancer, "Section Two: Instructions for Coding, Outcomes: (Recurrence Data), *FORDS: Facility Oncology Registry Data Standards: 2016,* i-3 & 321-333, https://www.facs.org/-/media/files/quality-programs/cancer/ncdb/fords-2016.ashx.

40 Personal correspondence between Sandra Kwong and Jacquie Ostrom, April 13, 2011.

41 Daniel J. Fitzgibbons, "A Decade After the Woburn Toxic Waste Case, Chemist Still Ponders Truth, Justice," July 23, 2019, https://www.umass.edu/pubaffs/chronicle/archives/00/08-25/decheke41.html; Agency for Toxic Substances and Disease Registry, "Male Breast Cancer Results," https://www.atsdr.cdc.gov/sites/lejeune/malebreastcancerstudy.html.

42 American Cancer Society, "Female Breast Cancer Incidence, 2010–2014," *Breast Cancer Facts and Figures*, 2017–2018, 6, https://www.cancer.org/content/dam/cancer-org/research/cancer-facts-and-statistics/breast-cancer-facts-and-figures/breast-cancer-facts-and-figures-2017-2018.pdf.

43 Edwin Silverberg and Roald N. Grant, "Cancer Statistics 1970," American Cancer Society, https://acsjournals.onlinelibrary.wiley.com/doi/pdf/10.3322/canjclin.20.1.10.

44 R. Siegel, J. Zou and Z. Jemal, "Cancer Statistics 2014," *CA: A Cancer Journal for Clinicians* 64, no. 1 (January/February 2014): 9-29, https://doi.org/10.3322/caac.21208.

45 A. Patrick Schneider 2nd et al., "The Breast Cancer Epidemic: 10 Facts," *The Linacre Quarterly* 81, no. 3 (2014): 244-77, https://doi.org/10.1179/2050854914Y.0000000027.

46 Estelle Sommeiller and Mark Price,"The New Gilded Age: Income Inequality in the US by State, Metropolitan Area, and County," Economic Policy Institute, July 19, 2018, https://www.epi.org/publication/the-new-gilded-age-income-inequality-in-the-u-s-by-state-metropolitan-area-and-county/.

47 NAACCR, Annual Report to the Nation, 2020, https://www.naaccr.org/annual-report-to-the-nation/.

48 "NAACCR Age-Adjusted Incidence Rates and 95% Confidence Intervals, 2000 US Standard Population By Age At Diagnosis; Female Breast, All Races, Female, U.S. Combined 2012-2016", custom report for Busting Breast Cancer from NAACCR, 2012.

49 A. J. Redig and S. McAllister, "Breast Cancer as a Systemic Disease: A View of Metastasis," *Journal of Internal Medicine* 274, no. 2, (2013): 113-26, https://doi.org/10.1111/joim.12084.

50 American College of Surgeons, National Cancer Database 2017; Judith A Malmgren et al., "Differential Presentation and Survival of De Novo and Recurrent Metastatic Breast Cancer Over Time: 1990-2010," *Breast Cancer Research and Treatment* 167, no.2 (2018): 579-590, https://doi.org/10.1007/s10549-017-4529-5.

51 Charlotte Bath, "Increase in Advanced Breast Cancer among Younger Women Is Small but Significant, and Trend Is Likely to Continue," May 1, 2013, https://www.ascopost.com/issues/may-1-2013/increase-in-advanced-breast-cancer-among-younger-women-is-small-but-significant/.

52 Archie Bleyer and H. Gilbert Welch, "Effect of Three Decades of Screening Mammography on Breast-Cancer Incidence," *The New England Journal of Medicine* 2371998-2005, (November 22, 2012): https://doi.org/10.1056/NEJMoa1206809; Also see: Chapter 5.

53 Since de novo metastatic cancer denotes that one or more metastatic tumors have been found, rather than one or more early-stage primary tumors in the breast, NCI and other government data bases are actually counting women, in this instance, not a woman's primary tumors.

54 R.H. Johnson, F.L. Chien and A. Bleyer, "Incidence of Breast Cancer With Distant Involvement Among Women in the United States, 1976 to 2009," *JAMA: Journal of the American Medical Association* 309, no.8 (2013):800–05, https://doi.org/10.1001/jama.2013.776.

55 Monte Morin, "Breast Cancer Among Young Women Increasing," *Los Angeles Times*, February 26,2013, https://www.latimes.com/health/la-xpm-2013-feb-26-la-sci-breast-cancer-younger-women-20130227-story.html.

56 American College of Surgeons National Cancer Database, https://www.facs.org/quality-programs/cancer/ncdb.

57 Ibid.

58 T. Takeshita et al., "Late recurrence of breast cancer is associated with pro-cancerous immune microenvironment in the primary tumor," *Scientific Reports* 9, no.16942 (2019), https://doi.org/10.1038/s41598-019-53482-x.

59 Nick Mulcahy, "The Mystery of a Common Breast Cancer Statistic," *Medscape*, March 14, 2020, https://www.medscape.com/viewarticle/849644#vp_1; Marc Hurlbert, "Where is the Data? The Epidemiology of Metastatic Breast Cancer," *Huffington Post*, October 6, 2017, https://www.huffpost.com/entry/where-is-the-data-the-epi_b_12311030; Kate Pickert, "Why the Women Most Likely to Die of Breast Cancer have Gotten the Least Attention," *Time*, Oct 1, 2019, https://time.com/5689570/metastatic-breast-cancer-research-treatment/.

60 T.N. Seyfried and L.C. Huysentruyt, "On the Origin of Cancer Metastasis," *Critical Reviews in Oncogenesis* 18, no. (2013): 43-73, https://doi.org/10.1615/critrevoncog.v18.i1-2.40; E. Cho, et al., "Breast Cancer Cutaneous Metastasis at Core Needle Biopsy Site, *Annals of Dermatology* 22, no. 2 (2010): 238-40, https://doi.org/10.5021/ad.2010.22.2.238; N.M. Hansen et al, "Manipulation of the Primary Breast Tumor and Incidence of Sentinel Node Metastases From Invasive Breast Cancer," *The Archives of Surgery: JAMA* 139, June 2004, 634-39; https://doi.org/10.1001/archsurg.139.6.634; K, Shyamala et al., "Risk of Tumor Cell Seeding Through Biopsy and Aspiration Cytology," *Journal of International Society of Preventive & Community Dentistry* 4, no.1 (2014): 5-11. https://doi.org/10.4103/2231-0762.129446; Isaiah J. Fidler, "The Pathogenesis of Cancer Metastasis: The 'Seed and Soil' Hypothesis Revisited, Perspectives," *Nature Review/Cancer* 3, June 2003, https://doi.org/10.1038/nrc1098; G. Szalayova et al., "Human Breast Cancer Biopsies Induce Eosinophil Recruitment and Enhance Adjacent Cancer Cell Proliferation," *Breast Cancer Research Treatment* 157, no. 3 (June 2016), 461-74, https://doi.org/10.1007/s10549-016-3839-3.

61 Abdulaziz Alsaif, "Breast Cancer Recurrence After Sentinel Lymph Node Biopsy," *Pakistan Journal of Medical Sciences* 31, no. 6 (2015): 1426-31. https://doi.org/10.12669/pjms.316.8427.

62 A.B. Mariotto, et al., "Estimation of the Number of Women Living with Metastatic Breast Cancer in the United States," *Cancer Epidemiology, Biomarkers and Prevention* 26, no.6 (June 2017): 809-15, https://doi.org/10.1158/1055-9965.

63 Commission on Cancer, "Cancer Registry Quality Control," *Optimal Resources for Cancer Care: 2020 Standards, Effective January 2020*, 57, https://www.facs.org/-/media/files/quality-programs/cancer/coc/optimal_resources_for_cancer_care_2020_standards.ashx.

64 N Berkowitz, S Gupta and G Silberman, "Estimates of the Lifetime Direct Costs of Treatment for Metastatic Breast Cancer," *Value In Health* 3, no.1(2000):23-30, doi: 10.1046/j.1524-4733.2000.31003.x.

65 Joyce O'Shaughnessy, "Treatment Advances in Solid Tumors During the Past Decade: Benchmark Studies Impacting Survival and Quality of Life," *The Oncologist* 10, no. S3 (October 2005): 20-9, https://doi.org/10.1634/theoncologist.10-90003-20.

66 A. J. Redig and S. McAllister, "Breast Cancer as a Systemic Disease: A View of Metastasis," *Journal of Internal Medicine* 274, no. 2 (2013): 113-26, https://doi.org/10.1111/joim.12084.

67 Nick Mulcahy, "The Mystery of a Common Breast Cancer Statistic," Medscape, March 14, 2020, https://www.medscape.com/viewarticle/849644; Takeshita et al., "Late recurrence of breast cancer is associated with pro-cancerous immune microenvironment in the primary tumor."

68 M.C. van Maaren et al., "Ten-Year Recurrence Rates for Breast Cancer Subtypes in the Netherlands: A Large Population-Based Study," *Cancer Epidemiology* 144 (October 28, 2018): 26-72, https://doi.org/10.1002/ijc.31914; Also see: Y. M. Geurts et al., "Patterns and Predictors of First and Subsequent Recurrence in Women with Early Breast Cancer," *Breast Cancer Research and Treatment* 165, no.3, (2017): 709-20, https://doi.org/10.1007/s10549-017-4340-3.

69 Katarzyna Pogoda et al., "Analysis of Pattern, Time and Risk Factors Influencing Recurrence in Triple-negative Breast Cancer Patients," *Medical Oncology* 30, no.1 (2013): 388. https://doi.org/10.1007/s12032-012-0388-4.

70 B.C. Haffty et al., "Locoregional Relapse and Distant Metastasis in Conservatively Managed Triple Negative Early Stage Breast Cancer," *Journal of Clinical Oncology* 24, no.36 (December 20, 2006): 5652-57, https://doi.org/10.1200/JCO.2006.06.5664.

71 Ibid.

72 Triple-Negative Breast Cancer Foundation, "TNBC Forum," https://forum.tnbcfoundation.org.

73 Sumayah Al-mahmood et al., "Metastatic and Triple-negative Breast Cancer: Challenges and Treatment Options," *Drug Delivery and Translational Research* 8, no. 5 (2018): 1483-1507, https://doi.org/10.1007/s13346-018-0551-3.

74 Joshua Emerson Smith, "California's Effort to Improve Cancer Registry Signals Shift to Preventative Care," California Health Report, September 14, 2015, https://www.calhealthreport.org/2015/09/14/californias-efforts-to-improve-cancer-registry-signals-shift-to-preventative-care/.

75 Bernie Sanders, with Huck Gutman, *Outsider in the House* (Brooklyn, NY: Verso, 1997) 156. Also see Sanders's and Gutman's revised 2015 edition of the book.

76 The legislation is available at https://www.cdc.gov/cancer/npcr/npcrpdfs/publaw.pdf.

77 Sanders and Gutman, *Outsider in the White House*, 155.

78 Public Law 102-515—Cancer Registries Amendment Act, October 24, 1992, 102nd Congress 106 STAT, 3372, https://www.cdc.gov/cancer/npcr/npcrpdfs/publaw.pdf.

79 Diane Mapes, "New Study Estimates Number of U.S. Women Living with Metastatic Breast Cancer, May 17, 2017, Fred Hutch New Service, https://www.fredhutch.org/en/news/center-news/2017/05/new-nci-study-estimates-metastatic-breast-cancer-rates.html.

80 Mary Engel, "Beth Caldwell's impact on metastatic breast cancer: By living—and dying—out loud, @CultPerfectMoms gave a voice to #stage4 that will not be silenced," *Fred Hutch News Service*, November 3, 2017, www.fredhutch.org/en/news/center-news/2017/11/beth-caldwell-impact-metastatic-breast-cancer.html.

10 BUSTING BREAST CANCER'S ACTION AGENDA

Individual women in the US are clearly under siege by an unnecessary breast cancer epidemic. Individual women also form the only group in the US today with the self-interest and now, with enough knowledge, to stop this unnecessary scourge. This can happen as one woman at a time uses the five simple breast cancer prevention steps described in this book. *Busting Breast Cancer's Action Agenda*, however, describes seven steps the US government can take to support women on their individual prevention journeys. Six of these items are straightforward administrative changes or requests for funds to launch primary prevention education campaigns. The final and 7th agenda item requests funding for a number of clinical trials that can evaluate the ability of metabolic therapies to help prevent or lower current recurrent metastatic breast cancer rates.

Each of these agenda items requires a specific agency within the federal government to place women's breast cancer prevention needs before the ongoing profit goals of the pharmaceutical industry and other commercial partners in today's booming breast cancer screening, diagnosis and treatment business. Women's groups on the local, state and federal levels may be the only forces interested in implementing this entire agenda. This means...*none of these agenda items will happen until women demand that such lifesaving and inexpensive changes take place!*

Action #1:

Remove the National Academy of Medicine (NAM) from its current control over our federal DGAs and RDAs.
Replace this powerful industry lobby with an independent objective panel of nutritional and functional medicine experts.

Background:
The National Academy of Medicine (NAM), one of the most powerful corporate lobbies in Washington, is funded by the processed food, pharmaceutical, medical, agribusiness, and chemical industries. Congress continues to informally give NAM the final authority over the legally mandated periodic

revisions to our federal Dietary Guidelines for Americans (DGAs) and our Recommended Daily Allowance for Vitamins and Minerals (RDAs). NAM's self-serving DGAs and RDAs have subsequently been funded and enforced by the US government for the past two decades, helping create today's expanding obesity epidemic and our vitamin D3 deficiency epidemic. Both of these preventable situations directly contribute to today's breast cancer epidemic. Under the powers of the National Nutrition Monitoring and Research Act of 1990, Section 102 8 (B), the Secretary of Health and Human Services oversees the administration of this law. The Secretary, therefore, has the power to replace NAM's oversight control with objective and independent nutritionists and functional medicine experts, i.e., individuals who do not have financial ties to any of the industries that annually fund NAM today. **For further background, see <u>Chapter 2</u> and <u>Chapter 3</u>.**

Action #2:

Request $7.4 million or more in funding from the Breast Cancer Research Program (BCRP) to establish the multi-year *National Safe Contraceptives/Safe HRT Campaign*.

This national education project will finally inform and educate women and health practitioners about the Penninger-Glimcher team's 2010 landmark discovery of how the progestin chemical in all contraceptive drugs, some IUDs, and some HRT drugs, initiates and accelerates breast cancer in current users. *The National Safe Contraceptives/Safe HRT Campaign* is primary prevention at its best. This campaign includes a contraceptive counseling component to help interested women safely and swiftly find equally effective and affordable, reversible or permanent hormone-free contraceptives and helps postmenopausal women find natural alternatives for relief of menopausal symptoms.

Using guidelines that can be developed by national independent breast cancer prevention and education organizations such as Breast Cancer Prevention Partners and Breast Cancer Action, this education campaign can significantly reduce breast cancer incidence in women of all ages. BCRP funding can enable a diverse network of existing women's health groups at the national, regional, state and local levels to implement this campaign for safe contraceptives and safe HRT options.

Background:

The BCRP's mission, with it $150 million annual budget, is "to challenge the scientific community to design research that will address the urgency of ending breast cancer. Specifically, the BCRP seeks to accelerate high-impact research with clinical relevance, encourage innovation and stimulate creativity, and facilitate productive collaborations...Considering the current breast cancer landscape and the BCRP's mission to end breast cancer, the BCRP seeks applications that address...overarching challenges, preventing breast cancer (primary prevention) and identifying determinants of breast cancer initiation, risk, or susceptibility..."

In 2012 the national Breast Cancer Research Program (BCRP) awarded Dr. Josef Penninger its annual $7.4 million Innovator Award, in recognition of the importance of the groundbreaking 2010 Penninger-Glimcher Study that discovered exactly how the progestin chemical, found in all hormonal contraceptives today and in progestin HRT drugs, can initiate the creation and accelerate the progress of breast cancer in current progestin drug users. The BCRP fully understands the ground-breaking primary prevention significance of this 2010 discovery, making them the perfect federal funding source for the national Safe Contraceptives/Safe HRT Campaign. **For further background see Chapter 4.**

Action #3:

Request that the Secretary of Health and Human Services or the FDA director reclassify hormone-free IUDs, restoring them to their original classification as *medical devices.*

This single administrative change will allow US women access to safer, better-fitting and affordable hormone-free IUDs. It will also reduce many low income or uninsured women's forced dependence on currently less expensive, but risky, progestin-based contraceptive drugs.

Background:

In 1999, the FDA re-classified long-popular inexpensive and hormone-free IUDs (medical devices) as "pharmaceutical drugs." This administrative move blocked any additional hormone-free IUD makes, models and sizes from entering the US market. Under their new classification as a "pharmaceutical drug," all new IUDs were now required to undergo prohibitively expensive ten-year double-blind placebo clinical studies before being allowed to be sold on the US market. Such costly trials have served to block any newer, safer and inexpensive progestin-free IUDs from the US market. This 1999 reclassification also created a monopoly market for the Paragard, still the single existing hormone-free IUD sold in the US. Over the past few decades the cost of a single Paragard IUD (manufactured for less than $5) has now risen to the exorbitant monopoly price of $800, not including the $200 insertion fee charged by clinics!

Once the FDA returns the Paragard copper coil and all other hormone-free IUDs to their original FDA classification as "medical devices," this single stroke of the FDA's pen will immediately drop the price of all hormone-free IUDs to competitive prices under $50@, as dozens of makes, models and sizes of safe and affordable hormone-free IUDs manufactured and sold in Europe since 1999, are made available to US women. This single administrative change will enable millions of younger women to afford to safely switch off of today's risky progestin contraceptive drugs. **For further background, see Chapter 4.**

Action #4:

Require the FDA to allow government health insurance plans and private health insurers to cover annual thermography screening for the diagnosis of cancer-causing breast *inflammation*.

Background:
Breast inflammation is the most significant early signal or precursor to the development of DCIS (stage 0) and invasive breast cancer (stages I-IV). Thermography is the best way for women to annually monitor the amount of inflammation in their breast tissue. Once breast inflammation is identified, a woman can begin to mitigate or eliminate this inflammation, using Busting Breast Cancer's prevention steps. **For further background, see Chapter 5.**

Action #5:

The Safe Breast Screening and Diagnostic Project:

This is a national primary prevention campaign to inform and teach women the benefits of regular breast self-exams (BSEs) and having regular clinical breast exams (CBEs).

Part I:
Request NIH funding to conduct objective clinical studies that illustrate the ability of breast self-exams (BSEs) and clinical breast exams (CBEs), including the use of new elastography technologies, to identify significant breast masses, especially in obese and overweight women, in women with larger breasts, and in women with dense breast tissue.

Part II:
Request that the BCRP fund a primary prevention campaign to inform and teach women the benefits of BSEs, breast massage, and CBEs as a safe and effective way for most women of all ages to regularly screen for fast-growing, potentially dangerous, palpable breast tumors.

Part III:
Request the FDA to approve federal and private health insurance coverage for ultrasound tumor diagnostic testing of any palpable breast masses, without first requiring physicians to order an invasive and potentially dangerous mammogram for the patient.

Background:
The radiology industry continues to control federal medical insurance regulations that require each woman to have a mammogram before being able to have an ultrasound breast screening or ultrasound diagnostic exam. In addition, the Komen Foundation, the largest supporter of community-based breast cancer groups and family planning clinics, refuses to fund any organization for any programs if they mention, educate or offer any services related to breast self-exams! The American Cancer Society also instructs women not to have regular clinical breast exams! This misinformation coming from these organizations, both heavily funded by the radiology industry, must be countered with federally funded programs that offer women factual and supportive information about the benefits of regular radiation-free breast massage, regular breast self-exams and having regular clinical breast exams. **For further background, see Chapter 5.**

Action #6:

Share all currently mandated recurrent metastatic breast cancer incidence data with the US public.

Background:

Today's data on recurrent metastatic breast cancer (rMBC) incidence, reported to the industry-based Commission on Cancer (CoC), and collected from physicians by each state cancer registry, continue to be withheld from the US public. This is an unacceptable practice. The CoC mandates that physicians and cancer centers immediately report each of their patients' breast cancer recurrence data to state cancer agencies and to the CoC. Published peer-reviewed clinical studies report that 20–40 percent of all women treated for early-stage invasive breast cancer in the US go on to develop recurrent metastatic breast cancer (rMBC), an early death sentence for each woman. These critical recurrence numbers should be immediately released to the US public. **For further background, see <u>Chapter 9.</u>**

Action #7:

Fund clinical studies to establish the most effective therapies for treating all types of breast cancer diagnoses.

Background:

The incidence of recurrent metastatic breast cancer appears to be increasing each year throughout the United States. In order to effectively manage all types of metastatic breast cancer cases, metabolic cancer clinics in Turkey, Egypt, and Hungary are now using various evolving metabolic protocols (inexpensive and nontoxic) to successfully manage this stage IV disease.[1] At the same time, many individual breast cancer patients worldwide, facing all stages, and all types of cancers, are pioneers, as they continue to use various metabolic protocols that often offer cancer patients effective disease management, along with the ability to achieve optimal health. There is no longer a need to hope; more hope continues to arrive for more patients in the form of nontoxic metabolic therapies.

But such clinical results, currently known to only a limited number of scientists, clinicians and patients, must now be established as an option for all breast cancer patients through CoC-approved and/or NCI-approved clinical trials. Such clinical studies, funded by the NCI, can establish the importance of using only metabolic therapies in the effective management of all stages of breast cancer, while also significantly reducing rMBC rates. Additional clinical trials can evaluate the efficacy of combining mainstream therapies with metabolic therapies. Separate sets of such comparative trials can also evaluate the exclusive use of metabolic protocols in the treatment of DCIS (stage 0 or non-invasive breast cancer). Finally, leading scientists and clinicians involved in the development and implementation of today's metabolic therapies must be given responsibility for the design and management of all trials that include any types of metabolic therapies, with CoC and NCI oversight. **For further background, see Chapter 1 and Chapter 7.**

Taking Action:

As mentioned, each of these agenda items requires a specific agency within the federal government to place women's breast cancer prevention needs before agencies' current habits of funding predominantly blockbuster drugs, or diagnostic and treatment procedures. Each of these prevention-based action items also requires existing women's health and breast cancer groups, ad hoc coalitions, along with small groups of concerned individuals to contact their elected representatives, write letters to the President and First Lady, the Secretary of Health and Human Services, the Breast Cancer Research Program and other agencies to help effect these changes. All such requests must also be publicized in electronic and print media. The squeaky wheel gets the oil. Let's all begin to squeak wherever we go, until Busting Breast Cancer's seven action steps are taken.

CHAPTER ENDNOTES

1   Ahmed M.A. Elsakka et al., "Management of Glioblastoma Multiforme in a Patient Treated With Ketogenic Metabolic Therapy and Modified Standard of Care: A 24-Month Follow-Up," *Frontiers in Nutrition* 5, no.20 (March 29, 2018): https://doi.org/10.3389/fnut.2018.00020; T.N. Seyfried et al., "Press-pulse: A Novel Therapeutic Strategy for the Metabolic Management of Cancer," *Nutrition and Metabolism* 14, no.19 (2017), https://doi.org/10.1186/s12986-017-0178-2; Mehmet Salih Iyikesici et al., "Efficacy of Metabolically Supported Chemotherapy Combined with Ketogenic Diet, Hyperthermia, and Hyperbaric Oxygen Therapy for Stage IV Triple-Negative Breast Cancer." *Cureus* 9, no.7 e1445 (July 7, 2017), https://doi.org/10.7759/cureus.1445. T.N. Seyfried, et al., "Consideration of Ketogenic Metabolic Therapy as a Complementary or Alternative Approach for Managing Breast Cancer," *Frontiers in Nutrition* 7, no. 21, (March 2020): 1-11, https://doi.org/10.3389/fnut.2020.00021.

CONCLUSION
CARING FOR OURSELVES EFFECTIVELY AND BUSTING THIS UNNECESSARY EPIDEMIC

"Real progress in the cancer war will be realized only after the cancer field breaks its addiction to the genetic theory and recognizes the centrality of mitochondrial damage in the origin and progression of the disease."

—Dr. Thomas N. Seyfried, The Metabolic Theory of Cancer: On the Origin, Management and Prevention of Cancer

"The sense of pleasing herself has been a very rare experience for most women; and when they attain it, it is a new found joy."

—Dr. Jean Baker Miller, Toward a New Psychology of Women

When I first heard about the new metabolic understanding of cancer, along with the importance of mitochondria within this new approach, I quietly had to confide to myself that I was not sure if mitochondria lived inside a cell, or outside a cell, let alone what this five-syllable word was supposed to do, and was the word *mitochondria* singular or plural? If mitochondria respired, was respiration different from breathing? If these little power batteries preferred to feed off of ketones, rather than the glucose we gobble up all day long, what are ketones, what do they do, and where do these ketones come from?

Gradually, I began to relax as I came to realize that any basic questions I needed to ask, as I tried to understand the bare bones of this metabolic approach to cancer, could be clearly answered. These answers were biological facts that science has understood for years. Our mitochondria, their prehistoric structure, and many of their functions, are part and parcel of today's accepted evolutionary biology that makes each of us tick. However, no one, until recently, had paid attention to one of our mitochondria's many abilities. This is the fact that when mitochondria suffocate and are no longer able to process healthy, life-giving oxygen, they can undergo a zombie-like transformation. Instead of dying as they begin to suffocate, they are able to revert back to using their prehistoric operating system; they become like their ancestors, glucose-guzzling fermenting bacteria! At this point, instead of dying, the mitochondria signal to their cell's nucleus to activate genes that now create the chaotic cascade of events we called *cancer*. Who knew?

Today's mainstream cancer industry has not yet embraced this concept that the mitochondria control the onset, the acceleration and the demise of each cancer cell. And so, the forces driving this industry cannot explain, for example, why one woman develops breast cancer, when another does not. Today's cancer industry, having gone down the wrong road for over fifty years, now finds it very hard to even think about retooling its current production line. Doing so would mean replacing a financially successful "standard of care" machine with much less profitable products. Therefore, today's cancer industry continues trying to figure out why one woman develops breast cancer, but another never does. Without understanding the precise origin of that first cancer cell, however, the industry is unable to educate anyone, including themselves, on effective cancer prevention steps.

Busting Breast Cancer is the good news book that women have been hoping and waiting for. The five simple prevention steps described in these past chapters are able to help us protect our breast cells' mitochondria, those tiny but mighty power batteries, from suffocation. This means that we finally have the necessary knowledge to keep breast cancer out of our bodies. Alleluia.

As I first ventured into the field of breast cancer prevention twelve years ago, I just kept asking my two basic questions: "Why does one woman develop breast cancer, but another never does? How can I keep breast cancer from developing in my body?" Too many of my friends were getting sick, and too many of my friends had already died, once their early breast cancer diagnoses turned metastatic.

Instead of hearing factual or biologically-based explanations, as I began my research, all I heard from our national breast cancer authorities, including Susan G. Komen for the Cure, the American Cancer Society, and the message conveyed by the multitudes of pink ribbons that appear every October, was a single statement: "Make sure to have a mammogram each year to see if you have developed a tumor yet." This is not cancer prevention; I knew that much. I have too many dead friends to prove it.

Once a breast tumor is diagnosed and a women asks her physician, "Why me?" the response is often, "Maybe it was just your turn," or, "I guess you are just the unlucky one," or, "Do you have a family history?" Physicians can say little more, as no one in today's medical schools or cancer centers has yet been allowed to teach our oncologists, radiologists, surgeons and family practitioners how the health of our mitochondria determine why and how one woman develops breast cancer, but another woman never does.

Today's cancer industry is little more than a narrow-minded, centrally regulated, government-subsidized, expanding and highly profitable monolithic industry. The idea of "first do no harm" has been thrown by the wayside as breasts are mutilated and amputated, as hair follicles are poisoned and fall out. Women are erroneously told, "Healthy cells must sometimes be destroyed in order to stop the bad guys."

Clinical studies that compare the use of *only* metabolic cancer treatments that starve cancer cells to death, without first subjecting patients to today's brutal "standard of care treatments" (radiation, surgical mutilation, and chemotherapy), are currently not allowed to take place in the US. The industry, protected by its own governing body, the Commission on Cancer, maintains iron-fisted control over what treatments are allowed or required. Physicians can lose their state medical licenses if they stray from the industry's dogmatic path of "standard of care" treatments.

An estimated 120 women die every day in the US while undergoing today's standard of care treatment for their metastatic breast cancer diagnoses, while more than 1600 people continue to die in the US each day while being treated with these same standard of care treatments for all types of cancer. This adds up to over a half million children and adults who are being unnecessarily sacrificed each year in the US alone, all because of an exclusive, misguided, rigid and powerful industry that continues to ban trials of any new, even biologically proven, metabolic cancer approaches and treatments.

Dr. Seyfried's stunning 2012 biological treatise, *Cancer as a Metabolic Disease: On the Origin, Management and Prevention of Cancer*, details how a person's initial cancer cell actually develops from that cell's suffocating mitochondria. Biologists, oncologists, and other scientifically minded individuals can read his textbook, happily venturing into the weeds of historical and recent biological knowledge; knowledge that continues to be ignored by today's mainstream cancer leaders. In his book, the Boston College professor, an award-winning biologist trained in genetics, grounded by fifty years of pre-clinical or laboratory work, much of it focused on the nature of metastatic tumors and on a variety of rare genetic diseases, has collected hundreds of scientific papers published over past decades that together explain how and why that first cancer cell does not begin with a mutating nuclear gene, but with our suffocating mitochondria. His textbook also describes the importance of managing cancer diagnoses by blocking cancer cells from processing or fermenting their favorite fuels, glucose, along with glutamine.

Glutamine is an essential amino acid that our bodies are able to make in huge quantities, as it is one of the most important amino acids required to maintain optimal health. Targeting this important cancer cell fuel to eliminate cancer cells can be difficult to achieve without depleting a patient's healthy cells' need for a continuous supply of this important amino acid. Dr. Seyfried, with the support of leading biochemists in the field of mitochondrial proteins within solid tumors, is now developing effective protocols to solve this problem.[1]

Since I first reached out to Dr. Seyfried in 2013, he has continued to generously offer me his guidance and collegial support. His mentoring has given me the information and the courage needed to complete this book. Reading Travis Christofferson's 2014 book, *Tripping Over the Truth: How the Metabolic Theory of Cancer Is Overturning One of Medicine's Most Entrenched Paradigms*, helped me further grasp the most important steps within this new understanding of how cancer develops. Christofferson's compelling narrative follows Dr. Seyfried's journey as the biologist, his students and lab staff uncover those earlier-published, but long-ignored and now-forgotten studies that clearly illustrate how, in each step within the cancer formation process, our cells' mitochondria call the critical shots.

The Breast Cancer Prevention Steps

In 2013, when I first heard about Dr. Seyfried's book detailing the complete theory of cancer as a metabolic disease, I had already spent a few years poring over breast cancer prevention studies from around the world. These were mainly epidemiological or statistical studies, done by hundreds of researchers that together offered overwhelming quantitative evidence that chronic obesity, different levels of radiation exposure, the progestin chemical in contraceptive drugs and in some IUDs and some HRT drugs, along with unbalanced or toxic estrogen levels (not estrogen *per se*!) often found in our food, and those chemical-like estrogens found in personal care products, cosmetics and plastics in the US today, along with a person's chronic low vitamin D3 blood levels, were somehow all helping create or enable those first breast cancer cells to develop in more and more women. Of course, none of these researchers were able to connect their statistical findings directly to breast cancer's biological origin; Dr Seyfried's 2012 book, had not yet been published.

Today, each of Busting Breast Cancer's chapters is constructed using a distillation of decades of epidemiological knowledge, securely placed within the metabolic theory, to create five effective biology-based and statistically proven prevention steps. Without the work of Dr. Seyfried and his expanding team of metabolic researchers, and without the statistical findings of these hundreds of breast cancer epidemiologists included in these chapters, *Busting Breast Cancer* could not have been written.

Here's a quick recap of the five simple breast cancer prevention steps one more time (please see Chapters 2 through 6 for full details). Begin by burning off that batch of excess fat from your body, especially around your middle. This can immediately ratchet down that inflammation now pulsating throughout your breast cells and probably the rest of your body, every day, all day. Second, raise your vitamin D3 blood level above 60 ng/ml by adding in enough supplements, fat loss, sunshine and/or indoor tanning. Now your immune system is powered up enough to stop the development of even the fastest-growing breast cancer cells.

Third, take time to thoughtfully move away from your progestin birth control drugs or progestin-laced IUD, and instead choose a hormone-free

IUD, or another hormone-free contraceptive option. The award-winning Penninger-Glimcher 2010 study, still being kept hush-hush from the public, finally shows how the progestin in these drugs begins the process of initiating and accelerating breast cancer in current users.

Also, have an estrogen balancing and an estrogen metabolite test, to figure out whether your hormones are currently imbalanced or in balance! This is important for all women: premenopausal, perimenopausal, and postmenopausal. Then explore natural ways to end the discomforts that accompany imbalanced or fluctuating hormones. There is rarely a need to resort to dangerous progestin drugs, at any age.

Fourth, begin to choose personal care products, cosmetics and foods that contain only natural, non-GMO ingredients to help keep toxic chemicals out of your body. Begin a gentle exercise practice, enjoy regular infrared saunas or high-sweat exercises, and practice intermittent fasting as you fill your body with clean, filtered water. All of these choices can help detoxify the cells throughout your breasts and the rest of your body, clearing out the cellular "exhaust," generated by high-carbohydrate (high starch and glucose) eating and by the variety of chemicals and excess hormones your body is probably absorbing every day.

Fifth, say goodbye to those brutal and invasive mammogram machines. Instead, make sure to enjoy breast massage and do a lot of breast self-exams. Also have an annual clinical breast exam, hopefully with a practitioner who utilizes the new hand-held SureTouch elastography scanner. Finally, having an anually regulation thermogram or infrared imaging thermogram, each using updated, but very different technologies, can identify any precancerous breast inflammation. This gives you a clear signal if your breast cells are inflamed; that's a first step toward developing DCIS or invasive breast cancer. Let your annual thermography report be your wake-up call to begin all of these nourishing early breast cancer prevention practices. Become proactive!

If a suspect lump is discovered, find a health practitioner who is willing to order any one of the many ultrasound breast diagnostic tests now available. There is no longer any need to subject yourself to painful and potentially harmful old-fashioned or "new and improved" radiation-based mammograms. That single mammogram report can open you up to a new life, filled with being overdiagnosed and overtreated, leading to an increased risk of developing recurrent metastatic breast cancer. No wonder Switzerland is considering a nationwide ban on all current and future mammogram clinics, with Canada and the Scandinavian countries not far behind! These are all countries with some form of nonprofit Medicare-like national healthcare system that puts a woman's welfare before industry's desire for expanding profits.

Thankfully, adopting all of these prevention-based lifestyle changes might also help you stay calmer, which, by itself, helps keep the insides of your cells cleansed of toxic levels of stress hormones. Most important, your daily meditation time enables you to shut out external stimuli and helps you notice and connect with your own breath. Meditation practice can lower your body's toxic cortisol hormone levels for at least a part of each day. Meditation is clearly the most important way to nurture and protect your breasts' mitochondria. Who knew?

Preventing rMBC: A Sixth Prevention Step to Consider

We are told that an average of 20–40 percent of the women who are treated for an early-stage breast cancer diagnosis, using today's mandated standard of care therapies, go on to develop recurrent metastatic breast cancer; still an early death sentence for all. Physicians, cancer centers, state cancer registries, the National Cancer Institute, along with investors and managers within our mainstream cancer industry, know these recurrent metastatic numbers very well. After all, metastatic breast cancer drugs fuel the fastest-growing segment of today's booming breast cancer industry, expected to enjoy a 9% CAGR for the coming years. Would rMBC rates decrease sharply if breast biopsies were halted?

The concept that a breast biopsy can initiate recurrent metastatic breast cancer, as described in Chapter 1 and Chapter 9, is the most controversial research included in this book. The studies explaining, describing and calculating this phenomenon continue to mount. But are these studies included in medical school curricula today?

Meanwhile, the number of annual rMBC diagnoses in the US remains hidden from public view, too embarrassing to share. But this growing number of women who are going on to develop rMBC can no longer be ignored. These are all women who have developed this early death sentence of recurrent metastatic breast cancer, *only after* they were "successfully treated" for an early-stage breast cancer diagnosis. So long as the number of women being rediagnosed each year with recurrent metastatic breast cancer is kept out of the public eye, *today's mandatory "standard of care" breast biopsies must remain suspect.*

The Busting Breast Cancer Journey to Activism

Friends, family, funders and creditors continued to grumble because it took me twelve years to independently research and write this book. There was always something more to learn, process, and then write and rewrite, before I felt ready to share this work with others. Many financial supporters lost hope, while new supporters arrived; excited at what I was discovering. But still, I found myself falling deeper into debt, while also feeling guilty about not finishing this work sooner. Finally, I simply surrendered to the uncertainties of this unusual project. Apparently, its completion could or would only happen in its own time.

If you have read through this book, you may have found yourself surrendering to the information within one chapter, but not in another. As a result, you may be willing to adopt one or a few of these five prevention steps. This is wonderful. But if you also decide to share your new prevention choices with others, be prepared! Most of *Busting Breast Cancer's* lifestyle changes, while "simple" to adopt, are not always "simple" for other to accept. Most of these changes require that you go against today's breast cancer authorities. Most of these effective guidelines run counter to the oncology, radiology, and pharmaceutical industries' beliefs. Most of these steps go against today's federal guidelines on "best" nutrition practices, "best" vitamin D3 guidelines, "best" contraceptive options, "best" breast screening and best tumor diagnostic practices.

Watch out when you share any of these prevention practices out loud; hold yourself steady. Friends, strangers, and physicians may laugh and point fingers, while some will walk away in disdain, their noses sniffing in the air.

Nevertheless, I hope you will take this information on the road, sharing the good news of how most breast cancer can be prevented. It is so important to help yourself and to also help another woman understand effective ways to stop the development of breast cancer at any point during one's life.

> "Harriet Tubman, an escaped African-American slave, did not simply make her way to the North and settle in for a comfortable life. She understood that slavery is as much a mind-set as it is a situation. To free herself internally, she devoted the rest of her life to freeing others. She once said, 'I freed a thousand slaves. I could have freed a thousand more if only they knew they were slaves.' She understood that even when literal freedom is granted, it may not mean the former slave is truly free. There is an internal game change that has to take place. One way to make this internal shift is to become an activist on behalf of others. When you change your perception of yourself from slave to activist, you transform from victim to heroine."
>
> *Regena Thomashauer, Pussy: A Reclamation*

As more women choose to use *Busting Breast Cancer's* five simple prevention steps and share these choices with others, we can each help lower today's unnecessary breast cancer epidemic, one woman at a time. I invite every reader to join me in this effective breast cancer prevention work, our newfound joy.

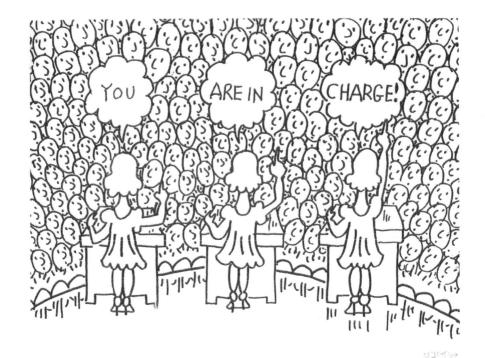

Phyllis Yampolsky 2014 ©

CONCLUSION ENDNOTES

1   Christos Chinopoulos and Thomas N. Seyfried, "Mitochondrial Substrate-Level Phosphorylation as Energy Source for Glioblastoma: Review and Hypothesis," *American Society for Neurochemistry* 10, no. 1759091418818261 (2018): 1-27, https://doi.org/10.1177/1759091418818261.

ACKNOWLEDGMENTS

Without this massive group of supporters, this grassroots-powered book would never have been possible.

My first acknowledgement goes to Mary Lou Tierney, *Busting Breast Cancer's* project manager. Without her guidance, discipline, good will and love, this book would never have made it into and through production and into your hands today. I also remain in awe of *Busting Breast Cancer's* designer, Tessa Magnuson of Align Graphic Design. Her work is always beautiful, creative and impeccable. And special thanks to that one editor, out of many, who took the "nastiness" out of my writing!

I also especially want to thank everyone who has donated their time and their dollars over the past twelve years because they believed in the possibilities of this project, which in fact only begin now with the publication of this book. Special thanks also go to Joan Loomis Hastings and Jane Lothrop Gardiner, whose steadfast personal belief in me and strong financial support enabled me to begin and complete this work.

Each person included here—as well as those inadvertently forgotten—has been important in the creation of this book. Hopefully, *Busting Breast Cancer* can now launch a grassroots movement that brings about effective change in both the prevention and treatment of this unnecessary twenty-first century disease.

In gratitude:

Foundations:

Foundation For Metabolic Cancer Therapies, Rapid City, SD

Community Foundation of the Florida Keys, Key West, FL

Essex County Community Foundation, Danvers, MA

Shirley Freeman and Harvey Server Environmental Fund, Key West, FL

Lloyd Symington Foundation, San Anselmo, CA

The Benevity Community Impact Fund, Hudson, OH

The Catherine F. and James H. Stentzel Foundation, Key West, FL

Organizations:

29 Concord Condominium Trust, Cambridge, MA

7th Wave Design, Key West, FL

Align Graphic Design, LLC, Pembroke NH

Annie Appleseed Project, West Palm Beach, FL

Archer Insurance, Beverly, MA

Beyond Pink, Spokane, WA

Blue Pencil Consulting

Cannon Murray Law, LLC, Gloucester, MA

Common Crow, Glouceser, MA

Coastal Auto, Manchester, MA

Cure To Cancer Summit

DCIS-411

Debra Lunt Hair Salon, Beverly Farms, MA

Dixie Mills, MD, Boston, MA

Duckworth's Bistrot, Gloucester, MA

Edits Made Easy

Energy Bits LLC, Boston MA

Fifteen Walnut Tavern, Hamilton, MA

Girl Friday Productions

Headline Hair and Nails, Key West, FL

Healing Way Center, Andover, MA

Healthy Spirit, Lexington, MA

I Read Labels For You

Keto Evangalist

Keto Mojo

Ketonix

Key West Women's Club

Latitude Design, Beverly, MA

Lisa Traevis, OD, Ipswich, MA

Lumina Hair Salon, Reading, MA

Manchester Community Center, Manchester, MA

Mariposa, Manchester, MA

Metabolic Health Summit

North Shore Business League

Organic Café, Beverly, MA

Organic Rainbow, Beverly, MA

Papalia Home Services, Boxborough, MA

Penta CPA, Hamilton, MA

Praxis Performance and Wellness, Beverly, MA (formerly ClubXcel)

Robert Blake, DDS, Beverly Farms, MA

Rocky Neck Cultural Center, Gloucester, MA

small fish-design, Gloucester, MA

Sugar Apple, Key West, FL

Sunbanque Tanning, Gloucester, MA

Adrea Brier

Jo Broderick

Bob Brown

Connie Brown

Dina Brown

Stephen Brox

Dawn Buchanan

Delores Bujalski

Katie Bull

Lorraine Bunker

Paula Burchart

Donnie Burgess

Stanislaw Burzynski

Stephen Butterfield

Rick Cacace

Rich & Rita Calnan

Kirsten Cameron

Joyce Cannon

Eleanor Carcuru

Amy Carlin

CeAnn Carney

Abra Carotenuto

Melissa Carrier

Joan Cayen

Terry Cellucci

Jenni Ceppi

Roberta Chadis

Travis Christofferson

Lori Clegg

Jim Clyde

Kathy Coakley

Brian Cocierman

Jennifer Cofer

Yuliya Cohen

Sharon Cohen;

Barb Coleman

Lynne G. Comb

Nancy Connoll

Lauren Coogan

Ann Cook

Mary Cooke

Marie Coppola

Al Costanza

Phoebe Coues

Jay Couzens

Liva Cowan

Nany Cowan

George Craig

Sheila Cran-Barry

Bonnie Crane

Sarah Creighton

Christine Cronin

Kimberly Cross

David Crowley

Melissa Cruz

Timmie Cullen

Laura Cutler

Dona D'Ambrosia

Michael Dallas

John Dalpe

Susan Daly

Christian Daoust

Susan Davis

Mary Dawson

Judy Dean

Fran Decker

Lisa DeConto

Louise & Joe DePino

Debora Desherbin

Delores Dickey

Deb Dickinson

Jane Hall Diehl

Sarah Dodd

Glenda Donovan

David Doucette

Christine Drewyer

Geri Duffy

Melanie Dukas

MaryKay Dyer

Mary Eagen

Jean Earle

Karuna Eberl

Georgia Ede MD

Rachel Edelman

Barbara Elliott

Eric Elloie

Laura Ells

Ingrid Emerick

Jane Eonos

Curtis Ersing MD

Adele Ervin

Laura Esserman
MD

James Eves

Donald Ewing

Denice Fabien

Mona Faherty

Jen Falconer

Tricia Fallon

Maureen Fallon

Martha Farmer

Dame Amelia
Fawcett

Myrna Fearer

Marian Feinberg

Ruth Felton;

Patricia Fenton

Susie Field

Mary Ann Fisher

Laurie Fleming

Roxanne Fleszar

Ann Fonfa

Murray Forbes

Sarina Fordice

Anna Forkan

Alice
Forrest-Peschel

Rosemary Fortin

Lydia Foster

Carol Fournier

Marleny Franco

Coleen Franzel

Stewart Fredenksen

Joyce Frederick

Shirley Freeman

Seth Friedman

Claudia Frost

Julia Frost

Belinda Fuch

Marissa Fulmer

Sally Garber

Jane & Charlie
Gardiner

Kim Gaskins

Carlene Gaspar

Robin Gaston

Kathleen Gayron

Sue Gee

Susan George

Anne Gero

Pamela Giarratana

Suzanne Gilbert

Debbie Gilliss

Jim Glefencs

Christina Godshalk

Jonas Goldberg

Eric Goldscheider

Dina Gomery

Michael J. Gonzalez

Nina Goodick

Nancy Goodman

Flash Gordon

Christine Gorham

Richard Graham

Michael Graves

Jon Gray

Deborah Greel

Diane Green

Tim Green

Cheryl Grey

Johanna Griffith

Martha Grubbins

Claude Guerlain

Gale Guild

Mad Jack Gunn

Laurie Gwynne

Judy Hadley

Donald & Nancy
Halgren

Lisa Hall

Michael Halpern

Meagan Hanna

Jamie Hanna

Carolyn Hanna

Carolyn Hardin

Ellen Hardy

Jon Hare

Carol Harkin

George Harrington

Susan Harrington

Ann Harrison

Linda & Richard
Harvey

Wil Hastings

Joan Loomis
Hastings

Patricia Hawkins

Mary Hayes

Mary Healy

Bob Heineman

Elba Herrera

Margaret & Ken
Herriott

Rose Herron

Lee Herter

Sheila Hill

Karen Hillien

Deborah
Hochhauser

Michael Holick MD
PhD

Debora Holland

Linda Holt

Nancy Hopkins

Beth Horne

David Howard

Pam Howard

Joanie Howe

Denny Howley

Rhonda Htoo

Luke Huber, ND

Robert M. Hull, Jr.

Marion Humberson

Betty Hutchins

Kendra Hutchinson

Monique Illona

Lori Incropera

Tim Ingraham

Sharon Jackson

Heidi Jackson-Dean

Nancy Javaris

Carol Johns

Karen Johnson

Anna Judd-Edwards

Miriam Kalamian

Elly, Karin &
Joel Katz

Stuart Kaufman

Craig Kayser

Maryann Keating

Johanna Keefe

Elsa Keefe

Susan Kelly

Jens Ker-Jensen

Will Keyser

Kyle Khani

Lynn Kimball

Sue Kinzie

Richard Klein

Norma Klobucher

Patty Knaggs

David Knoll

Johanna Krelich

Allyn Krieger-
Fiedler ND

Helmut Krieger

Carmen Kruczynski

Ray Krzyzek

Michele Kulick

Judy Kumar

David Lachapelle

Nijole Ladd

Ben LaGuer

Ray Lamont

Janet Landry

Lisa Landy

Kathy Lanford

Tom Lang

Bob Laniak

Steve LaPierre

Maryann Laraia

Kitty Coolidge
  Lastavica, MD

Martha Lazarus

Peter Leando

Carol LeBlanc

Darrow Lebovici

Diane Lee

Tracie Lee

Claire Leggett

Lysa Leland

Caroline Lena

Stacy Lewis

Sho Litchenstein

Lisa Lillelund

Sigrid Lindo

Ron Lipkowitz

Lauren Liss

Bettie J. Little

Susan Livingston

Leslie Lobell

Sheri Lohr

Pauli Loomis

Sally Loring

Nancy Loring

Holly Loring

Deborah Lowery

Debora Lunt

Cindi Luppi

Maureen Lussier

Ben Lynch

Peter Lyons

Lisa Maccario

Lela Maciboba

Annie MacMillian

Tony Maczura

Victoria Madeya

Axel Magnuson

Lindsay Malboeuf

Marie Mancinelli

Christine Mangano

Lee Mantoni

Donna Markussen

Mary Marlow

Kris Maroney

Jane Marshall

Kristen Martin

Annamarie Martin

Sophia Martz

Mary Beth Massilon

Marianne
  Masterson

Jean Matlack

Joseph C. Maroon,
  MD

Bruce Matt

Matuschka

Tim Mayo

Katrina
  Mayo-Smith

Ann McCardle

Gail McCarthy

Charlie McCarthy

Bill & Jane
  McConnell

Robin McQueen

Mark McDonough

Jill McFadgen

Laurie McFarlane

Nancy McGonegan

Alma McLaughlin

Roger McNeise

Jenna McTiernan

Connie McVicker

Kara Mears

Susan Mears

Therese Melden

Luise Mendelso

Dion Mermegas

Jennifer Messier

Melissa Meyers

Kate Miano

Constance Miller

Carol Miller

Stuart Miller

Debbie Milne

David Minkoff MD

Patti Mitchell

Ann Marie Mitchell

Allison Moir-Smith

Christine Moore

Mari Morgen

Kathy Moriconi

Carol Morse

Gar Morse

Pam Morss

Charles Movalli

May Mumma
Ohman

Natalie Munoz

Kris Munroe

Maria Murphy

Bridget Murray

Ed Murray

Lace Murray

Ramona Murray

Marcia Musgrave

Steve Mushkin

Deanna Naddy

Lynn Nadeau

Janak Nathan MD

Ayatolla (Steve)
Nazemi, MD

Linda Nearing

Deborah Nelson

Elizabeth Neumeier

John Newbury

Katharine Newhall

Angie Nicastro

Patricia
Niedzwiecki

Trinie & Jens
Nielson

Gail Norris

Kirstin Nussgruber

Ellen Nylen

Mike O'Connor

Patty O'Connor

Lee O'Leary

Judith Olsen

Sigrid Olsen

Peter & Charlene
Onanian

Pyore Oo

Myint Oo, MD

Alex Osterhaut

Jacquie Ostrom

Kristen Overlock

Sydney Owens

Rosalie Padre

Mary Palermo

Maryanne
Pappenikou

Joanna Parisi

LuAnn Pasciak

Michael Patti

Joann Patton

Linda Paul

Peter Peckarsky

Georgia Pepper

Rachel Perlmutter

Penny & Michael
Pesatauro

Joseph Peterson MD

Victoria Philip

Julie Pierce

Stella Pierce

Scott Pitt

Loree Pitts

Deborah Pitts

Sonya Podrebarac

Angela Poff

Marcia Polese

Diana Policaro

Mary Carlin Porter

Jane Potter

Janet Powers

Ann Powers

Patricia Prijatel

Ann Pulver

Tina Puppe

Susan Quateman

Diane Quijada

Carol Raineville,

Sandra Randall

Eric Rayman, ND

Sherry Read

Freda Gould
  Rebelsky

Duane Reed

Donna Reid

Jessica Reinis

Tom & Del Riquier

Leanne Robinson

Jaime Rodriquez

Christine Roe

Saskia Roell

Karen Roller

Todd Rolli

Matt Rose

Anne Rosenfeld

Margaret Ross

Leslie Rothwell

Heather Ryan

Melissa Ryan

Pamela Ryan

Greg Sacca

Nina Samoiloff

Denice Samolchuk

Fay Sargent

Jackie Sargent

Gail Sarofeen

Diane Schaeffer

Ruth Scheer

Ron Schrank

Anna Schutz

Sylvia Scofield

Linda Scott

Dannette Scott

Stella Mae Seamans

Tom Sears

Sherrill Sellman ND

Jo Sephus

Jo Sephus

Jay Severin

Catherine Shannon

Rawy Shediac

Diane Shen

Toby Symington

Mary Waters
  Shepley

Donna Shields

Judi Shipman

Shelly Shuka

Barb Sienkiewicz

Dorothy Sieradzki

Robert Singleton

Pat Slade

Peg Slocum

Martha Smeallie

Nancy Smith

Shona Smith

Russell Smith

Nora Smith

Jody
  Smith-Williams

Margaret Somer

David Somerville

Kathryn Soucy

Joanne Southgate

Louise Southwell

Lucy Sprague

Kathy Staab

Ashara Stansfield

Barbara Steele

Cathy Stentzel

Jane Stephens

Evy Stewart

Betty Stone

Rocky Stone

Mike Storella

Susan Storm

Krista Stotz

Ron Straka

Fred Studier

Lynda Surdam

Gail Swajue

Cheryl Swansburg

Martha Swanson

Ron Swanson

Jocelyn Tan MD

Susan Taomina

Ken Tarr

Lori Tharps

Mark Thayer

Rachel Theriault

Lindsay Thomas

Pam Thorne

Libby Thorne

Sue Thorne

Robin Tiro-Kinnon

David Tory

Helen Tory

Jemma Tory

Polly Townsend

Pamela Tucker

Stacey Tully

Eleanor Tutein

Meg Twohey

Ric & Deb Upton

Julie Van Fleet

Joan van Roden

Keith & Joan
   Vangeison

Lawrence Vincent

Lisa & Eoin Vincent

Gloria Vinson

Ute Von Haller

Judi Vost

Sylvia Vriesendorp

Anil Wadia

Bobbie Wagg

Mary Jo Wagner

Susan Wagner

Anne Walker

Julie Wallace

Julie Wallace

Julie Ward

Margaret Ward

James Watson

Iris Weaver

Suzanne Weinman

H Gilbert Welch MD

Jane Welch

Dave Weldon

Mary Ann Wenniger

Brittanie Wesley

Marian Werner

Alex Westerhoff

Candace Wheeler

Alexandra J. White

Nita White

Steve & Linda
   Willard

Ross Williams

Doris Williams

Linda Williams

Jodie Smith

Williams

Alan Wilson

Kathy Wilson

Liz Wilson

Sara Wilworth Dyer

Nasha Winters ND

Alice Winthrop

Betsy Wittemann

Joy Wood

Vincie Woodhams

Margo Woods

Roger Worden

Betsy Works

Edwina Yezierski

Azzie Young

George Yu MD

Lisa Zafran

Phyllis Zampolski

Kelly Zanal

Nancy Zare

Carol Zoppel

ABOUT THE AUTHOR

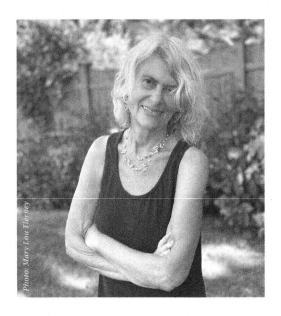

Photo: Mary Lou Tierney

Susan Wadia-Ells describes herself as a cultural change agent. Educated in organizational behavior, cross-cultural communication, political economy and women's studies, she identifies problems common to women, finding creative ways to improve these situations. She describes her life as "often finding myself in the right place, at the right time, with the right plan and the right support to move ahead and get the job done."

While working at Polaroid during the 1970s, she soon organized fellow women employees, demanding equal job opportunities, pay and benefits, before being appointed corporate affirmative action manager.

During the 1990s, a number of close friends were diagnosed with early-stage breast cancer; each was "successfully treated" for their invasive tumors, but later diagnosed with recurrent metastatic breast cancer, giving each an early death sentence. By 2008, Dr. Wadia-Ells had begun researching statistical studies on what was causing so much breast cancer throughout the US. Her column, *Honest Health*, published by the *Gloucester (MA) Daily Times* starting in 2009, questioned mammograms; castigated the use of sunscreen and birth control drugs, and warned against growth hormones in meat and dairy.

In 2013 she discovered the eminent geneticist Thomas N. Seyfried's groundbreaking text, *Cancer as a Metabolic Disease*, that finally pieced together large chunks of ignored basic biological knowledge. His findings described the development of early-stage and recurrent metastatic cancer. This knowledge meant Dr. Wadia-Ells could begin teaching women the straightforward biology behind the causes and development of breast cancer. Now she could write a book that would describe how to effectively protect oneself from developing this unnecessary disease.

Dr. Wadia-Ells has also studied and worked in Iran, India, Brazil, Zimbabwe, and the Conch Republic of Key West. She holds a BA from Hood College, a graduate degree in political economy from The Fletcher School (Tufts), and a PhD in Women's Studies from the Union Institute. Her earlier books include: *Birth Control Drugs and Breast Cancer: Learn the Terrible Truth* (Book Baby) and *The Adoption Reader: Birth Mothers, Adoptive Mothers and Adoptive Daughters Tell Their Stories* (Seal Press). Dr Wadia-Ells has one son, Anil, and lives in Manchester-by-the-Sea, Massachusetts.

Made in United States
Orlando, FL
19 May 2023

33267647R00212